AIDS Clinical Review 1992

AIDS Clinical Review 1992

edited by

PAUL VOLBERDING • MARK A. JACOBSON

*University of California—San Francisco, and
San Francisco General Hospital
San Francisco, California*

MARCEL DEKKER, INC.   New York • Basel • Hong Kong

Library of Congress card number: 89-642413

ISBN: 0-8247-8739-0

ISSN: 1045-2877

This book is printed on acid-free paper.

Marcel Dekker, Inc.
270 Madison Avenue, New York, New York 10016

Current printing (last digit):
10 9 8 7 6 5 4 3 2 1

PRINTED IN THE UNITED STATES OF AMERICA

Preface

As the AIDS epidemic has progressed, we have been impressed with the growing number and variety of clinicians—physicians, nurses, administrators, microbiologists, therapists, and epidemiologists—who are dealing directly with patients suffering from HIV disease. We are most impressed by the unslakable curiosity of these clinicians, by their persistent desire to be apprised of the newest clinical developments, and by their eagerness to provide the most current, state-of-the-art therapy. The AIDS epidemic has generated a new subspecialty of medicine for these clinicians, one that combines elements of virology, infectious diseases, oncology, dermatology, neurology, epidemiology, psychiatry, and the social sciences. The need to disseminate this logarithmically growing body of information is more than matched by the immense enthusiasm of these clinicians to learn more about HIV disease. Since 1989, the *AIDS Clinical Review* has met a growing need for a single-volume yearly update for these clinicians in which some of the most important and controversial clinical issues are dissected and discussed in depth.

AIDS Clinicial Review 1992 is the fourth in a series of yearly volumes that focuses on specific areas in which important new advances have occurred in the epidemiology, diagnosis, therapy, and prevention of HIV infection and HIV-associated complications. Although less encyclopedic than a conventional textbook, the *Review* has the advantage of more rapid publication. All the chapters in this year's review were written within nine months of publication, an interval that compares favorably with that for a review article published in a major medical journal. However, unlike a series of review articles, the *Review* offers a larger perspective and the possibility of interdisciplinary insights.

Each *Review* author is a clinical investigator who has published recent original work on his or her topic. The authors critically examine the latest relevant clinical research, especially articles and abstracts published in the past year, and discuss results of their own recent investigations, as well as reviewing new, unpublished data. They also identify important research questions that future investigations should attempt to answer. Thus, some of the most important progress in HIV clinical research has been identified and is presented in this single-source reference for the worldwide clinical community that deals directly with HIV infection and disease.

Four chapters in this year's *Review* focus on epidemiological and natural history issues regarding HIV infection and disease. In one of the most important chapters ever published in this *Review*, Patrick Li and E. K. Yeoh synthesize dramatic new developments regarding the spread of HIV infection into Southeast Asia and the Indian subcontinent. This chapter is the first comprehensive review of these epidemiological data to be published; the worldwide health, social, and economic implications of these developments are staggering. Nancy Hessol and Susan Buchbinder summarize the current state-of-the-art understanding of the predictive value of clinical and laboratory markers for HIV disease progression. Constance Wofsy et al. critically evaluate recent studies regarding the transmission, epidemiology, and natural history of HIV infection in women; and Donald Northfelt and Joel Palefsky discuss important new advances in our understanding of the interaction between HIV and human papillomavirus (HPV) infection, with an emphasis on the role HPV may play in HIV-related anogenital malignancies.

Three chapters emphasize new developments in the diagnosis and treatment of AIDS-associated opportunistic infections. Clark Inderlied and Carol Kemper summarize the current state of knowledge regarding disseminated *Mycobacterium avium* complex infection; Mark Jacobson reviews the use of a newly FDA-licensed intervention, foscarnet therapy, for opportunistic cytomegalovirus, herpes simplex virus, and varicella-zoster virus disease; and Peter Mariuz and Benjamin Luft discuss recent advances in the management of toxoplasmic encephalitis.

Two chapters focus on the latest developments in antiretroviral therapy. A comprehensive current update on antiretroviral drug therapy, including new data on the use of combination agent regimens, is provided by Victoria Johnson; and an overview of recent data regarding use of quantitative virological techniques to monitor response to antiretroviral therapy is given by David Katzenstein and Mark Holodniy.

In addition, four chapters emphasize specific areas that may be of interest to many readers. Carl Grunfeld and Donald Kotler describe our evolving understanding of the pathophysiology of the AIDS-wasting syndrome; Deborah and John Greenspan present an overview of the natural history and management of HIV-associated oral complications; James Kahn, Donald Northfelt, and Steven Miles review current understanding of the pathogenesis and optimal management of Kaposi's sarcoma; and Judy Macks and Donald Abrams discuss the growing problem of emotional "burnout" in AIDS health care providers.

Our heartfelt thanks are due to the *Review*'s authors. These overworked investigators took additional time away from their family, friends, and sleep to make their contributions to this volume. We are confident their efforts will improve the care of patients with HIV disease.

Paul Volberding
Mark A. Jacobson

Contents

Contents

Contributors

Donald I. Abrams, M.D.   Assistant Director, AIDS Activities, San Francisco General Hospital, and Associate Professor of Clinical Medicine, University of California—San Francisco, San Francisco, California

Susan P. Buchbinder, M.D.   Chief, Clinical Studies Section, Research Branch, AIDS Office, San Francisco Department of Public Health, and Assistant Clinical Professor, Department of Medicine, University of California—San Francisco, San Francisco, California

Judith B. Cohen, M.P.H., Ph.D.   Research Epidemiologist and Director, AWARE, Division of AIDS/Oncology, Department of Medicine, University of California—San Francisco, and San Francisco General Hospital, San Francisco, California

Rebecca Coleman, Pharm.D.   Assistant Clinical Professor, Department of Clinical Pharmacy, University of California—San Francisco, and AIDS Program, San Francisco General Hospital, San Francisco, California

Ruth Greenblatt, M.D.   Assistant Professor, Department of Medicine, University of California—San Francisco, and San Francisco General Hospital, San Francisco, California

Deborah Greenspan, B.D.S., D.Sc.   Clinical Professor, Department of Stomatology, University of California—San Francisco, San Francisco, California

John S. Greenspan, B.D.S., Ph.D., F.R.C.Path.   Professor and Chairman, Department of Stomatology, University of California—San Francisco, San Francisco, California

Carl Grunfeld, M.D., Ph.D.   Associate Professor of Medicine, Department of Medicine, University of California—San Francisco, and Department of Veterans Affairs Medical Center, San Francisco, California

Nancy A. Hessol, M.S.P.H.   Assistant Chief, Research Branch, AIDS Office, San Francisco Department of Public Health, San Francisco, California

Mark Holodniy, M.D.   Clinical Assistant Professor of Medicine, Stanford University School of Medicine, Stanford, and Acting Chief, Infectious Disease Section, Palo Alto Veterans Affairs Medical Center, Palo Alto, California

Clark B. Inderlied, Ph.D.   Associate Professor and Director, Clinical and Molecular Microbiology Laboratory, Department of Pathology and Laboratory Medicine, Children's Hospital Los Angeles, and University of Southern California School of Medicine, Los Angeles, California

Mark A. Jacobson, M.D.   Assistant Professor of Medicine in Residence, University of California—San Francisco, and Clinical Director, AIDS Program, San Francisco General Hospital, San Francisco, California

Victoria A. Johnson, M.D.   Assistant Professor, Division of Infectious Diseases, Department of Medicine and Microbiology, University of Alabama at Birmingham, Birmingham, Alabama

James O. Kahn, M. D.   Assistant Clinical Professor, Department of Medicine, University of California—San Francisco, and San Francisco General Hospital, San Francisco, California

David A. Katzenstein, M.D.   Associate Medical Director, Center for AIDS Research, Stanford University Medical Center, and Assistant Professor of Medicine, Division of Infectious Diseases, Department of Medicine, Stanford University School of Medicine, Stanford, California

Carol A. Kemper, M.D.   Associate Director, AIDS Program, Division of Infectious Diseases, Stanford University School of Medicine, Stanford, and Santa Clara Valley Medical Center, San Jose, California

Joyce A. Korvick, M.D.   Medical Officer, Division of AIDS, National Institute of Allergy and Infectious Diseases, National Institutes of Health, Bethesda, Maryland

Donald P. Kotler, M.D.   Associate Professor of Clinical Medicine, Department of Medicine, College of Physicians and Surgeons, Columbia University, and St. Luke's-Roosevelt Hospital Center, New York, New York

Patrick C. K. Li, M.B., B.S. (Hong Kong), M.R.C.P. (U.K.)   Senior Medical Officer, Medical A Unit, Queen Elizabeth Hospital, Hong Kong

Benjamin J. Luft, M.D.   Associate Professor, Division of Infectious Diseases, State University of New York at Stony Brook, Stony Brook, New York

Judy A. Macks, M.S.W., L.C.S.W.   Partner, Organization Consultant and Trainer, JKRAssociates, San Francisco, California

Peter R. Mariuz, M.D.   Instructor in Medicine, Division of Infectious Diseases, State University of New York at Stony Brook, Stony Brook, New York

Steven A. Miles, M.D.   Associate Professor of Medicine, University of California—Los Angeles, Los Angeles, California

Donald W. Northfelt, M.D.   Assistant Clinical Professor, Cancer Research Institute and AIDS/Oncology Division, University of California—San Francisco, and San Francisco General Hospital, San Francisco, California

Nancy S. Padian, M.P.H., Ph.D.   Assistant Adjunct Professor, Department of Epidemiology and Biostatistics, University of California—San Francisco, and San Francisco General Hospital, San Francisco, California

Joel M. Palefsky, M.D., C.M.   Assistant Professor of Laboratory Medicine, Department of Medicine and Stomatology, University of California—San Francisco, San Francisco, California

Constance B. Wofsy, M.D.   Professor of Clinical Medicine, University of California—San Francisco, and Co-Director, AIDS Activities Program, San Francisco General Hospital, San Francisco, California

Eng Kiong Yeoh, F.R.C.P. (Edin.), F.R.C.P. (Lond.), F.R.C.P. (Glasg.)   Director of Operations, Hospital Authority, Hong Kong

Current Epidemiological Trends of HIV Infection in Asia

Patrick C. K. Li
Queen Elizabeth Hospital, Hong Kong

Eng Kiong Yeoh
Hospital Authority, Hong Kong

I. INTRODUCTION

When AIDS was first identified in the early 1980s, most cases were reported from America, Europe, and Africa, and very few patients were detected in Asia (1) (Table 1). Epidemiologists at that time differentiated three geographical patterns of HIV transmission (2). Asian countries were classified as belonging to pattern III, with most cases resulting from use of imported contaminated blood products or sexual contact with persons from pattern I or II countries. This prevailing concept was reflected in the tendency of many Asian countries to classify their patients as "imported" or to impose travel restrictions on HIV-infected individuals (3).

With better understanding of the epidemiology of AIDS and as the course of the epidemic in Asia unfolded, it became recognized that the differentiation of distinct geographical patterns of HIV transmission was an oversimplification of the pandemic. Countries initially showing one predominant pattern of HIV transmission might evolve into a different pattern with time, and the main groups of individuals infected by HIV

Table 1 Cumulative Number of AIDS
Cases Reported to WHO from Asia by
Year

Year	Number reported
1981	3
1982	3
1983	11
1984	18
1985	49
1986	132
1987	253
1988	403
1989	664
1990	1078
1991	1254

were more determined by the existence and degree of various high-risk
behaviors responsible for its spread. Asian countries that had implemented sentinel surveillance programs were able to detect HIV infection
among most of the population groups recognized to be at increased risk
(Table 2).

Table 2 Patterns of HIV Transmission in Asia

	Number of countries doing testing	Number of countries reporting infection	Percentage
Male homosexuals	16	14	88
Male STD patients	15	12	80
Female sex workers	17	9	53
Drug injectors	17	11	65
Hemophiliacs	13	11	85
Transfusion recipients	14	10	71
Blood donors	18	11	61
Pregnant women	13	6	46

Countries surveyed: Brunei, China, Hong Kong, India, Indonesia, Japan, Macao, Malaysia, Mongolia, Myanmar, Nepal, Philippines, Republic of Korea, Singapore, Sri Lanka,
Taiwan, Thailand, Vietnam.

II. THE MAGNITUDE OF THE PROBLEM

Although only 1254 AIDS patients were reported from Asia as of January 1, 1992 (1,4), constituting less than 1% of the global total, this by no means represents the true extent of the epidemic. In view of the poorly developed surveillance system and the limited diagnostic experience and facilities in many countries, it is believed that considerable underdiagnosis and under-reporting have occurred. In addition, some HIV-infected individuals with profound immunodeficiency might have died of other causes or infections not usually associated with AIDS and thus have not been counted (5).

It was also recognized that the number of AIDS patients only reflected the prevalence of infection in Asia in the early 1980s. While most countries in Asia still reported a small number of AIDS patients (1), more recent reports of the number of HIV-infected individuals indicate a more serious extent of the infection in Asia. Even the detected HIV-infected individuals might represent only the tip of the iceberg, as such numbers are heavily influenced by the extent of HIV testing in each country as well as the willingness of the infected individuals to come forward for testing. For example, the official estimates of the number of HIV-infected individuals are now 200,000–400,000 for Thailand (6) and 250,000 for India (7). The World Health Organization (WHO) estimates that as of mid-1991, over one million infections might have occurred in Asia (8).

Attempts to assess the current magnitude of the epidemic in Asia are hindered by the fact that only limited serosurveillance data are available from the countries of the region and there are only crude estimates of the size of the at-risk population. Even with such limited information, the potential magnitude of the problem is evident. For example, in Thailand the official estimate of the number of commercial sex workers was 150,000, but nongovernmental organizations believe the true number could be as many as 800,000 (9,10). In Bombay, India, alone, there are an estimated 100,000–300,000 female sex workers (7,11,12). In China, where prostitution is illegal and hence no accurate estimate of the number of sex workers is available, 85,866 cases of sexually transmitted diseases were reported in 1988 (13), indicating indirectly that a sizable number of sex workers are present.

Little information is available on homosexual practice in the region, primarily because of its illegal status in many countries, as well as the attached social stigma. There is also a general lack of large-scale KABP (knowledge, attitude, belief, practice) study on the general population, so that little is known about the sexual preference of the population at large. A partner-relations survey of Thai men between the ages of 15 and

49 showed that 17% had premarital sex and another 11.5% had extramarital sex (14). In this study, 77% of men reporting sexual contact outside their regular relationships had used commercial sex within the past 12 months. Only 3.5% reported homosexual activity. It is estimated that there are between 3–8 million customers of the sex service industry in Thailand (15). Dr. A. S. Paintal, director general of the Indian Council for Medical Research, estimated in 1990 that 100,000 acts of sexual intercourse occurred with infected female sex workers every day in Bombay (11). These anecdotal reports highlight the immense potential for HIV to spread through heterosexual contact in Asia.

The increasing importance of heterosexual transmission could lead to involvement of sectors of the population not previously considered to be at risk. In a serosurveillance study of male Thai military recruits aged 20–22, 2% were found to be HIV-positive, with a seroprevalence of up to 10% in recruits from the northern part of Thailand (9,15). Another study in Madras, India, revealed a high prevalence of sexually transmitted diseases (17%) among housewives (16), which reflected the level of promiscuity of their husbands, raising a warning for the possibility of perinatal transmission of HIV.

Apart from sexual transmission, sharing of contaminated needles and syringes has become an important channel for HIV transmission in Asia. There are many drug users in countries near the "Golden Triangle" and along the routes of drug trafficking (17-20). In Bangkok alone, there are an estimated 80,000 drug users, of which over 80% are injectors (17). When needed availability is scarce, as in prisons, in countries where needles are only available on prescription, or where needle possession is illegal, sharing of equipment for drug injection is common.

III. HIV-1 AND HIV-2

Most of the infections reported from the region have been due to HIV-1. In December 1989, a Sri Lankan who had traveled to Africa was identified to be infected with HIV-2 (19). More recently, detection of HIV-2 infection was reported from Tamil Nadu and Bombay, India, among local STD patients and prostitutes, as well as foreign students from Kenya (21–23). Dr. Y. O. Shin from the Republic of Korea also reported two patients who had traveled to Africa with co-infection by HIV-1 and HIV-2. Although HIV-2 infection is still relatively uncommon in Asia, more serosurveillance studies have to be conducted to fully assess its prevalence and to monitor its trend. Such findings would have implications for the serodiagnosis of HIV infection and safeguarding the blood donation system.

IV. DEMOGRAPHIC PATTERN OF HIV INFECTION

There is a heavy male preponderance among the AIDS patients and HIV-infected individuals in most countries. However, a lower male-to-female ratio for HIV carriers has been noted in India, the Republic of Korea, Sri Lanka, and Thailand, while more infected women than men were identified from the Philippines, reflecting the relative importance of heterosexual transmission in these countries. The World Health Organization estimates that the overall rates of infection in Asia are 1:2500 for men and 1:3500 for women (24), which resembles closely the sex ratio in Africa.

While many of the initial AIDS cases reported from Asia were foreigners or local people who had traveled abroad, more and more countries have acknowledged the occurrence of AIDS and HIV infection among the indigenous populations. Once the spread of HIV in the local population had begun, the contribution of "imported" infection became insignificant.

The vast majority of HIV infection has occurred among the adult population, mainly resulting from sexual transmission and sharing of needles for drug injection. The few pediatric cases have been mostly due to use of contaminated blood products, but countries such as India, Japan, Malaysia, the Philippines, and Thailand have seen the emergence of perinatal transmission. Most infected babies were born of mothers who injected drugs or were infected through heterosexual transmission.

The exposure categories for the AIDS patients still show a predominance of homosexual transmission. This would be in keeping with the main trend in Asia in the early and mid-1980s. The pattern in the identified HIV-infected individuals shows a greater variation with some countries identifying large numbers of carriers infected through heterosexual transmission or sharing needles for drug injection. This correlates with the recent increasing trend of HIV infection in these groups in Asia and could be expected to lead to a drastic change in the pattern of exposure categories among AIDS patients in the coming years.

V. MODES OF TRANSMISSION

A. Sexual Transmission

Although homosexual men were the first group of individuals identified to be infected in the region, and most countries had reported infection in this group, seroprevalence studies are few in number. This is because of the absence of a well-defined homosexual community in most countries. Many studies were conducted on male sex workers. Although there has been a general rising trend, the rate of increase has been gradual and the seroprevalence reported does not exceed 10% (Table 3).

In contrast, the rate of spread of HIV among the heterosexual population has been much more rapid. The increase was first noted among female sex workers in Thailand and India. While there were very few infected women in these groups before 1988, an explosive increase in seroprevalence was noted in 1989. A study in Chiangmai from December 1989 to July 1990 demonstrated a seroconversion rate of 3.4 to 4.8% per person-month (31) and a follow-up study in August 1990 revealed a similarly high rate of 10% per month (32). The general seroprevalence in these

Table 3 HIV Seroprevalence in Male Homosexuals

Country	Date	No. positive/ no. tested	Percentage	Ref.
China	1985–1989	0/98	0	X.Q.Qi[e]
Hong Kong	1985–1988	5/261	1.9[a]	
		2/40	5.0[b]	
	1989–1991	4/122	3.3[a]	
		2/24	8.0[b]	
India				
Goa	1988	1/270	0.37	G. Petersen[e]
Madhya Pradesh	1988	0/157	0	G. Petersen[e]
Tamil Nadu	1991	3/185	1.6[c]	25
		3/4163	0.05[d]	25
Indonesia	1988–1990	0/73	0	19
Japan, Tokyo	1985–1989	12/669	1.79[a]	26
	1985–1989	12/117	10.26[b]	26
Mongolia	1988–1990	0/114	0	19
Myanmar	1985–1990	0/202	0	19
Philippines	1985–1989	4/1744	0.024	26
Singapore	1984–1989	24/1805	1.33	26
Taiwan	1989	33/1184	2.8	27
Thailand	1988	44/1885	2.3[c]	28
	June 1989		2.7 (0–4)[c]	29,30
	Dec. 1989		3.3[c]	29
	June 1990		5.3[c]	29

[a]Local.
[b]Foreigner.
[c]Male sex workers.
[d]Prisoners.
[e]Personal communication (unpublished data).

two countries is now in the range of 20–30%, with some localities reporting prevalence as high as 50–70% (5,9) (Table 4).

There are many reasons for the rapid spread of HIV among female sex
workers in Asia. The incidence of sexually transmitted diseases (STDs)
is high and their knowledge of AIDS, STDs, and their prevention has

Table 4 HIV Seroprevalence in Female Sex Workers

Country	Date	No. positive/ no. tested	Percentage		Ref.
China	1985–1989	0/28293	0		X.Q.Qi[c]
Hong Kong	1985–1991	2/13765	0.015		33
India	1986	10/3027	0.33		G. Petersen[c]
Bombay	1986–1990	145/1919	7.56		34
	Mar. 1988		1.6		34
	Jan. 1990		23		34
	1990	150/2000	30		34
Delhi	1988	1/701	0.14		35
New Delhi	1988	22/73	30.1		G. Petersen[c]
West Bengal	1986	1/897	0.11		11
Indonesia	1988–1990	0/7937	0		19
Japan	1985–1989	1/742	0.14		26
Malaysia	1985–1990	0/542	0		G. Petersen[c]
Mongolia	1988–1990	0/193	0		19
Myanmar	1985–1989	0/610	0		19
	1990	45/539	8.3		19
Philippines	1985–1987	20/25392	0.079		36
	1985–1989	64/111914	0.057		26
Rep. of Korea	1985–1990	12/1308209	0.001		37
Singapore	1984–1989	0/19386	0		26
Taiwan, Taipei	1988–1990	0/4079	0		38
Thailand	1988	17/6272	0.3		28
	June 1989		3.5	(0–44)[a]	39
			0	(0–5)[b]	39
	Dec. 1989		6.3	(0–43)[a]	39
			1.2	(0–10)[b]	39
	June 1990		9.3	(0–67)[a]	39
			1.2	(0–17)[b]	39
Bangkok	1989	34/1089	3.1		G. Petersen[c]
Chiangmai	1989	87/238	36.5		32
Vietnam	1991	0/2089	0		G. Petersen[c]

[a]Workers in brothels, hotels, teahouses (high class).
[b]Workers in other establishments (low class).
[c]Personal communication (unpublished data).

been inadequate (10,12,40). Because of economic and social pressure, they usually have little say on the use of condoms. Very often, they have to continue working despite menstruation or the presence of STDs, thereby making them more susceptible to HIV infection and more likely to pass it on to their clients. This situation is by no means confined to India and Thailand. Countries now seeing relatively low seroprevalence among their sex workers could see a similar rapid spread if an effective AIDS prevention program is not implemented.

A direct consequence of the escalating prevalence of HIV infection among female sex workers in India and Thailand has been a similar increase among the male patients of the STD clinics of these two countries. Most of these individuals were infected through the heterosexual route (Table 5). Although seroprevalence in general is still below 1%, a high rate of 18% was reported from northern Thailand. HIV-infected male STD patients from some Asian countries might report sexual contacts in the high-prevalence countries. However, since most of them also have had local sexual contacts, the possibility of a local source of infection cannot be ruled out. As some of them could have transmitted the infection to the local sex workers, such countries could expect to see a trend of increasing indigenous heterosexual spread of HIV in the next few years.

B. Drug Injection

Infection among drug injectors was reported mainly from 1988 onwards. The rapid trend of increase in seroprevalence in several countries is alarming. For example, in Thailand, the seroprevalence increased from 1% before February 1988 to 30% in September of the same year, with some cities reporting levels of infection up to 51% in June 1989 and 70% in June 1990 (39,46). Similarly, in the Manipur state of India before September 1989, there were no infected drug users detected. By June 1990, 54% of the intravenous drug users were found to be infected (47). Other countries such as Malaysia, Myanmar, and China are also seeing evidence of HIV infection among their drug injectors (Table 6). Countries such as Afghanistan, Bangladesh, Nepal, Pakistan, and Sri Lanka also have large heroin-using populations. Southwest Asian heroin from the "Golden Crescent" is mainly used, and the inhalation route is more common (55). The potential for HIV to spread in these countries could increase should there be a shift to injection by the heroin-using population.

The rapid spread of HIV among the drug injectors is probably related to the frequency of needle sharing, especially among new drug users, those

Table 5 HIV Seroprevalence in Male Sexually Transmitted Disease Clinic Patients

Country	Date	No. positive/ no. tested	Percentage		Ref.
China	1985–1989	1/5685	0.018		X.Q.Qi[a]
Hong Kong	1985–1988	12/76522	0.016		33
	1989–1991	27/53820	0.050		33
India					
Agra	1987–1990	3/297	1.01		41
Delhi	1988	0/4572	0		35
Madras and	1987		0.5		42
Madurai	1988		0.6		42
	1989		1.1		42
	1990		1.2		42
Tamil Nadu	1987–1988	2/7284	0.027		43
	1989–1990	7/5824	0.12		43
Vellore	1986–1988	9/2215	0.41		44
Mongolia	1988–1990	0/1778	0		19
Myanmar	1985–1989	36/6722	0.54		19
	1990	25/1334	1.87		19
Nepal	1988–1990	7/5115	0.14		19
Sri Lanka	1986–1991	2/3542	0.08		19
Taiwan, Taipei	1988–1990	42/41666	0.10		38
Thailand	June 1989		0	(0–10)	39
	Dec. 1989		2	(0–17)	39
	June 1990		2.5	(0–22)	39
Chiangmai	June 1990	36/200	18		45
Vietnam	1987–1988	0/728	0		26

[a]Personal communication (unpublished data).

confined in prisons, and where the law-enforcing agency precludes the possibility of possessing clean needles (40). The high infection rate among drug injectors has serious implications, as they are a potential source of heterosexual transmission.

C. Blood and Blood Products

In the mid-1980s, a high prevalence of HIV infection was detected among the hemophiliac patients in countries using clotting factor concentrates imported from pattern I countries (26,27,33,56,57). With the availability of donor-screened and heat- or chemically treated products, the risk to hemophiliac patients should be markedly reduced.

Table 6 HIV Seroprevalence in Drug Users

Country	Date	No. positive/ no. tested	Percentage		Ref.
Bahrain	1991	25/858	2.9		48
China	Oct. 1989	146/1167	12.5		13
Hong Kong	1985–1991	1/5919	0.017		33
India, Manipur	1986–1989	0/2322	0		49
	1989–1990	765/1412	54		49
	1986–1991	1080/2600	41.5		50
	1989–1990	910/2326	39		51
	June 1990	844/1564	54		47
	Nov. 1990	1016/2324	43.7		19
Indonesia	1988–1990	0/211	0		19
Japan	1985–1989	1/2753	0.036		26
Malaysia	1985–1988	0/4948	0		26
	1988–1989	52/2344	2.2		26
Myanmar	1985–1989	54/313	17		19
	1990	440/701	63		19
	1989	176/441	39.9		G. Petersen[a]
Nepal	1990	1/446	0.22		19
Singapore	1984–1989	0/498	0		26
Taiwan					
Kaohsiung	1989	0/390	0		52
Taipei	1988–1990	5/1209	0.41		38
Thailand	before Feb. 1988		1		46
	Feb. 1988		4		46
	Sept. 1988		30		46
	June 1989		39	(0–51)	39
	Dec. 1989		30.1	(0–66)	39
	June 1990		31.4	(0–70)	39
	Mar. 1988		15.6		17
	Sept. 1988		42.7		17
	Apr. 1989		44.6		17
	Nov. 1989		38.5		17
Bangkok	Apr. 1988		15.6		53
	Oct. 1988		42.7		53
	Apr. 1989		44.6		53
Chiangmai	1989	15/61	24.6		G. Petersen[a]
Hat Yai Hospital	1988–1989	148/1823	15.7		54
Vietnam	1987–1988	0/184	0		26

[a]Personal communication (unpublished data).

Blood donors constituted a convenient group for conducting HIV surveillance, and consequently considerable information has accumulated concerning this group. The prevalence is in general very low but recently an increasing trend has been reported from India and Thailand, especially among paid blood donors (Table 7). Seroprevalence rates of up to 3–7% have been reported in these two countries, raising concern over the potential for transfusion-related HIV infection.

At present, apart from countries such as Brunei, Hong Kong, Japan, Macao, Malaysia, Republic of Korea, Singapore, Thailand, and Vietnam, many other Asian countries still rely on paid donors or are unable to afford the cost of screening all blood donors before blood is used for transfusion. With a rising prevalence of infection among the blood donors, there is an urgent need for such countries to institute a voluntary blood donation system and to implement universal screening of blood donors.

Because of the low prevalence of HIV infection among blood donors, the infection rate of transfusion recipients also has been low in general. Transfusion-associated HIV infection was mainly reported from India and Thailand (50,56,57,66), the two countries with a higher seroprevalence among the blood donors. A cause for concern was raised by a report from northern Thailand where some individuals were infected following transfusions of HIV-screened blood (66). This was probably due to HIV-infected individuals in the "window period" slipping through the screening process, and this possibility would be greater in high-incidence areas.

Another potential channel of HIV transmission shown to be important in developing countries in Africa and eastern Europe has been the use of improperly sterilized needles in the health-care setting. While no outbreak similar to the incidents in Rumania (67) or the Soviet Union (68) has been reported in Asia, some countries in the region have been unable to afford the use of disposable syringes and needles and do not have adequate facilities for sterilization of used instruments. Such a setting could result in HIV transmission when improperly sterilized needles are used for treatment of STDs or tuberculosis, both of which are associated with HIV infection.

D. Perinatal Transmission

In the early period of the AIDS epidemic, most Asian countries saw the infection mainly affecting the male population and hence perinatal transmission of HIV was infrequent. With the rising trend of HIV infection among female sex workers and the increasing importance of heterosexual

Table 7 HIV Seroprevalence in Blood Donors

Country	Date	No. positive/ no. tested	Percentage		Ref.
China	1985–1989	0/43109	0		X.Q.Qi[c]
Hong Kong	1985–1989	10/658574	0.0015[b]		
	1990–1991	7/284947	0.0025[b]		
India	1989–1990	5163/852272	0.61		19
Agra	1988–1990	50/1479	3.38[a]		41
Bombay	1989	440/18305	2.4[a]		58
		140/99361	0.14[b]		58
Delhi	1989	4/1700	0.24[a]		59
		0/8000	0[b]		59
	1989–1991	28/26746	0.10[a]		60
		7/52956	0.01[b]		60
Manipur	1986–1991	28/808	3.47		50
	1989–1990	22/731	3.01		51
New Delhi	1988	37/12795	0.29		G. Petersen[c]
Vellore	1986–1988		0.19[b]		61
Indonesia	1987–1989	0/27300	0		19
Japan	1987		0.0001[b]		62
	1990		0.0003[b]		62
Tokyo	1987		0.0004[b]		62
	1990		0.0007[b]		62
Mongolia	1988–1990	0/29543	0		19
Myanmar	1985–1989	70/14418	0.49		19
	1990	193/38701	0.50		19
Nepal	1988–1990	1/8533	0.012		19
Philippines	1985–1989	0/3756	0		26
Rep. of Korea	1985–1990	18/3472658	0.0005		37
Singapore	1984–1989	10/231535	0.004		26
Sri Lanka	1988–1990	1/85843	0.0012		63
Taiwan	1985–1989	86/550000	0.02		G. Petersen[c]
Thailand	1988–1989	343/274776	0.12		64
	June 1989		0.28	(0–3.7)	39
	Dec. 1989		0.23	(0–7.7)	39
	June 1990		0.46	(0–4.7)	39
Bangkok	1987		0.006		46
	1988		0.047		46
	1989		0.083		46
Chiangmai	June 1989		3.7		46
	Dec. 1989		6.8		46
	1990	10/289	3.46		45
Phayao	Dec. 1989		7.4		46
Vietnam	1988–1990	0/5513	0		65

[a]Paid donors.
[b]Voluntary donors.
[c]Personal communication (unpublished data).

transmission in many Asian countries, a larger number of women are becoming infected. These include not only sex workers and female drug injectors, but the spouses of male STD patients (5,19,39,69). If the AIDS epidemic in Asia continues in the same direction as that in Africa, more children born with HIV infection as well as "AIDS orphans" will emerge in the next decade.

VI. CLINICAL MANIFESTATIONS

Limited information is available concerning the clinical manifestations of AIDS and HIV infection in Asia. This relates to the small number of patients and the lack of diagnostic facilities in some countries. Only a few clinical series have been reported and no autopsy studies are available to date. Most of the opportunistic infections reported are similar to those seen in the developed countries (70–73) (Table 8).

Table 8   Clinical Manifestations of AIDS in Asia

	Hong Kong	Singapore	Philippines	Thailand
Number	52	19	11	75
Cryptosporidium	4%	5%	18%	4%
Isospora	2%	5%	—	—
Pneumocystis	48%	53%	73%	26%
Toxoplasma	8%	—	—	2%
Cytomegalovirus	21%	21%	18%	4%
Herpes simplex	8%	16%	27%	4%
Varicella-zoster	19%	32%	—	6%
Cryptococcus	12%	11%	9%	2%
Candida	8%[a]	11%[a]	55%	30%
Histoplasma	—	—	—	8%
Penicillium	8%	—	—	4%
Melioidosis	—	—	—	2%
M. tuberculosis	12%	5%	45%	20%
M. avium	13%	—	18%	2%
Salmonella	4%	5%	18%	4%
Kaposi's sarcoma	13%	21%	9%	—
Non-Hodgkin's lymphoma	4%	11%	9%	—
Tumors (not specified)	—	—	—	9%
AIDS dementia	—	—	18%	7%

[a]Oral candidiasis not included.

Mycobacterial infections appear to be an important opportunistic pathogen in this locality. In addition, a peculiar fungus called *Penicillium marneffei* was found in a significant proportion of the AIDS patients in Hong Kong and Thailand. This fungus had previously been identified only among residents of Southeast Asia or tourists to that region. More clinical and autopsy studies are urgently needed to better define the pattern of opportunistic diseases specific for Asia in anticipation of the future increase in number of AIDS patients.

VII. PROJECTION OF AIDS IN ASIA

From the serosurveillance data described in the previous sections, a general increasing trend in seroprevalence is evident, with the most rapid increase being found among intravenous drug users and female sex workers. Heterosexual transmission and sharing contaminated needles and syringes for drug injection would be the two most important routes of transmission in Asia.

The preponderance of heterosexual transmission and the rapid increase in seroprevalence is reminiscent of the rapid spread of HIV in sub-Saharan Africa in the early 1980s. In fact, the potential for HIV to spread would be even greater for Asia, in view of the fact that its adult population of 500 million is nearly twice that of sub-Saharan Africa (225 million) (7). WHO projected that by the mid- to late 1990s, more Asians than Africans could become infected with HIV each year (6).

The rapid rate of spread of HIV in Asia resulted in WHO's need to repeatedly revise its estimate of the number of infected individuals in the region. In 1989, WHO estimated that there were 100,000 HIV carriers in Asia and Oceania (74). In 1990, this estimate was revised to 500,000 for Asia alone (75), and in 1991 the number was increased to 1–1.5 million (8). In late 1988, the WHO Delphi survey projected that 1.5 million HIV-infected individuals would be present in Asia by the year 2000 (74). In 1991, it was projected that by the mid-1990s, there will be over 2.5 million HIV-infected individuals in Asia out of a global total of 15 million. By the year 2000, around 250,000 AIDS cases could be reported annually from Asia (8).

When their number of AIDS patients was small, Asian countries had a chance to learn from the mistakes and experiences of countries in the other continents. Unfortunately, instead of laying down solid prevention programs based on informing their populations about AIDS and reaching and counseling individuals practicing high-risk behavior, many countries wasted time tracking down and deporting HIV-infected foreigners or waiting for the number of cases to increase before taking action. Many countries were also handicapped by their scarce health-care resources, which needed to cope with many other diseases of public concern, as well as the lack of adequate health education and social support infrastructure. Information concerning local sexual practice and drug-injection behaviors are generally lacking or inadequate.

With the anticipated explosive increase in the number of AIDS and HIV-infected patients in many developing countries in Asia, significant impact on the demography, economy, and social stability could result. With the many similarities in the epidemiology, rate of spread of HIV, and the health-care and socioeconomic structures of most Asian and African countries, an equally gloomy outlook is inevitable should the current trend in Asia continue. For example, India has projected that the under-5 mortality will increase from 166/1000 in 1988 to 185/1000 by the year 2000 (76), wiping out the decline in mortality achieved over the past three decades. The impact on the demography of the population of Asia would become most evident in the second decade of the next century (6).

VIII. CONCLUSIONS

While many countries in Asia did not take the opportunity to learn from the experience with the AIDS epidemic in the other continents, a number of lessons can be learned from the unfolding course of AIDS in Asia. First of all, it proved beyond any doubt that AIDS was not confined by geographical boundaries. Any person, of whichever sex, age group, nationality, or social background, can become prey to HIV. Asia also illustrated the possibility that HIV, once introduced into a community and given the right kind of behavior facilitating its spread, could spread explosively.

The predominant pattern of HIV transmission is most dependent on the prevailing type of high-risk activity—whether unprotected homosexual or heterosexual contact or sharing needles and syringes for drug injection. For example, the main pattern of transmission is drug injection in northern India, whereas in other parts of the country, it is mainly through heterosexual contact. As the experience in Thailand demonstrated, certain groups of individuals might be predominantly affected initially, spreading to other groups with time, and ultimately involving people not previously recognized as belonging to risk groups. The HIV epidemic has shifted in quick succession from male homosexuals to drug injectors, then to female sex workers. The clients of the sex industry and finally their wives and children will likely be next.

With the projected number of HIV-infected individuals in Asia and the ill-equipped health-care infrastructure and resources in many countries, the impact of AIDS will not be confined to the medical community but could lead to potentially devastating social, economic, and political problems. No country, government, or individual group can win the battle against AIDS on its own. Countries should cast away the idea of preventing foreigners with HIV infection from bringing in the infection or isolating carriers who have been identified within the countries. AIDS has already arrived in Asia, and such discriminatory measures could only give a façade of preventing the spread of AIDS. They would only be tackling the tip of the iceberg while permitting HIV to permeate clandestinely until the time bomb is detonated. What is needed are attitudes of frank acceptance of the existence and threat of AIDS, and the motivation of people practicing high-risk activity to modify their behavior. For such efforts to be successful, close collaboration and cooperation between international bodies, governments, nongovernmental organizations, and persons with AIDS will be crucial.

ACKNOWLEDGMENTS

The authors would like to thank the following persons for their assistance in supplying valuable information in the preparation of this article: Dr. G. Petersen (Western Pacific Region, WHO), Dr. N. K. Shah (South East Asian Region, WHO), Dr. H. Dyer (Burroughs Wellcome), Dr. M. F. Ferreira (Macao), Dr. X. Q. Qi (People's Republic of China), Dr. E. Hernandez (Philippines), Dr. Y. O Shin (Republic of Korea), and Dr. R. Chan (Singapore).

REFERENCES

1. World Health Organization. Update: AIDS cases reported to Surveillance, Forecasting and Impact Assessment Unit (SFI), Office of Research (RES), Global Programme on AIDS, January 1, 1992.

2. Mann JM. The global picture of AIDS. Keynote address, Fourth International Conference on AIDS, 1988, Stockholm, Sweden. WHO/GPA/DIR/88.2.

3. World Health Organization. Tabular information on legal instruments dealing with HIV infection and AIDS. WHO/GPA/HLE/91.1.

4. World Health Organization. Acquired immunodeficiency syndrome (AIDS) data as at 1 October 1991. Weekly Epidemiological Record 1991; 66:289–90.

5. Parvi KM. Status of AIDS/HIV in India. Virus Information Exchange Newsletter 1991; 8:54-6.

6. World Health Organization. AIDS in the 1990s—Meeting the challenge. WHO Press, 12 October, 1991.

7. Global Programme on AIDS. Current and future dimensions of the HIV/AIDS pandemic. A capsule summary. WHO/GPA/RES/SFI/91.4, April 1991.

8. Chin J. Present and future dimensions of the HIV/AIDS pandemic. Keynote address, Seventh International Conference on AIDS, 1991, Florence, Italy. Virus Information Exchange Newsletter 1991; 8:74-80.

9. Viravaidya M. Confronting, a culture at risk: a curbside view of AIDS education and prevention in Thailand. Proceedings of AIDS in Asia and the Pacific Conference, Canberra, August 5-8, 1990:63-7.

10. Sittitrai W. Multi-stage interventions for sex workers in Thailand. Proceedings of AIDS in Asia and the Pacific Conference, Canberra, August 5-8, 1990:165-71.

11. Anonymous. India: Prostitutes and the spread of AIDS. Lancet 1990; i:1332.

12. Watsa MC. AIDS: intervention strategies for prostitution—India. Proceedings of AIDS in Asia and the Pacific Conference, Canberra, August 5-8, 1990:171-5.

13. Qi XQ. Cultural and social issues in the transmission of IIIV in China. Proceedings of AIDS in Asia and the Pacific Conference, Canberra, August 5-8, 1990:89-92.

14. Sittitrai W, et al. The survey of partner relations and risk of HIV infection in Thailand (Abstracts). Seventh International Conference on AIDS, Florence, June 16-21, 1991:MD4113.

15. Ungphakorn J. The impact of AIDS on women in Thailand. Proceedings of AIDS in Asia and the Pacific Conference, Canberra, August 5-8, 1990: 151-4.

16. Ravinathan A, Ravinathan R, Meeran M, et al. Oral contraception, IUD, condom use and man to woman heterosexual transmission of STD/HIV infection (Abstracts). Seventh International Conference on AIDS, Florence, June 16-21, 1991:MD4232.

17. Sakuntanaga P. Intervention strategies relating to injecting drug behaviour—Thailand. Proceedings of AIDS in Asia and the Pacific Conference, Canberra, August 5-8, 1990:134-6.

18. Hong Kong Government. Central Registry of Drug Abuse. Twenty-seventh report (1981-1990).

19. World Health Organization South-East Asia Regional Office. Situation of HIV/AIDS in the countries of the South-East Asia Region (compilation of unedited reports received from countries). SEA/RC44/Inf.2.

20. Ismail NSN. Intervention strategies relating to injecting drug behaviour—Malaysia. Proceedings of AIDS in Asia and the Pacific Conference, Canberra, August 5–8, 1990:139–41.

21. Rubsamen-Waigmann H, Briesen HN, Maniar JK, et al. Spread of HIV-2 in India (Correspondence). Lancet 1991; 337:550–1.

22. Rubsamen-Waigmann H, Pfutzner A, Scholz C, et al. Spread of HIV-2 in India (Abstract). Seventh International Conference on AIDS, Florence, June 16-21, 1991:MC3291.

23. Sehgal S. HIV-2 infection in North India (Abstract). Seventh International Conference on AIDS, Florence, June 16–21, 1991:MC3249.

24. Chin J. Global estimates of AIDS cases and HIV infection: 1990; AIDS 1990; 4(suppl 1):S277–83.

25. Ravinathan R, et al. HIV seroprevalence among the homosexuals of Tamilnadu & effects of condom-skills training on AIDS prevention (Abstract). Seventh International Conference on AIDS, Florence, June 16–21, 1991:WC3074.

26. World Health Organization Western Pacific Regional Office. AIDS Report. Virus Information Exchange Newsletter 1989; 6:160–8.

27. Chuang CH. Current status of HIV infection in Taiwan (Abstract). Fifth International Conference on AIDS, Montreal, June 4–9, 1989:G501.

28. Traisupa A, Teerathum C, Tharavanich S, Saengsue S. Seroprevalence of antibody to human immunodeficiency virus HIV-1 in a high risk group in 4 provinces with tourist attractions. Thai AIDS J 1990; 2:57–63.

29. Thongcharoen P. HIV infection in Thailand. Virus Information Exchange Newsletter 1991; 8:57.

30. Ungchusak K, Thanprasertsuk S, Sriprapandh S, et al. First national seroprevalence survey of HIV-1 infection in Thailand, June 1989 (Abstract). Sixth International Conference on AIDS, San Francisco, June 21–24, 1990:FC99.

31. Sawanpanyalert P, Ungchusak K, Thanprasertsuk S, Akarasewi P. Seroconversion rate and risk factors for HIV-1 infection among low-class female sex workers in Chiangmai, Thailand: a multi cross-sectional study (Abstract). Seventh International Conference on AIDS, Florence, June 16–21, 1991: WC3097.

32. Siraprapasiri T, Thanprasertsuk S, Rodklay A, et al. Risk factors for HIV among prostitutes in Chiangmai, Thailand. AIDS 1991; 5:579–82.

33. Li PCK, Lee SH, Saw TA, et al. Epidemiology of HIV infection in Hong Kong (Abstract). Seventh International Conference on AIDS, Florence, June 16–21, 1991:MC3284.

34. Bhave GG, Wagle UD, Tripathy SP. HIV sero-surveillance in promiscuous females of Bombay, India (Abstract). Sixth International Conference on AIDS, San Francisco, June 21–24, 1990:FC612.

35. Singh YN, Malaviya AN, Tripathy SP, et al. HIV serosurveillance among prostitutes and patients from a sexually transmitted disease clinic in Delhi, India. J Acq Immun Def Synd 1990; 3:287–9.

36. Hayes CG, Manaloto CR, Basaca-Sevilla V, et al. Epidemiology of HIV infection among prostitutes in the Philippines. J Acq Immun Def Synd 1990; 3:913–20.

37. Choi KH, Kim MS, Catania J, et al. First HIV seroprevalence survey in South Korea (Abstract). Seventh International Conference on AIDS, Florence, June 16–21, 1991:MC3235.

38. Lin HC, Shi YH. Seroprevalence of HIV-I among clients attending STD clinic in Taipei (Abstract). Seventh International Conference on AIDS, Florence, June 16–21, 1991:WC3142.

39. Ungchusak K, Thanprasertsuk S, Vichai C, et al. Trends of HIV spreading in Thailand detected by national sentinel serosurveillance (Abstract). Seventh International Conference on AIDS, Florence, June 16–21, 1991:MC3246.

40. Sittitrai W. HIV transmission and interventions in Thailand: socio-economic and cultural issues. Proceedings of AIDS in Asia and the Pacific Conference, Canberra, August 5–8, 1990:81–7.

41. Patil SA, Shivraj U, Sengupta KK, et al. Serosurveillance of high risk groups for the prevalence of HIV-1 infection in Agra, India. Virus Information Exchange Newsletter 1991; 8:22–3.

42. Kandaswami J, Ravinathan R, Padmarajan S, et al. Sero-epidemiological study of HIV infection in two major centres of south India (Abstract). Seventh International Conference on AIDS, Florence: June 16-21, 1991:MC3302.

43. Williams J, Raja DA, Venkatram MK. HIV seropositivity among genital HSV patients attending the STD Clinic, Government Rajaji Hospital, Madurai, Tamil Nadu, India. Virus Information Exchange Newsletter 1991; 8: 65–6.

44. Mathai R, Prasad PVS, Jacob M, et al. HIV seropositivity among patients with sexually transmitted diseases in Vellore. Indian J Med Res 1990; 91: 239–41.

45. Kunanusont C, Weniger BS, Foy H, et al. Modes of transmission for the high rate of HIV infection among male STD patients and male blood donors in Chiangmai, Thailand (Abstract). Seventh International Conference on AIDS, Florence, June 16–21, 1991:WC3086.

46. Thongcharoen P. AIDS in Southeast Asia: Thailand. Med Prog 1990; July: 19–22.

47. Ramalingaswami V. The implications of AIDS in developing countries. Keynote address. Seventh International Conference on AIDS, Florence, Italy, 1991.

48. Fulayfil R, Baig ZHB. Prevalence of HIV antibodies in high risk groups, Bahrain (Abstracts). Seventh International Conference on AIDS, Florence, June 16–21, 1991:MD4161.

49. Naik TN, Sarkar S, Singh HL, et al. Intravenous drug users—a new high-risk group for HIV infection in India. AIDS 1991; 5:117–8.

50. Singh NB, Singh YI, Singh HL. Increasing incidence of HIV infection in Manipur—a north-eastern state of India. Virus Information Exchange Newsletter 1991; 8:66.

51. Singh NB, Singh YI, Singh HL. Epidemic of HIV infection among intravenous drug users in Manipur, India. Virus Information Exchange Newsletter 1991; 8:20.

52. Chung DC, Ko YC, Chen CJ, et al. Seroepidemiology of hepatitis B virus, hepatitis D virus, and human immunodeficiency virus infections among parenteral drug abusers in southern Taiwan. J Med Virol 1989; 28:215–8.

53. Vanichseni S, Sakuntanaga P, et al. Results of three seroprevalence surveys for HIV in IVDU in Bangkok (Abstract). Sixth International Conference on AIDS, San Francisco, June 21–24, 1990:FC105.

54. Bogird C, Jongpaiboolpathna J. HIV infection among intravenous drug users: a study at Hat Yai Hospital 1988–1989. Thai AIDS J 1989; 1:83–7.

55. Gammelgaard J. Availability and pattern of abuse of heroin. Proceedings of AIDS in Asia and the Pacific Conference, Canberra, August 5–8, 1990: 131–3.

56. De M, Banerjee D, Chandra S, Bhattacharya DK. HBV and HIV seropositivity in multi-transfused haemophilics and thalassaemics in Eastern India. Indian J Med Res 1990; 91:63–6.

57. Singh YN, Bhargava M, Malaviya AN, et al. HIV infection in Asian Indian patients with haemophilia and those who had multiple transfusion. Indian J Med Res 1991; 93:12–4.

58. Apte SV, Joshi SH, Dumasia AN, Patil RS. Prevalence of anti-HIV antibodies among blood donors in Bombay (Abstract). Sixth International Conference on AIDS, San Francisco, June 21–24, 1990:FC611.

59. Singh YN, Malaviya AN, Tripathy SP, et al. Human immunodeficiency virus infection in the blood donors of Delhi, India. J Acq Immun Def Synd 1990; 3:152–4.

60. Singh YN, et al. HIV infection in the blood donors of Delhi, India: 1 1/2 years' experience. J Acq Immun Def Synd 1991; 4:1008–9.

61. Singhvi A, Pulimodd RB, John TJ, et al. The prevalence of markers of hepatitis B and human immunodeficiency viruses, malarial parasites and microfilaria in blood donors in a large hospital in South India. J Trop Med Hyg 1990; 93:178–82.

62. Shimizu M. Safe blood in low prevalence areas—Japan. Proceedings of AIDS in Asia and the Pacific Conference, Canberra, August 5–8, 1990:146–7.

63. DeZoysa N. Safe blood in low prevalence areas—the Sri Lankan experience and perspective. Proceedings of AIDS in Asia and the Pacific Conference, Canberra, August 5–8, 1990:142–4.

64. Nuchprayoon C, Tanprasert S, Chumnijarakij T. HIV screening in donated blood—a reflection of AIDS epidemiology in Thailand. Thai AIDS J 1990; 2:87–98.

65. Tuyen BQ. Safe blood in low prevalence areas—some experience in Viet Nam. Proceedings of AIDS in Asia and the Pacific Conference, Canberra, August 5–8, 1990:144–5.

66. Chanarat P, Thongkrajai P, Kulapongs P. The possibility of HIV transmission via anti-HIV-negative blood in polytransfused beta-thalassemia patients in northern Thailand. Vox Sanguinis 1990; 58:224–5.

67. Bradley H, Popovivi F, Jezek Z, et al. Risk factors for HIV infection among abandoned Romanian children (Abstract). Seventh International Conference on AIDS, Florence, June 16–21, 1991:ThD109.

68. Pokrovsky VV, Eramova EU. Nosocomial outbreak of HIV infection in Elista, USSR (Abstract). Fifth International Conference on AIDS, Montreal, June 4-9, 1989:WA05.

69. Sankari SS, Solomon S. Trends of HIV infections in antenatal/infertility clinic—an ominous sign (Abstract). Seventh International Conference on AIDS, Florence, June 16–21, 1991:WC3236.

70. Chew SK, Chan R, Monteiro EHA, Sng EH. Human immunodeficiency virus in Singapore—the first 50 cases. Singapore Med J 1990; 31:587–91.

71. Li PCK, Yeoh EK, Lee SS, et al. Clinical manifestations of AIDS in Hong Kong (Abstract). Seventh International Conference on AIDS, Florence, June 16–21, 1991:MB2453.

72. Monzon OT, Basaca-Sevilla V, Hayes C, et al. The spectrum of clinical disease among Filipino cases (Abstract). Fifth International Conference on AIDS, Montreal, June 4-9, 1989:TBP377.

73. Tanphaichitra D. Three patterns of AIDS in the topics: an overview (Abstract). Seventh International Conference on AIDS, Florence, June 16–21, 1991: MB2452.

74. Mann JM. Global AIDS into the 1990s. Keynote address, Fifth International Conference on AIDS, Montreal, Canada. WHO/GPA/DIR/89.2, 1989.

75. Merson MH. Global AIDS prevention and control. Proceedings of AIDS in Asia and the Pacific Conference, Canberra, August 5–8, 1990:27–30.

76. Ramachandran P. Impact of AIDS on women and children. Proceedings of AIDS in Asia and the Pacific Conference, Canberra, August 5–8, 1990:122–30.

2

Predictors of HIV Disease Progression in the Era of Prophylactic Therapies

Nancy A. Hessol
San Francisco Department of Public Health,
San Francisco, California

Susan P. Buchbinder
San Francisco Department of Public Health and University of
California San Francisco, San Francisco, California

I. INTRODUCTION

As we enter the second decade of the AIDS epidemic, there is still no cure for HIV infection, but a tremendous amount has been learned about disease progression. What once was an observational approach to monitoring HIV disease progression has now turned into an active course of early intervention using antiviral and prophylactic therapies to prevent HIV-related disease and death. As our approach to managing HIV infection changes, so must our thinking about predictors of HIV disease progression. In this chapter we begin by addressing the effect of antiviral and prophylactic therapies on AIDS and survival. We then highlight current information on predictors for HIV disease progression. Finally, we address the role of cofactors in HIV disease progression and, when applicable, contrast the old data with the new.

II. EFFECT OF ANTIVIRALS AND PROPHYLAXIS ON HIV DISEASE PROGRESSION

Zidovudine (AZT) was approved for treatment of patients with AIDS or severe ARC in March 1987 after it was shown in a randomized clinical trial to significantly decrease mortality and the frequency of opportunistic infections (1). Similarly, in 1989, the Centers for Disease Control (CDC) recommended prophylaxis against *Pneumocystis carinii* pneumonia (PCP) in HIV-infected persons with previous PCP or low CD4 + counts (<200 cells/ mm³ or <20%) after clinical trials demonstrated that prophylaxis significantly reduced the risk of PCP (2,3). Over time, use of these agents has increased in HIV-infected populations, and this trend can be expected to continue (4-7).

Questions have been raised about the impact of these agents on the "natural history" of HIV infection, including the duration of the latency period (time from HIV infection to AIDS), survival time after an index AIDS diagnosis, and the relative frequency of specific HIV-related diseases. It is important to reassess the predictive power of previously defined markers of HIV disease progression, as antiviral and prophylactic therapies become more widely available and are utilized earlier in infection.

Various attempts have been made to assess the impact of therapies on HIV disease progression rates outside of clinical trials. Using data from the Multicenter AIDS Cohort Study, it was demonstrated that use of zidovudine and PCP prophylaxis was associated with significant reductions in progression from one clinical stage to the next (8). Although analyses that compare nonrandomized groups are subject to confounding, these results suggest that efficacy can be demonstrated outside of clinical trials.

Other investigators have compared HIV disease progression rates before and after FDA approval of zidovudine. One study found weak (but not statistically significant) evidence that the latency period has been lengthening since 1987 and suggested that zidovudine was one of several plausible explanations (9). Using data from the San Francisco City Clinic Cohort Study (SFCCCS), investigators found that Kaplan-Meier progression curves from seroconversion to AIDS and death were much lower than projected curves based on pre-1987 data (10). Again, zidovudine use is only one of several possible explanations; in fact, nearly half of the men infected prior to 1981 in the SFCCCS who had not developed AIDS had reported never taking zidovudine or PCP prophylaxis. Thus, zidovudine may be only one of several factors that slow HIV disease progression.

Investigators have also attempted to assess the impact of therapies on AIDS incidence in the United States. While incidence rates have continued to rise, the rate of rise slowed in the middle of 1987, the year zidovudine was approved by the FDA (11). This "leveling" of incidence occurred primarily in homosexual/bisexual men not using intravenous drugs, and was most marked in urban epicenters (San Francisco, New York, Los Angeles) and in white men. Because these were the groups with the highest rates of utilization of zidovudine, these trends are assumed to be indirect evidence of the impact of antiviral therapies.

Mathematical models also support the effect of zidovudine on AIDS incidence. Investigators have found a deficit in the United States AIDS incidence in homosexual men, hemophiliacs, and transfusion recipients; they were able to account for a large portion of the deficit through estimates of zidovudine use in these groups and its expected impact on the latency period (5,12). They reported that other explanations, including a decrease in rates of new HIV infection, revision of the CDC AIDS case definition in 1987, and reporting delays accounted for a much smaller portion of the deficit in their models. Other investigators have countered that these alternative explanations may, in fact, contribute to the AIDS deficit (13,14). It is likely that several factors are responsible for the observed trends in AIDS incidence.

Zidovudine is also expected to lengthen survival following an AIDS diagnosis. Since 1986, there has been a significant increase in survival, particularly in persons first diagnosed with PCP (15,16). Using data linking zidovudine use with demographics and survival time after AIDS, one study demonstrated in multivariable analysis that 2-year survival was greater in persons who had used zidovudine than in those who had not (17). While this offers further evidence that zidovudine may be responsible for improving recent trends in survival, the study also points to inequities in access to zidovudine. Women, ethnic minorities, and persons 45 years of age or older were significantly less likely to receive zidovudine after an AIDS diagnosis than were non-Hispanic white men 30 years of age or younger. It is imperative that these inequities be addressed and that future studies assess the impact of prophylactic therapies on HIV disease progression in these groups.

As additional antiviral and prophylactic agents are developed and utilized, it will be important to assess the impact of these agents on HIV disease progression, AIDS, and survival. It is therefore necessary to reevaluate laboratory and clinical predictors of HIV disease progression in the context of antiviral and prophylactic therapies, as this may be one of our most useful strategies for targeting and evaluating specific interventions. It is also important to explore other factors in addition to therapies that contribute to delayed progression; such factors may direct us to new areas of research for therapies and vaccines.

III. LABORATORY PREDICTORS OF HIV DISEASE PROGRESSION

Laboratory markers remain among the most important predictors of HIV disease progression. Laboratory markers of HIV disease progression that have consistently proven to be important are T-cell subsets, neopterin, beta-2 microglobulin, and, to a lesser extent, p24 antigen. Most prospective studies of HIV-infected individuals showed a less favorable outcome for persons with a low absolute CD4 + lymphocyte count (18-23). In general, studies that have evaluated CD4 + counts as a predictor of HIV disease development have found that CD4 + cell counts of less than 200 are associated with poorer prognosis.

In addition to a low absolute CD4 + count, some prospective studies have found an association between other T-cell measurements and increased progression rates. These measurements include the rate of decline in absolute CD4 + counts (24-26), a low proportion of CD4 + lymphocytes (23,26), a low total lymphocyte count (23,26), an increased absolute number of CD8 + suppressor cells (27), and/or a low CD4 + /CD8 + ratio (23).

Some studies have demonstrated an unfavorable prognosis for persons with p24 antigenemia (28-30). However, other studies have found that in multivariable analysis, p24 antigen is not a good independent predictor of AIDS (23,31,32). A possible reason for the lack of consistency between studies evaluating p24 antigen is that p24 antigenemia is uncommon in AIDS-free HIV-infected individuals (33). This low prevalence of p24 antigenemia in AIDS-free individuals, however, makes p24 antigen a useful measure for monitoring response failure to antiviral agents such as zidovudine (34,35), dideoxycytidine (36,37), and dideoxyinosine (38,39). The studies have also used changes in the level of HIV antigenemia to provide an index of the antiviral effect of treatment.

The prognostic significance of elevated beta-2 microglobulin (23) and elevated serum neopterin concentrations (23,30) has been confirmed in several studies. In studies of homosexual men, however, these two markers are highly correlated with each other so that in multivariable analysis only one marker is generally determined to be an independent predictor of progression. In users of intravenous drugs, beta-2 microglobulin has not been a good prognostic indicator (40,41). In addition to its use as a prognostic marker, beta-2 microglobulin, like p24 antigen, has been followed for antiviral response (42).

Several studies have also shown that quantitation of viral load correlates with clinical manifestations of HIV infection (43-47). Viral isolation of HIV has been measured from a variety of sources, including RNA and DNA through polymerase chain reaction tests, peripheral blood mononuclear cells, plasma culture, and serum p24 antigen. Additional epidemiological studies that are prospective in design are needed in order to determine whether viral titers are prognostic for HIV disease progression or merely markers of current status.

Other laboratory measures that have been suggested to be predictive of progression to AIDS in HIV-infected individuals include increased serum immunoglobulins (48), the presence of interferon alpha (49), elevated immune complexes (23), and serum-soluble interleukin-2 receptor (23,50). An additional laboratory measure that has been predictive of survival in people with AIDS is a low hemoglobin level (51). Mathematical models that include at least one serum marker in addition to T-cell subsets tend to have a greater prognostic value that either alone. However, the addition of multiple serological markers has diminishing benefits.

IV. CLINICAL PREDICTORS OF HIV DISEASE PROGRESSION

Despite increasing reliance on laboratory predictors of HIV disease progression, HIV-related clinical symptoms continue to provide important prognostic information. Recent studies have been able to define more clearly those clinical signs and symptoms that serve as independent predictors of progression to AIDS, when controlling for laboratory markers such as CD4+ counts.

Oral candidiasis and constitutional symptoms (idiopathic fever, night sweats, diarrhea, weight loss) have been repeatedly found to be the strongest clinical predictors of progression to AIDS, even when adjusting for CD4+ count (20,52-54). Hairy leukoplakia, particularly when detected by trained examiners, may be found in relatively healthy HIV-infected persons and thus appears to be a significant but less strong predictor of development of AIDS (54). Other HIV-related symptoms are found to occur more frequently in HIV-infected persons but do not provide independent prognostic information, including generalized lymphadenopathy and herpes zoster (20,55).

Interestingly, both severity and duration of symptoms associated with acute seroconversion may predict a more rapid rate of progression to AIDS (56,57). Although this information may be of limited value in clinical or epidemiological settings in which this information is obtained retrospectively, it does raise intriguing questions about potential virological or immunological mechanisms governing HIV disease progression.

Clinical symptoms may also independently predict survival following an AIDS diagnosis. In one study, fever and thrush independently predicted survival following an AIDS diagnosis when adjusting for CD4+ count and use of zidovudine (58).

A recent study in HIV-infected homosexual men without AIDS found that clinical conditions could not be used to predict CD4+ cell counts (59). The authors concluded that clinical and serological parameters may provide important prognostic information, but cannot be used to reliably determine the level of CD4+ cells.

Clinical predictors provide prognostic information independent of laboratory markers; however, laboratory markers have been shown to have greater prognostic significance in several studies where both clinical and laboratory predictors were included in multivariable analyses. The relative importance of laboratory predictors in relationship to each other, especially those that may be different measurements of the same biological or immunological response, is crucial in determining their true predictive value.

V. COFACTORS FOR HIV DISEASE PROGRESSION

In addition to use of therapies and prophylaxis to prevent or delay HIV disease progression, other factors may be influential in determining the course of HIV infection. A cofactor for HIV disease progression can be defined as a parameter that, if present, can alter the natural course of disease progression. The most significant cofactor associated with HIV disease progression is age of the infected individual. Several studies have now shown an association between older age and more rapid progression to HIV disease (60-62). Older adults also had a more rapid decline in CD4+ counts than young adults, suggesting that prophylaxis against opportunistic infections be started earlier in older adults.

Several studies have evaluated the association between viral infections and progression time to AIDS. Among the viral cofactors studied are cytomegalovirus (63-65), human herpes virus-6 (65), Epstein-Barr virus (65), hepatitis B, and hepatitis C (66). Although in vitro interactions between HIV and other viruses have been well demonstrated, in vivo evidence for increased disease progression is conflicting at best. A few studies have shown an increase in progression to AIDS associated with histories of other sexually transmitted diseases (57,67), while other studies have not found this association (68).

A controversial area is whether or not women have a faster progression to AIDS and death than men. There continue to be reports from Nairobi on women prostitutes who progressed to HIV disease very rapidly (69). It is not clear, however, whether this rapid progression is associated with gender or other factors, such as nutrition, medical care, and exposure to sexually transmitted diseases. Early studies of survival time from AIDS diagnosis to death in women, compared to men, did find that women had a shorter survival (70). However, two recent studies examining survival from AIDS diagnosis to death found there was no statistical difference between survival time in heterosexual men and survival time in women (71,72). By comparing survival among similar risk groups (i.e., heterosexually transmitted HIV infection), the investigators were able to control for confounders, such as socioeconomic status, ethnicity, and presenting AIDS diagnosis.

One area speculated to be a potential cofactor for HIV disease progression is nutrition, but few studies have been done. One study in homosexual men (73) and another study in Rumanian children (74) found that poor nutrition was associated with more rapid HIV disease progression. A recent report found that high serum copper and low serum zinc levels were predictive of progression to AIDS (75). However, the temporal relationship between nutrition and illness remains unclear, and it may be that the disease causes the nutritional problems rather than the other way around.

Another controversial cofactor is whether psychosocial factors play a role in HIV disease progression. A recent study found that depression and lack of social support was associated with shorter survival time following an AIDS diagnosis (76). In contrast, another recent study found that stressful life events did not appear to alter HIV disease progression time (77).

Among the cofactors recently studied that were not associated with HIV disease progression were current intravenous drug use (78,79) and cigarette smoking (80,81). These results contrast with previous reports on intravenous drug users (82) and cigarette smoking (83). In general, the more recent studies were better designed and analyzed and should be regarded as more definitive.

An area of considerable laboratory interest has been genetic influences on HIV disease progression. Most of the work has evaluated the role of host HLA frequencies and the association with clinical and immunological status (84-87). As laboratory techniques improve and are standardized, it will be easier to compare results from the various studies.

VI. CONCLUSION

In the 1990s, HIV infection is increasingly being viewed as a manageable chronic disease rather than as an immutable terminal illness. As the arsenal of prophylactic and therapeutic drugs continues to grow, HIV-infected individuals will live longer with an improved quality of life. Predictors and cofactors of HIV disease progression will become increasingly important for developing and evaluating new therapies and targeting early intervention strategies. The challenge for the 1990s will be to provide all HIV-infected individuals with access to quality health care and social services, a necessary prerequisite for rapid dissemination of new interventions.

REFERENCES

1. Fischl MA, Richman DD, Grieco MH, et al. The efficacy of azidothymidine (AZT) in the treatment of patients with AIDS and AIDS-related complex: a double-blind placebo-controlled trial. N Engl J Med 1987; 317:185–91.

2. Leoung GS, Feigal DW, Montgomery AB, et al. Aerosolized pentamidine for prophylaxis against *Pneumocystis carinii* pneumonia. N Engl J Med 1990; 323: 769–75.

3. Hirschel B, Lazzarin A, Chopard P, et al. A controlled study of inhaled pentamidine for primary prevention of *Pneumocystis carinii* pneumonia. N Engl J Med 1991; 324:1079–83.

4. Lang W, Osmond D, Samuel M, Moss A, Schrager L, Winkelstein W. Population-based estimated of zidovudine and aerosol pentamidine use in San Francisco: 1987-1989. J Acquir Immun Defic Syndr 1991; 4:713–16.

5. Rosenberg PS, Gail MH, Schrager LK, et al. National AIDS incidence trends and the extent of zidovudine therapy in selected demographic and transmission groups. J Acquir Immun Defic Syndr 1991; 4:392–401.

6. Holmberg S, Conley L, Buchbinder S, et al. Therapeutic and prophylactic drug use by homosexual men in 3 U.S. cities. VII International Conference on AIDS. Vol. 2. Florence, Italy, June 16-21, 1991:303.

7. Graham NMH, Zeger SL, Kuo V, et al. Zidovudine use in AIDS-free HIV-1-seropositive homosexual men in the Multicenter AIDS Cohort Study (MACS), 1987-1989. J Acquir Immun Defic Syndr 1991; 4:267–76.

8. Graham NMH, Zeger SL, Park LP, et al. Effect of zidovudine and *Pneumocystis carinii* pneumonia prophylaxis on progression of HIV-1 infection to AIDS. Lancet 1991; 338:265–9.

9. Taylor JMG, Kuo JM, Detels R. Is the incubation period of AIDS lengthening? J Acquir Immun Defic Syndr 1991; 4:69–75.

10. Buchbinder S, Hessol N, O'Malley P, et al. HIV disease progression and the impact of prophylactic therapies in the San Francisco City Clinic Cohort: a 13-year follow-up. VII International Conference on AIDS. Vol. 2. Florence, Italy, June 16-21, 1991:33.

11. CDC. HIV prevalence estimates and AIDS case projections for the United States: report based upon a workshop. MMWR 1990; 39(No RR-16):1–31.

12. Gail MH, Rosenberg PS, Goedert JJ. Therapy may explain recent deficits in AIDS incidence. J Acquir Immun Defic Syndr 1990; 3:296–306.

13. Brookmeyer R. Reconstruction and future trends of the AIDS epidemic in the United States. Science 1991; 253:37–42.

14. Segal M, Bacchetti P. Deficits in AIDS incidence. J Acquir Immun Defic 1990; 3:832–6.

15. Lemp GF, Payne SF, Neal D, Temelso T, Rutherford GW. Survival trends for patients with AIDS. JAMA 1990; 263:402–6.

16. Harris JE. Improved short-term survival of AIDS patients initially diagnosed with *Pneumocystis carinii* pneumonia, 1984-1987. JAMA 1990; 263:397–401.

17. Moore RD, Hidalgo J, Sugland BW, Chaisson RE. Zidovudine and the natural history of the acquired immunodeficiency syndrome. N Engl J Med 1991; 324:1412–16.

18. Goedert JJ, Biggar RJ, Melbye M, Mann DL, Wilson S, Gail MH, Grossman RJ, DiGioia RA, Sanchez WC, Weiss SH, Blattner WA. Effect of T4 count and cofactors on the incidence of AIDS in homosexual men infected with human immunodeficiency virus. JAMA 1987; 257:331–4.

19. Kaplan JE, Spira TJ, Fishbein DB, Bozeman LH, Pinsky PF, Schonberger LB. A six-year follow-up of HIV-infected homosexual men with lymphadenopathy: evidence for an increased risk of developing AIDS after the third year of lymphadenopathy. JAMA 1988; 260:2694–7.

20. Moss AR, Bacchetti P, Osmond D, Krampf W, Chaisson RE, Stites D, Wilber J, Allain JP, Carlson J. Seropositivity for HIV and the development of AIDS or AIDS-related condition: three-year follow-up of the San Francisco General Hospital cohort. Br Med J 1988; 296:745–50.

21. Schecter MT, Craib KJP, Le TN, Willoughby B, Douglas B, Sestak P, Montaner JSG, Weaver MS, Elmslie KD, O'Shaughnessy MV. Progression to AIDS and predictors of AIDS in seroprevalent and seroincident cohorts of homosexual men. AIDS 1989; 3:347–53.

22. De Wolf F, Lange JMA, Houweling JTM, et al. Numbers of CD4 + cells and the levels of core antigens and antibodies to the human immunodeficiency virus as predictors of AIDS among seropositive men. J Infect Dis 1988; 158: 615–22.

23. Fahey JL, Taylor JMG, Detels R, et al. The prognostic value of cellular and serologic markers in infection with human immunodeficiency virus type 1. N Engl J Med 1990; 322:166–72.

24. Detels R, English PA, Giorgi JV, et al. Patterns of CD4+ cell changes after HIV-1 infection indicate the existence of a codeterminant of AIDS. J Acquir Immun Defic Syndr 1988; 1:390–5.

25. Phillips AN, Lee CA, Elford J, Janossy G, Timms A, Bofill M, Kernoff PBA. Serial CD4 lymphocyte counts and development of AIDS. Lancet 1991; 337: 389-92.

26. Burcham J, Marmor M, Dubin N, Tindall B, Cooper DA, Berry G, Penny R. CD4+ is the best predictor of development of AIDS in a cohort of HIV-infected homosexual men. AIDS 1991; 5:365–72.

27. Anderson RE, Shiboski SC, Royce R, Jewell NP, Lang W, Winkelstein Jr W. CD8+ T lymphocytes and progression to AIDS in HIV-infected men: some observations. AIDS 1991; 5:213–5.

28. Pedersen C, Nielsen CM, Vestergaard BF, Gerstoft J, Krogsgaard K, Nielsen JO. Temporal relation of antigenaemia and loss of antibodies to core antigens to development of clinical disease in HIV infection. Br Med J 1987; 295:567–9.

29. Allain JP, Laurian Y, Paul DA, et al. Long-term evaluation of HIV antigen and antibodies to p24 and gp41 in patients with hemophilia: potential clinical importance. N Engl J Med 1987; 317:1114–21.

30. Sheppard HW, Ascher MS, McRae B, Anderson RE, Lang W, Allain J-P. The initial immune response to HIV and immune system activation determine the outcome of HIV disease. J Acquir Immun Defic Syndr 1991; 4:704–12.

31. Fernandez-Cruz E, Desco M, Montes MG, Longo N, Gonzalez B, Zabay JM. Immunological and serological markers predictive of progression to AIDS in a cohort of HIV-infected drug users. AIDS 1990; 4:987–94.

32. Phillips AN, Lee CA, Elford J, Webster A, Janossy G, Griffiths PD, Kernoff PBA. p24 antigenaemia, CD4 lymphocyte counts and the development of AIDS. AIDS 1991; 5:1217–22.

33. MacDonell KB, Chmiel JS, Poggensee L, Wu S, Phair JP. Predicting progression to AIDS: combined usefulness of CD4 lymphocyte counts and p24 antigenaemia. Am J Med 1990; 89:706–12.

34. Chaisson RE, Allain JP, Leuther M, Volberding PA. Significant changes in HIV antigen level in the serum of patients treated with azidothymidine. N Engl J Med 1986; 315:1610–11.

35. Jackson GG, Paul DA, Falk LA, et al. Human immunodeficiency virus antigenaemia in the acquired immunodeficiency syndrome and the effect of treatment with zidovudine. Ann Intern Med 1988; 108:175–80.

36. Yarchoan R, Perno CF, Thomas RV, et al. Phase I studies of 2′,3′-dideoxy-cytidine in severe human immunodeficiency virus infection as a single agent and alternating with zidovudine (AZT). Lancet 1988; 1:76–81.

37. Merigan TC, Skowron G, Bozzette SA, et al. Circulating p24 antigen levels and responses to dideoxycytidine in human immunodeficiency virus (HIV) infections: a phase I and II study. Ann Intern Med 1989; 110:189–94.

38. Lambert JS, Seidlin M, Reichman RC, et al. 2′,3′-Dideoxyinosine (ddI) in patients with the acquired immunodeficiency syndrome or AIDS-related complex; a phase I trial. N Engl J Med 1990; 322:1333–40.

39. Cooley TP, Kunches LM, Saunders CA, et al. Once-daily administration of 2′,3′-Dideoxyinosine (ddI) in patients with the acquired immunodeficiency syndrome or AIDS-related complex; a phase I trial. N Engl J Med 1990; 322: 1304–5.

40. Flegg PJ, Brettle RP, Robertson JR, Clarkson RC, Bird AG. Beta-2 micro-globulin levels in drug users: the influence of risk behaviour. AIDS 1991; 5: 1021–4.

41. Zangerle R, Fuchs D, Reibnegger G, Fritsch P, Wachter H. Markers for disease progression in intravenous drug users infected with HIV-1. AIDS 1991; 5:985–91.

42. Jacobsen MA, Bacchetti P, Kolokathis A, et al. Surrogate markers for survival in patients with AIDS or AIDS related complex treated with zidovudine. BMJ 1991; 302:73–8.

43. Levy JA, Shimabukuro J. Recovery of AIDS associated retrovirus from patients with AIDS or related conditions and from healthy individuals. J Infect Dis 1985; 152:734–8.

44. Spira TJ, Kaplan JE, Feorino PM, Warfield D, Fishbein B, Bozman LH. HIV viraemia as a prognostic indicator in homosexual men with lymphadenopathy syndrome. N Engl J Med 1987; 317:1093–4.

45. Paul DA, Falk LA, Kessler HA, et al. Correlation of serum HIV antigen and antibody with clinical status in HIV-infected patients. J Med Virol 1987; 22: 357–63.

46. Coombs RV, Collier AC, Allain JP, et al. Plasma viraemia in human immuno-deficiency virus infection. N Engl J Med 1989; 321:1626–30.

47. Escaich S, Ritter J, Rougier P, Lepot D, Lamelin J-P, Sepetjan M, Trepo C. Plasma viraemia as a marker of viral replication in HIV-infected individuals. AIDS 1991; 5:1189–94.

48. Polk BF, Fox R, Brookmeyer R, et al. Predictors of the acquired immuno-deficiency syndrome developing in a cohort of seropositive homosexual men. N Engl J Med 1987; 316:61–66.

49. Buimovici-Klein E, Sonnabend JA, Lange M, Friedman-Klein AE, Klein RJ, Vilcek J. Predictors of AIDS in homosexual men. N Engl J Med 1987; 317:245.

50. Osmond DH, Shiboski S, Bacchetti P, Winger EE, Moss AR. Immune activation markers and AIDS prognosis. AIDS 1991; 5:505–11.

51. Steinberg JP, Spear JB, Murphy RL, et al. Predictors of outcome in AIDS patients receiving zidovudine. J Acquir Immun Defic Syndr 1989; 2:229–34.

52. Fischl MA, Richman DD, Hansen N, Collier AC, Carey JT, Para MF. The safety and efficacy of zidovudine (AZT) in the treatment of subjects with mildly symptomatic human immunodeficiency virus type 1 (HIV) infection: a double-blind placebo-controlled trial. Ann Intern Med 1990; 112:727–37.

53. Phair J, Munoz A, Detels R, Kaslow R, Rinaldo C, Saah A. The risk of *Pneumocystis carinii* pneumonia among men infected with human immunodeficiency virus type 1. N Engl J Med 1990; 322:161–5.

54. Katz MH, Greenspan D, Westenhouse J, et al. Progression to AIDS in HIV-infected homosexual and bisexual men with hairy leukoplakia and oral candiasis: results from three San Francisco epidemiologic cohorts. AIDS, in press.

55. Murray HW, Godbold JH, Jurica KB, Roberts RB. Progression to AIDS in patients with lymphadenopathy or AIDS-related complex: reappraisal of risk and predictive factors. Am J Med 1989; 86:533–8.

56. Pedersen C, Lindhardt BO, Jensen BL, et al. Clinical course of primary HIV infection: consequences for subsequent course of infection. Br Med J 1989; 299:154–7.

57. Phair J, Detels R, Jacobsen L, Rinaldo C, Saah A, Munoz A. AIDS within five years of seroconversion. VII International Conference on AIDS. Vol. 1. Florence, Italy, June 16-21, 1991:47.

58. Saah A, Hoover D, Munoz A, Detels R, Phair J, Rinaldo C, Vermund SH. The correlates of survival after diagnosis of AIDS. VII International Conference on AIDS. Vol. 1. Florence, Italy, June 16-21, 1991:83.

59. Lifson AR, Hessol NA, Buchbinder SP, Holmberg SD. The association of clinical conditions and serologic tests with CD4 + lymphocyte counts in HIV-infected subjects without AIDS. AIDS 1991; 5:1209–15.

60. Goedert JJ, Kessler CM, Aledort LM, et al. A prospective study of human immunodeficiency virus type 1 infection and the development of AIDS in subjects with hemophilia. N Engl J Med 1989; 321:1141–8.

61. Operskalski EA, Transfusion safety study group. Transfusion transmitted HIV infection: rate of progression to AIDS. VII International Conference on AIDS. Vol. 1. Florence, Italy, June 16-21, 1991:68.

62. Phillips AN, Lee CA, Elford J, et al. More rapid progression to AIDS in older HIV-infected people: the role of CD4+ T-cell counts. J Acquir Immun Def Syndr 1991; 4:970-5.

63. Jackson JB, Erice A, Englund JA, Edson JR, Balfour HH Jr. Prevalence of cytomegalovirus antibody in hemophiliacs and homosexuals infected with human immunodeficiency virus type 1. Transfusion 1987; 28:187-9.

64. Webster A. Cytomegalovirus as a possible cofactor in HIV disease progression. J Acquir Immun Def Syndr 1991; 4(Suppl.1):S47-52.

65. Thompson C, Salvato P, Morrow J, Ragsdale D, Kotarba J. Active herpes virus infection and T and B cell dysfunction in HIV progression. VII International Conference on AIDS. Vol. 1. Florence, Italy, June 16-21, 1991:324.

66. Tagger A, Ribero ML, Grossi A, et al. Vertical transmission of HIV and HCV infections in infants born to HIV and HCV seropositive mothers. VII International Conference on AIDS. Vol. 1. Florence, Italy, June 16-21, 1991:301.

67. Hessol NA, Barnhart L, O'Malley P, et al. The natural history of HIV infection in a cohort of homosexual and bisexual men: cofactors for disease progression, 1978-1989. V International Conference on AIDS, Montreal, Canada, June 4-9, 1989:96.

68. Coates RA, Farewell VT, Raboud J, et al. Cofactors of progression to acquired immunodeficiency syndrome in a cohort of male sexual contacts of men with human immunodeficiency virus disease. Am J Epidemiol 1990; 132:717-22.

69. Anzala AC, Plummer FA, Wambugu P, et al. Incubation time to symptomatic disease and AIDS in women with a known duration of infection. VII International Conference on AIDS. Vol. 1. Florence, Italy, June 16-21, 1991:84.

70. Rothenberg R, Woelfel M, Stoneburner R, et al. Survival with the acquired immunodeficiency syndrome: experience with 5,833 cases in New York City. N Engl J Med 1987; 317:1297-1302.

71. Ellerbrock TV, Bush TJ, Chamberland ME, Oxtoby MJ. Epidemiology of women with AIDS in the United States, 1981 through 1990. JAMA 1991; 265:2971-5.

72. Royce RA, Tu X, Pagano M. Gender differences in survival after AIDS diagnosis: US surveillance data. VII International Conference on AIDS. Vol. 1. Florence, Italy, June 16-21, 1991:331.

73. Baum MK, Beach R, Mantero-Atlenza E, Fletcher M, Rosner B, Eisdorfer C, Shor-Posner G. Predictors of change in immune function: longitudinal analysis of nutritional and immune status in early HIV-1 infection. VII International Conference on AIDS. Vol. 1. Florence, Italy, June 16-21, 1991:329.

74. Luzi G, Ferrara M, Messaroma I, et al. Immunological and virological parameters in AIDS children from Rumania. VII International Conference on AIDS. Vol. 1. Florence, Italy, June 16-21, 1991:301.

75. Graham NMH, Sorensen D, Odaka N, et al. Relationship of serum copper and zinc levels to HIV-1 seropositivity and progression to AIDS. J Acquir Immun Def Syndr 1991; 4:976–80.

76. Caumartin S, Joseph JG, Chmiel J. Premorbid psychosocial factors associated with differential survival time in AIDS patients. VII International Conference on AIDS. Vol. 1. Florence, Italy, June 16-21, 1991:324.

77. Kessler RC, Foster C, Joseph J, Ostrow D, Wortman C, Phair J, Chmiel J. Stressful life events and symptom onset in HIV infection. Am J Psychiatry 1991; 148:733–8.

78. Giovanni R, Pezzotti P, Lazzarin A, et al. Risk of developing AIDS after HIV seroconversion in injecting drug users: analysis of early markers of disease evolution. VII International Conference on AIDS. Vol. 1. Florence, Italy, June 16-21, 1991:33.

79. Massimo Galli, Musicco M, Gervasoni C, et al. No evidence for a role of continuing intravenous drug injection in accelerating disease progression in HIV-1 positive subjects. VII International Conference on AIDS. Vol. 2. Florence, Italy, June 16-21, 1991:67.

80. Craib KJP, Schechter MT, Le TN, et al. Effect of cigarette smoking on CD4 count and progression to AIDS in a cohort of homosexual men. VII International Conference on AIDS. Vol. 1. Florence, Italy, June 16-21, 1991:325.

81. Burns DN, Kramer A, Yellin F, et al. Cigarette smoking: a modifier of human immunodeficiency virus type 1 infection? J Acquir Immun Defic Syndr 1991; 4:76–83.

82. Weber R, Ledergerber B, Opravil M, Luthy R. Cessation of intravenous drug use reduces progression of HIV-infection in HIV+ drug users. VI International Conference on AIDS. Vol. 1. San Francisco, California, June 20-24, 1990:142.

83. Royce RA, Winkelstein W, Bacchetti P. Cigarette smoking and incidence of AIDS. VI International Conference on AIDS. Vol. 1. San Francisco , California, June 20-24, 1990:143.

84. Mann DL, Murray C, Yarchoan R, Blattner WA, Goedert JJ. HLA antigen frequencies in HIV-1 seropositive disease-free individuals and patients with AIDS. J Acquir Immun Defic Syndr 1988; 1:13–7.

85. Steel CM, Ludlam CA, Beatson D, et al. HLA haplotype A1 B8 DR3 as a risk factor for HIV-related disease. Lancet 1988; 1:1185–8.

86. Kaslow RA, Duquesnoy R, Van Raden M, et al. A1, Cw7, B8, DR3 HLA antigen combination associated with rapid decline of T-helper lymphocytes in HIV-1 infection. Lancet 1990; 335:927-30.

87. Louie LG, Newman B, King M-C. Influence of host genotype on progression to AIDS among HIV-infected men. J Acquir Immun Defic Syndr 1991; 4:814–8.

3

Quantitative Virological Measures of Antiretroviral Therapy

David A. Katzenstein
*Center for AIDS Research, Stanford University Medical Center,
and Stanford University School of Medicine, Stanford, California*

Mark Holodniy
*Stanford University School of Medicine, Stanford,
and Palo Alto Veterans Affairs Medical Center,
Palo Alto, California*

I. INTRODUCTION

The pathogenesis of human immunodeficiency virus (HIV) infection is characterized by a progressive decline in immune function coupled with an increasing rate of virus replication and infection of CD4+ T cells (1,2). The ability to directly and indirectly assess virus replication by assays performed on blood cells or tissue, serum, and plasma has led to the concept of measurement of "virus load" as a marker for natural history and disease progression (3,4). These observations are being extended to clinical trials of antiviral drugs where changes in virus load are increasingly used to assess the potential efficacy of antiviral drugs and immunotherapeutic biologics. One quantitative virological assay, the measurement of an HIV core structural protein p24 antigen in the serum, has been used in a wide variety of clinical trials. Additional methods of quantification of virus load, including cell and plasma dilution microculture, flow cytometric enumeration of infected cells, and quantitative PCR studies of HIV RNA and DNA, have only recently been introduced (Table 1).

Table 1 Measurement of Virological Markers by Clinical and Immunological Stage of Disease

Virological markers	Asymptomatic		ARC	AIDS
	>500 CD4	<500 CD4		
p24 Antigen	−	−	+	+
Acid disassociated p24 antigen	+	+ +	+ +	+ +
Plasma culture	−	+	+ +	+ +
Cell culture	+	+ +	+ +	+ +
RNA PCR (plasma)	+	+ +	+ +	+ +
DNA PCR (cells)	+ +	+ +	+ +	+ +

−: <20% patients positive; +: 20-50% patients positive; + +: 50-90% patients positive.

In this review, we will discuss techniques in quantitative virology as they have been applied to clinical trials of antiviral drugs. It is important for the reader to bear in mind that the sensitivity and specificity of quantitative measures of virus load depend on the population of HIV-infected individuals studied, the variability of the specific assay, and the mechanism of action of the compound under study. Direct and indirect measurements of virus load promise to provide a guide to physicians in the treatment of individual patients as well as to investigators developing new drugs. However, despite the theoretical importance of a decrease in virus load as indicated by quantitative viral markers, they have not been accepted as the sole basis for either licensure or package insert indications for the use of a drug in HIV-infected patients.

The importance of measurements of virus load as well as the value of different methodologies will ultimately be determined by their ability to predict efficacy (or failure) of antiviral therapy. Animal models such as SCID-hu mouse have indicated that quantification of viral load could serve as a marker of response to antiretroviral efficacy. To date, validation of quantitative virological tests has been achieved mainly in studies of dideoxynucleoside analogs and interferon. In these studies it has been possible to correlate the results of tests of virus load with the maintenance of the health and well-being of HIV-infected individuals. As additional agents and combinations of antiviral drugs are used in clinical trials, further observations correlated to the prevention of disease progression will be key to the appropriate use of quantitative measures of virus load in HIV-infected patients.

II. HIV p24 ANTIGEN

The principle core protein of HIV, p24 antigen, is produced as a proteolytic cleavage product from p55, the precursor full-length gag protein of HIV (5,6). In addition to the incorporation of p24 into the core of virus particles (7), p24 antigen is expressed on the surface of virus-infected cells and accumulates in the culture supernatant of infected CD4+ lymphocytes and macrophages (8). In the cells of HIV-infected patients, p24 antigen has been detected within circulating cells by antibody staining using flow cytometry (9–11).

In the serum or plasma of some HIV-infected individuals, picogram quantities of p24 antigen may be detected using commercial ELISA assays. The prevalence of detectable p24 antigen depends largely on the stage of disease as determined by CD4+ cell number and clinical symptoms (12–15). In studies of the natural history of HIV infection, p24 antigen has been found in association with viremia in the plasma of patients with acute infection 2–4 weeks before the appearance of anti-HIV antibodies (16,17). Persistence of p24 antigenemia has been associated with rapid disease progression (18). Serum p24 antigen can be detected in 30–50% of patients with AIDS and ARC and fewer than 20% of asymptomatic subjects (12–15,19,20). It is important to note that the prevalence of detectable p24 antigen in African and African-American patients may be lower than in other ethnic groups based on a difference in the magnitude of anti-p24 antibody responses (21–23).

The sensitivity of the p24 antigen ELISA depends on the affinity of the capture and detection antibodies used in the assay relative to the affinity of competing anti-p24 antibodies present in the serum of HIV-infected individuals (24,25). Detection of picogram quantities of p24 antigen has been achieved by several commercial p24 antigen kits developed by different manufacturers (26–28). Recently, several investigators have shown that acid hydrolysis of serum, which denatures native anti-p24 antibodies, can increase the detection of p24 antigen by ELISA (29–33). Similarly, alcohol fractionation of plasma (12) and polyethylene glycol (PEG) precipitation of immune complexes (34,35) have been shown to concentrate p24 antigen. These studies suggest that p24 antigen in the serum of HIV-infected patients is complexed with anti-p24 antibodies. The increasing prevalence of detection of p24 antigen by ELISA in patients with AIDS and ARC may be attributed to increasing viral load and declining anti-p24 antibodies.

Patients with detectable p24 antigen are more likely to have infectious virus that can be cultured from plasma. A correlation between plasma virus titer and quantitative p24 antigen has been observed in several studies (4,36–38). However, the calculated amount of p24 contained in intact virus particles (100 pg/10^6 virions) is much greater than the observed number of virus particles by assays of infectivity or quantification of viral RNA (39). It is likely that most of the p24 antigen in the system results from excess production of core protein or the degradation of virus particles. In either case, the detection and quantification of serum p24 antigen provides a marker for viral load, but does not directly measure virus.

A. Clinical Trials

Measurement of p24 antigen has been reported in more than 30 clinical trials since 1987. Fluctuation in the levels of p24 antigen has been observed in natural history studies and among placebo recipients in several antiviral drug studies (40). Most investigators have required at least a 50% decline in quantitative p24 antigen or the complete suppression of detectable p24 as an indication of drug activity. In the initial placebo control trial of zidovudine (ZDV) in AIDS and ARC patients, 50% of the patients had detectable p24 antigen at enrollment. Among those with detectable antigen levels, after 16 weeks of drug administration, 59% of ZDV-treated patients and 7% of placebo recipients were p24 antigen-negative (41). This decline of p24 antigen in ZDV-treated patients was associated with increasing CD4 cell numbers and the prevention of clinical events in drug recipients. This suggested that p24 might be a surrogate marker for clinical response in AIDS and ARC patients receiving dideoxynucleoside compounds (42,43). Similar associations were observed in phase 1 trials in small numbers of AIDS and ARC patients treated with dideoxyinosine (44,45) and dideoxycytosine (46,47).

Measure of p24 antigen has also been used in trials of combination therapies to demonstrate an enhanced effect ZDV combined with alpha-interferon (48–50) and foscarnet (51). In addition, p24 antigen suppression may be useful in demonstrating the antiviral equivalence of different dose regimens and schedules of antiviral drugs using short-term trials with limited numbers of patients (43,52–54). Failure to demonstrate a change in p24 antigen in patients may be equally important as a rapid means to demonstrate lack of antiviral activity. Thus p24 measurements in phase 1 studies of suramin (55), dextran-sulfate (56), rifabutin (57), soluble recombinant CD4 (58), and ribavirin (59) provided important information that limited further use of these agents in larger trials.

Changes in p24 antigen in placebo-controlled efficacy trials of ZDV in asymptomatic (60) and mildly symptomatic patients (61) have also been observed. Fischl et al. (61) reported that 23% of mildly symptomatic patients had measurable p24 antigen at enrollment in ACTG 016. During the first 16 weeks of the study, a 50% decrease in quantitative p24 antigen was observed in 65% of patients taking ZDV as compared to 22% of placebo recipients. Similarly, new p24 antigenemia developed in 8% of placebo recipients as compared to 3% of ZDV-treated subjects (62). Among asymptomatic subjects in ACTG 019, Volberding et al. (60) found that only 2% of subjects enrolled in ACTG 019 were p24 antigen-positive. However, cross-sectional analysis of these patients demonstrated decreases in quantitative p24 antigen in drug recipients.

To date, unfortunately, results of p24 antigen assays performed in such trials have rarely been examined for a correlation with ultimate clinical outcome. The few studies in which serum p24 quantitative changes have been studied with regard to clinical outcome have failed to show a significant correlation (63).

The use of commercial ELISA kits has provided a simple marker of virus infection that has been useful in the evaluation of the potential antiviral efficacy of agents in phase 1 and 2 studies. Since the prevalence and magnitude of serum p24 antigen increases with stage of disease, quantification of p24 has been most practical in patients with AIDS and ARC and more difficult in studies of drugs in asymptomatic subjects. Recently, several investigators have confirmed the initial observations of a substantial increase in the magnitude and prevalence of detectable p24 antigen with acid pretreatment of serum (29–34). Resolution of the optimal buffering system to liberate p24 from immune complexes without degrading the antigen may allow application of p24 quantification to a much broader range of clinical studies and might improve correlation of p24 changes with clinical outcome.

III. HIV PLASMA CULTURE

Cell-free infectious HIV in the plasma of AIDS patients was first demonstrated by cocultivation of plasma with phytohemagglutinin-stimulated peripheral blood mononuclear cells (PBMC) from a normal donor (64). The initial method that demonstrated growth of HIV in culture (detection of reverse transcriptase activity in the culture supernatant) has largely been supplanted by p24 antigen detection by ELISA. Titers of infectious virus have been determined by culture of serial dilutions of plasma. Determination of p24 antigen production in the supernatant has been used to define the limiting dilution at which virus infection has occurred. Published studies of plasma viremia have used somewhat different methods, some of which may account for differences in the sensitivity of the assay (4,36–38,52,65–73). These differences have included the type of anticoagulant (heparin, EDTA, or acid citrate dextrose), the use of fresh or frozen plasma, centrifugation or filtration to remove platelets and debris, and ultracentrifugation of plasma to concentrate virus particles. The duration of culture has ranged from 2 to 6 weeks, and the frequency with which medium and donor cells have been replenished in the culture has varied.

Irrespective of differences in technique, frequency and titer of plasma viremia is increased with disease progression, decreasing CD4 cell numbers, and detectable p24 antigen. Comparison of p24 antigen detection and plasma culture has demonstrated that nearly all p24 antigen-positive patients are plasma virus-positive, and a significant number of p24 antigen-negative patients also have measurable plasma viremia. The frequency of detectable plasma viremia has varied from 56 to 100% of HIV-seropositive patients, however, nearly all patients with symptomatic HIV disease (AIDS and ARC) have been shown to have plasma viremia, whereas plasma viremia cannot be detected in the majority of asymptomatic subjects (36–38,52).

Although plasma viremia can be detected in most patients with AIDS and ARC, titers of infectious virus may depend on differences in the handling of samples and techniques used to detect and quantitate plasma virus. Sensitivity of detection of plasma viremia is likely to be increased by performing realtime cultures in which plasma is added to donor peripheral blood mononuclear cells (PBMC) within 4 hours of phlebotomy. One small study has suggested that low-speed centrifugation of cells, centrifugal enhancement, increases their sensitivity to plasma virus (74). While the use of fresh plasma prevents loss of infectivity due to freeze-thawing of samples, each time point in a longitudinal study must be titered on a different donor's PBMC. Because use of different donor's cells may result in up to a 100-fold difference in the titer of clinical virus isolates, the susceptibility of the donor cells to infection could be an important source variation in real-time assays (74). Conversely, freezing plasma and performing assays of longitudinal time points on the same donor cells may be problematic in that the stability of virus in frozen plasma and the loss of infectivity due to freeze thawing is not clearly defined. While each method introduces different problems, all of the published reports of plasma viremia in relation to drug therapy have used freshly cultured plasma.

Plasma culture has been studied in relationship to drug therapy in small numbers of individuals in published reports (4,37,38,48,52). Ho et al. showed that plasma virus titers declined more than 10-fold in seven patients treated with ZDV for 4 weeks while serial samples from untreated patients remained constant over 12–20 weeks (4). Similarly, Saag et al. found that plasma virus titers decreased in 8 patients following 16–40 weeks of ZDV treatment (37). In a study comparing three dose regimens of ZDV, Collier et al. reported that mean plasma virus titers declined nearly 100-fold in 12 patients after 12 weeks of treatment (52). In a recent study of plasma viremia, we found a fivefold difference in mean titer comparing 16 ZDV-treated and 24 untreated subjects with fewer than 250 CD4 cells/cu mm. In 45 patients studied prospectively, 26 of 45 had plasma viremia at baseline, and a decrease in titer was seen in 12 of 14 who tolerated treatment for 4 weeks (38). In a combination study of ZDV and alpha-interferon, a 10-fold decrease was shown in mean titers 6 and 12 weeks after the initiation of interferon treatment. The greatest decline in plasma titers, greater than 100-fold, was seen in three patients who received full-dose IFN-alpha for 12 weeks, and these patients had a return to their baseline titers after IFN-alpha was discontinued (48). In this study, the sensitivity of the assay may have been increased by ultracentrifugation of fresh plasma to concentrate virus particles from 10 ml of plasma.

Using current methodology, titration of infectious virus in plasma as a technique to demonstrate drug effect is likely to be useful only in patients with relatively advanced disease. The increase in ability to measure virus in patients with more advanced disease could be the result of increased virus replication, a change in the replication characteristics of virus that allow better recovery in vitro, or a decline in neutralizing antibodies that may prevent recovery of virus. The recovery of plasma virus may depend on each of these factors in addition to the characteristics of the target donor cells and techniques used to handle plasma. Nevertheless, in several small pilot studies, dideoxynucleoside therapy appears to decrease plasma viremia.

IV. HIV PBMC CULTURES

Cocultivation of patient PBMC with activated donor cells using supernatant reverse transcriptase (RT) activity and, more recently, p24 antigen detection, in culture supernatant to determine the endpoint is a widely used technique to obtain clinical virus isolates from patients. Improvements in cocultivation techniques have allowed the detection of HIV by cell culture in more than 90% of HIV-seropositive individuals (4,36). One approach to the quantitation of virus infection using cell culture has been the measurement of the time required to detect RT or p24 antigen production in flask cultures of 5–10 × 10^6 cells (50). In more recent studies, limiting dilution microculture techniques have been used to define the number of cells or the titer per million PBMC capable of producing p24 antigen in culture (4,75). As in studies of plasma viremia, differences in technique and the variable susceptibility of the primary donor PBMC poses a problem in the standardization of PBMC culture techniques.

A. Clinical Trials

Many of the clinical trials that have reported changes in cell culture of HIV have been performed at the National Institutes of Health (NIH) by investigators in the NIAID working with alpha-interferon. In a study of alpha-interferon in patients with Kaposi's sarcoma (KS), Lane et al. (76) found that three patients with more than 400 CD4 cells/mm^3 responded to treatment (with a decrease in tumor). These patients also had a greater than 75% decrease in p24 antigen followed by an increase in the time to peak RT in flask cultures (76). In a subsequent placebo-controlled trial of alpha-interferon in 34 asymptomatic subjects with more than 400 CD4 cells, 7 or 17 (41%) interferon recipients became culture-negative (defined as three sequential negative cultures) as compared to 2 of 17 (13%) of the placebo group (77). When interferon was combined with ZDV in patients with KS, Kovacs et al. reported that 6 of 12 patients became culture-negative on combined therapy (49). A similar effect of interferon and ZDV on recovery of HIV from the blood cells of patients with KS has also been observed in studies by Krown et al. (50).

V. GENE AMPLIFICATION

Another approach for detection and quantification of HIV is the use of molecular hybridization. These techniques make use of HIV-specific DNA or RNA probes to detect HIV genomic sequences contained within circulating blood cells or tissue. Because of the inherent insensitivity of direct hybridization, gene amplification through the use of the polymerase chain reaction (PCR) was successfully applied for the detection of HIV-specific nucleotide sequences contained within patient samples (78). With the advent of PCR, it has become possible to detect small numbers of HIV DNA or RNA copies. Initially PCR was used in the detection of HIV-specific sequences rather than quantification of viral copy number. PCR has been used to detect HIV RNA and DNA in plasma (79) and proviral HIV DNA and RNA in circulating mononuclear cells (80), spinal fluid (81), stool (82), semen (83), and other tissues (84-88). PCR has been widely applied to the detection of HIV proviral DNA for diagnosis in seropositive subjects (89,90), infants born to seropositive mothers (91,92), seronegative subjects at risk for HIV infection (93,94), and individuals with indeterminant Western blots (95,96). Detection of provirus in subsets of PBMC has been used to detect different phenotypes containing HIV proviral DNA in circulation (97–99).

A few studies have attempted to quantitate HIV viral load in subjects by PCR, either as proviral DNA or as viral mRNA. The level of sensitivity achieved in gene amplification is usually expressed as input copy number detected. Studies using 30 cycles of amplification of a HIV-specific sequence and hybridization with a specific probe have reported the ability to detect as few as three to five copies of input DNA with isotopically labeled probes (100) or 10 copies with a nonisotopic enzyme immunoassay (101). The number of HIV provirus copies contained in the sample DNA has been determined using a plasmid standard containing the sequence of interest (102). When a dilution series of known copy number of this standard is run in the same reaction as the clinical sample, the input copy number of the clinical sample can be determined. Quantification of provirus copy number or number of infected cells has also been achieved by limiting dilution PCR of PBMC with nested primers (103) and serial dilution of CD4 sorted cells (104). Quantitative changes have been shown with disease progression (3) and between AIDS and asymptomatic subjects (105). In addition, virion-associated RNA in serum has been quantitated after reverse transcription and PCR using an RNA standard curve (106).

The response to antiretroviral therapy is now only beginning to be studied by PCR. As stated earlier, plasma HIV viremia is only present in certain patients. We have reported that patients without demonstrable infectious virus may have HIV RNA present in plasma or serum (106). Recently we evaluated 72 patients in a cross-sectional study of HIV disease to determine the impact of ZDV therapy on plasma HIV RNA copy number. Thirty-nine subjects who were not currently receiving therapy had a mean copy number of 690 $\pm$ 360, compared to 33 subjects who were currently receiving ZDV who had a mean copy number of 134 $\pm$ 219/200 μl ($p <$ 0.05). In addition, 27 subjects were evaluated before and 1 month after the initiation of dideoxynucleoside therapy. Plasma HIV RNA copy number decreased from 540 $\pm$ 175 to 77 $\pm$ 35 after therapy ($p < 0.05$). Therefore, it would seem that HIV RNA levels in plasma might serve as a marker of viral load (107).

In other studies of therapeutic response, Karpas et al. (108) reported that serum HIV RNA and DNA levels fell to undetectable levels in 10 sub-

jects with advanced HIV disease after 2 months of passive immunoglobulin therapy, suggesting an immune therapy-based response in circulating
HIV RNA load. However, another study looking at quantification of HIV
proviral DNA in five AIDS patients who received immunoglobulin therapy
showed no significant decrease in provirus when compared to three patients
who were receiving placebo (109). In the latter study, HIV plasma RNA
was not measured. Ottman et al. (110) were successful in detecting HIV
RNA in plasma from 95% of subjects evaluated, including 24 of 25 subjects on ZDV. Bagnarelli et al. (111) examined 27 subjects, 5 of whom
were receiving ZDV therapy, and 4 of 5 had detectable plasma HIV RNA,
while 3 of these 4 had cellular HIV mRNA present as well. All of these
patients had CD4 cells below 200/mm^3, 3 of 5 were p24 antigenemic, and
the methodological approach involved ultracentrifugation to sediment
virus, enhancing virion-associated HIV RNA recovery. In addition, 40
and 35 cycles of amplification after reverse transcription were performed
by Ottman et al. and Bagnarelli et al., respectively. This method would
increase the sensitivity of such an assay to detect HIV RNA, but the ability
to show quantitative changes would be lost unless a limiting dilution were
performed. Mitsuya et al. (112) have reported an acute fall in plasma HIV
RNA in 10 of 11 subjects who received dideoxyinosine (ddI) for 8 weeks
or longer (112). A decrease was also seen in 7 patients who received ddI
for 46–70 weeks (113).

Quantification of HIV proviral DNA in circulating PBMC has been
studied to a greater degree than plasma or cellular HIV RNA. Lee et al.
(105) studied a single PBMC sample from 27 subjects and determined that
ARC and AIDS patients had more copies of HIV proviral DNA/10^6 cells
than asymptomatic patients (1245 vs. 213). Genesca et al. (114) confirmed
this finding in 25 patients where symptomatic subjects has a mean of 802
copies/10^5 PBMC, while asymptomatic subjects had a mean of 67 copies/
10^5 PBMC. Finally, Oka et al. (115) also confirmed that symptomatic
subjects have higher HIV proviral copy numbers in CD4 cells than asymptomatic subjects. However, asymptomatic subjects receiving ZDV had
the same mean proviral copy numbers as untreated asymptomatic subjects (115). Schnittman et al. (3) reported that the frequency of HIV-infected CD4 + T cells increased in those patients who developed HIV-related symptoms or AIDS, while in those patients who remained clinically
stable, the frequency of HIV-infected CD4 cells remained stable.

Gene amplification of HIV DNA has also been performed on PBMC
samples obtained from subjects receiving antiretroviral therapy. Several
studies have been published that describe the persistence of proviral signal

despite the subject having received antiviral therapy. In a study of 21 HIV-seropositive subjects, Hart et al. demonstrated HIV DNA by PCR in 3 of 3 subjects who were receiving ZDV (80). Oka et al. (115) evaluated 10 asymptomatic subjects who were on ZDV for a mean of 6.8 months and concluded that proviral DNA copy number was not significantly different than for asymptomatic subjects who were not receiving therapy (436 vs. 405/10^5 CD4 cells, respectively). In addition, 8 patients who had ARC or AIDS and who were receiving ZDV had a mean copy number of 892/10^5 cells (115). Their conclusion was that proviral copy number increased with advancing disease and was not altered by ZDV therapy. Pozansky et al. (116) evaluated the proviral HIV DNA copy number from CD4 cells from 9 HIV-seropositive subjects (2 asymptomatic, 3 ARC, 4 AIDS) by limiting dilution. All subjects had been receiving antiretroviral therapy. The frequency of cells containing proviral DNA ranged from 0.01 to 0.0001, and there was no relationship between proviral copy number, stage of disease, or CD4 count. McElrath et al. (99) studied 23 patients, 10 of whom were receiving ZDV. There was no difference in the ability to detect signals from patients on therapy compared to those not receiving therapy. In addition, 8 of these 10 patients had detectable signals by at least one primer pair in monocyte fractions obtained by cell sorting.

Finally, cellular mRNA levels have been measured in relation to antiviral therapy. Schnittman et al. (73) examined HIV mRNA levels in CD4 cells from subjects to analyze in vivo expression. Twenty-three of 49 subjects were receiving antiretroviral therapy. All of these subjects had at least one detectable HIV mRNA PCR product, implying active expression in the presence of antiviral therapy. Murphy et al. (117) evaluated 10 patients at baseline and then every 2 weeks following AZT therapy. Two patients had increases in *tat* mRNA and proviral DNA levels that were concordant with declining CD4 levels. Seven patients had no change in CD4 cell count, and one had an increase that corresponded with a decline in mRNA and DNA levels.

Most of these small series have obtained only one or two samples from patients. It has, therefore, been difficult to assess constancy of proviral copy number over time or whether PCR can serve as a useful marker in antiretroviral therapy. Constancy of proviral copy number was evaluated in 10 subjects on 3 consecutive days. Although copy number ranged from 80 to 16,000 μg DNA, a constant signal was observed over the 3 days in each patient (118). Donovan et al. (119) followed 6 patients who had multiple samples taken during a 5- to 14-month period while on ZDV therapy. One patient had a sample taken before starting therapy. Five of 6 had their first sample obtained within 4 months of initiating ZDV therapy. Five of 6 had a CD4 count under 250/mm^3, and 4 of 6 were p24 antigenemic. They found that proviral DNA copy number was consistent over time and was not reduced while on ZDV therapy. However, they did not have any untreated controls, and only 1 of 6 subjects had baseline samples obtained prior to the start of therapy. Oka et al. (120) followed 6 patients weekly who received beta-interferon daily for 4 weeks, and they saw no change in provirus copy number. Aoki et al. (121) studied 13 subjects, 2 with AIDS and 11 with ARC, who received ddI in a phase I trial. Patients were evaluated at baseline and then from 8 to 14 weeks after the start of therapy. Nine of 12 available patients showed a significant decrease in HIV proviral DNA copy number with ddI therapy. There were no untreated controls in this study. Israel et al. (122) looked at the response of provirus levels and their relationship to viral culture in 8 patients begun on ZDV therapy. After 4 weeks of therapy, provirus fell from 4.6/1000 PBMC to 0.28/1000. Plasma and PBMC TCID fell from 179/ml and 2131/10^6 to 5/ml and 11/10^6, respectively. Phenotypic ZDV resistance was detected 2-9 months posttherapy. In 3 of 5 subjects who developed resistance, mean PBMC and plasma TCID and provirus DNA copy number increased 70-, 9-, and 6-fold, respectively. We have also shown a decrease in proviral DNA (123) in 13 asymptomatic subjects studied over a 10- to 24-month period. In 4 untreated subjects there was no significant change in provirus levels over a mean period of 13 months. In 8 patients treated with ZDV and recombinant interleukin-2, proviral copy number fell significantly after 12 weeks of therapy. Subsequent courses, which included 12 weeks of ZDV alone or 4 weeks of IL-2 alone, did not significantly change the already depressed provirus copy number. Proviral copy number also remained depressed during drug-free washout periods between courses. Finally, a return of proviral copy number to baseline levels was observed after 7 months following discontinuation of therapy and having received no further therapy.

VI. FLOW CYTOMETRY

Determination and quantification of circulating blood leukocyte subsets by automated fluorescent activated cell sorting has been successfully applied to HIV disease. It is now clear that the T-helper cell, which is CD3 + CD4 + , is the main reservoir for HIV infection (97). For the past several years, phenotypic analysis for quantification of CD4 + and CD8 + cells has been used to monitor prognosis and response to antiretroviral therapy.

The development of AIDS-related diagnoses is directly correlated with a significant decline in CD4+ cells (124). In addition, clinical trials involving antiretrovirals have shown a short-term increase in CD4+ cells (42-45), which may not be sustained after long-term administration of such drugs (62). A recent review by Landay et al. outlines current and future applications of flow cytometry for HIV disease (125).

A recently developed assay measures cell-associated p24 antigen or p24 FCA (flow cytometric assay) by antibody staining of cells and detection of p24 antigen by flow cytometric analysis. Using this form of assay, Cory et al. were able to detect one HIV-infected cell/10,000 uninfected cells (9). Ohlsson-Wilhelm et al. (126) studied 55 HIV-positive subjects and found that p24+ cells ranged from undetectable to 13.6% (mean 2%). The range of infected cells was the same in asymptomatic subjects as those with AIDS. However, ZDV-treated subjects had much lower values. P24 FCA values were inversely related to the number of days to culture positivity and to absolute CD4 count (11). McSharry et al. (10) studied 85 subjects not on therapy. They found a range of 4-25% p24+ cells. There was a positive correlation between clinical status and number of p24+ cells and an inverse correlation between CD4 number and p24+ cells from subjects in CDC classes III and IV. An additional 95 subjects from CDC class IV who were receiving ZDV were also studied. When compared to subjects in CDC class IV not on ZDV, those receiving ZDV had a slight decrease in p24+ cells—10.8% vs. 8.4%, respectively. Nine subjects were analyzed over 6 months while on ZDV. There was consistency of p24 FCA over time. Ohlsson-Wilhelm et al. (126) looked at an additional 33 subjects who were receiving antiretroviral therapy and grouped them according to CD4 count: 18 with CD4 cells between 200-500/mm^3 (Group I) and 15 with less than 200/mm^3 (Group II). Group I had a much higher percentage of CD4+ cells than group II—20.1% vs. 9.9%. However, the absolute number of CD4+ cells that were p24 antigen-positive was reversed. Group I had 3.3% vs. 21.2% in group II, suggesting that the number of CD4+ cells expressing p24 antigen increases as a patient has declining CD4 counts. Although we are not given any information regarding the type or duration of antiviral therapy, the implication from this study is that in subjects with fewer than 200 CD4 cells/mm^3, a significant number of cells will contain p24 regardless of antiviral therapy.

VII. CONCLUSION

Although an ideal surrogate marker of virus replication in HIV infection has not been established, this is clearly an important objective in the design of clinical trials. Currently, measurement of p24 antigen is the most widely used and least expensive method to assess virus load. New methods to disassociate antigen from immune complexes and the development of more sensitive ELISA techniques will expand the applications of quantitative p24 antigen assays. As an increasing number of drugs are licensed and more candidate compounds move into clinical trials, quantitative measurement of p24 antigen is a technique that may be used to optimize the management of drug therapy in individual patients. Culture methods, quantification of plasma and cell associated virus, which depend on the use of primary donor cells, will most likely be limited to studies in a relatively small number of research laboratories. If cell lines can be found (or constructed) that consistently support the growth of clinical isolates, quantitative culture could play a larger role in clinical trials. Quantitative amplification of HIV-specific RNA and DNA directly measures virus and provirus without the uncertainties associated with virus growth in cell culture. However, the exquisite sensitivity of PCR and problems of cross-contamination, as well as the difficulties in standardizing methods to detect the products of amplification reactions, will limit the widespread application of PCR.

Application of these new methods of quantitative virology is circumscribed by our understanding of the natural history of HIV, current limits of the effectiveness of treatment, and the technical limitations of each of the assays. Thus far it has been possible to establish an association between increasing viral load and progression of disease as characterized by increasing symptoms and decreasing CD4 cell numbers. In the absence of treatment, infectious virus in plasma and cells, HIV RNA and DNA as measured by PCR, and serum p24 antigen have been shown to increase with stage of disease. In prospective studies of patients starting therapy, each of these measurements of virus load have been shown to decrease in patients treated with ZDV, other nucleoside analogs, or interferon (Table 2). Equally important is the observation that increasing virus load as measured by some of these methods may occur with withdrawal of drugs or the development of drug resistance.

The course of HIV infection is characterized by a long period of asymptomatic viral infection, the onset of symptoms related to immunodeficiency, and ultimately the development of AIDS. Traditionally, clinical trials of antiviral drugs and biologics have relied on comparison of the relative ability of the agent(s) under study to slow or prevent the development of disease and death. In view of the current recommendations that treatment for HIV infection should begin before the occurrence of symp-

Table 2 Changes in Virological Markers after Antiretroviral Therapy

Virological markers	ZDV	ddI	ddC	Interferon-α
p24 Antigen	+ +	+ +	+ +	+
Plasma culture	+ +	+ +	NR	+
Cell culture	±	NR	±	+
RNA PCR (plasma)	+ +	+ +	NR	NR
DNA PCR (cells)	+ +	+ +	NR	NR

±: <30% of patients responding; +: 30-50% of patients responding; + +: 50-90% of patients responding; NR: No results reported.

tomatic disease, there is a growing consensus that the evaluation of new agents should not depend solely on morbidity and mortality among patients participating in clinical trials. Several current clinical trials of anti-HIV treatment combine quantitative measurement of viral load with careful analysis of immunological responses. The goal is to provide rapid definition of the antiviral efficacy of compounds earlier in infection, without relying on clinical endpoints. Improvement in techniques to measure virus load will lead to clinical trial strategies that rapidly and directly assess the efficacy of new drugs, biologics, and combination therapies.

REFERENCES

1. Ho DD, Pomerantz RJ, Kaplan JC. Pathogenesis of infection with the human immunodeficiency virus. N Engl J Med 1987; 317:278-86.

2. Fauci AS. The human immunodeficiency virus: infectivity and mechanisms of pathogenesis. Science 1988; 239:617-22.

3. Schnittman SM, Greenhouse JJ, Psallidopolous MC, et al. Increasing viral burden in CD4+ cells from patients with human immunodeficiency virus (HIV) infection reflects progressive immunosuppression and clinical disease. Ann Intern Med 1990; 113:438-43.

4. Ho DD, Mougdil T, Alam M. Quantitation of human immunodeficiency virus type 1 in the blood of infected persons. N Engl J Med 1989; 321:1621-5.

5. Bryant M, Ratner L. Myristolation-dependent replication and assembly of human immunodeficiency virus 1. Proc Natl Acad Sci USA 1990; 87:523-7.

6. Chassagne J, Verelle P, Dionet C, et al. A monoclonal antibody against LAV gag precursor: use for viral protein analysis and antigenic expression in infected cells. J Immunol 1986; 136:1442-5.

7. Gelderblom HR, Hausmann EHS, Ozel M, et al. Fine structure of human immunodeficiency virus (HIV) and immunolocalization of structural proteins. Virology 1987; 156:171-6.

8. Laurent AG, Krust B, Rey MA, Montagnier L, Hovanessian AG. Cell surface expression of several species of human immunodeficiency virus type 1 major core protein. J Virol 1989; 63:4074-8.

9. Cory JM, Ohlsson-Wilhelm BM, Brock EJ, et al. Detection of human immunodeficiency virus infected lymphoid cells of low frequency by flow cytometry. J Immunol Methods 1987; 105:71-8.

10. McSharry JJ, Costantino R, Robbiano E, et al. Detection and quantitation of human immunodeficiency virus-infected peripheral blood mononuclear cells by flow cytometry. J Clin Micro 1990; 28:724-33.

11. Ohlsson-Wilhelm BM, Cory JM, Kessler HA, et al. Circulating human immunodeficiency virus (HIV) p24 antigen-positive lymphocytes: a flow cytometric measure of HIV infection. J Infect Dis 1990; 162:1018-24.

12. Wittek AE, Phelan MA, Wells MA, et al. Detection of human immunodeficiency virus core protein in plasma by enzyme immunoassay. Ann Intern Med 1987; 107:286-92.

13. Eyster EM, Ballard JO, Gail MH, et al. Predictive markers for the acquired immunodeficiency syndrome (AIDS) in hemophiliacs: persistence of p24 antigen and low T4 cell count. Ann Intern Med 1989; 110:963-9.

14. Cao Y, Valentine F, Hojvat S, et al. Detection of HIV antigen and specific antibodies to HIV core and envelope proteins in sera of patients with HIV infection. Blood 1987; 70:575-8.

15. Goudsmit J, DeWolf F, Paul DA, et al. Expression of human immunodeficiency virus antigen (HIV-Ag) in serum and cerebral spinal fluid during acute and chronic infection. Lancet 1986; 2:177-80.

16. Daar ES, Mougdil T, Meyer RD, Ho DD. Transient high levels of viremia in patients with primary human immunodeficiency virus type 1 infection. N Engl J Med 1991; 324:961-4.

17. Clark SJ, Saag MS, Decker WD, et al. High titers of cytopathic virus in plasma of patients with symptomatic primary HIV-1 infection. N Engl J Med 1991; 324:954-60.

18. Rinaldo C, Kingsley L, Neumann J, et al. Association of human immunodeficiency virus (HIV) p24 antigenemia with decrease in CD4 + lymphocytes and the onset of acquired immunodeficiency syndrome during the early phase of HIV infection. J Clin Microbiol 1989; 27:880-4.

19. MacDonell KB, Chmiel JS, Poggensee L, et al. Predicting progression to AIDS: combined usefulness of CD4 lymphocyte counts and p24 antigenemia. Am J Med 1990; 89:706-11.

20. Murray HW, Godbold JH, Jurica KB, Roberts RB. Progression of AIDS in patients with lymphadenopathy or AIDS-related complex: reappraisal of risk and predictive factors. Am J Med 1989; 86:533-8.

21. Baillou A, Barin F, Allain JP, et al. Human immunodeficiency virus antigenemia in patients with AIDS and AIDS related disorders: a comparison between European and African populations. J Infect Dis 1987; 156:830-3.

22. Katzenstein DA, Latif AS, Grace SA, et al. Clinical and laboratory characteristics of HIV-1 infection in Zimbabwe. J AIDS 1990; 3:701-7.

23. Lucey D, Hendrix C, Andrzejewski C, et al. Racial differences in p24 antibody titers and total serum IgG levels in North American persons with HIV-1 infection (Abstract M.C.3259) presented at the VII international Conference on AIDS, Florence Italy, June 16-21, 1991.

24. Allain JP, Laurian Y, Paul DA, et al. Long-term evaluation of HIV antigen and antibodies to p24 and p41 in patients with hemophilia. N Engl J Med 1987; 317:114-21.

25. McRae B, Lange JAM, Asher MS, et al. Immune response to HIV p24 core protein during the early phases of human immunodeficiency virus infection. AIDS Res Hum Retroviruses 1991; 7:737-43.

26. Healey DS, Maskill WJ, Neate EV, et al. A preliminary evaluation of five antigen detection assays. J Virol Methods 1988; 20:115-125.

27. Todak G, Klein E, Lange M, et al. A clinical appraisal of the p24 antigen test. (Abstract M.C.3112) presented at the VII International Conference on AIDS, Florence Italy, June 16-21, 1991.

28. Maniez M, Ferroni A, Dupressoir MV, et al. Evaluation of four commercial HIV-1 antigen assays (Abstract M.A. 1106) presented at the VII International Conference on AIDS, Florence Italy, June 16-21, 1991.

29. Vasudevachari MB, Salzman NP, Woll DR, et al. Clinical utility of an enhanced human immunodeficiency virus type-1 p24 antigen capture assay. Ann Intern Med (in press 1992).

30. Mathiesen T, Sundquist VA, Albert J, et al. Acid hydrolysis of serum samples to increase detection of HIV antigen. J Virol Methods 1988; 22:125-31.

31. Nishanian P, Huskins KR, Stehn S, et al. A simple method for improved assay demonstrates that HIV p24 antigen is present as immune complexes in most sera from HIV infected individuals. J Infect Dis 1990; 162:21-8.

32. Bollinger RC, Kine R, Francis H, et al. Acid hydrolysis and the sensitivity of p24 antigen detection for the evaluation of therapy in asymptomatic HIV-1 infected individuals (Abstract M.B.34) presented at the VII International Conference on AIDS, Florence Italy, June 16-21, 1991.

33. Winger EE, Reddy MM, Hargrove D, et al. A sensitive method for monitoring efficacy of anti-retroviral therapy in HIV infected individuals: a highly

sensitive p24 antigen assay (Abstract M.B.38) presented at the VII International Conference on AIDS, Florence Italy, June 16-21, 1991.

34. Fiscus S, Wallmark EB, Folds JD, et al. Detection of infectious immune complexes in human immunodeficiency virus type 1 (HIV-1) infections: correlation with plasma viremia and CD4 cell counts. J Infect Dis 1991; 164:765-9.

35. McHugh TM, Stites DP, Busch MP, et al. Relation of circulating levels of human immunodeficiency virus (HIV) antigen, antibody to p24, and HIV-containing immune complexes in HIV-infected patients. J Infect Dis 1988; 158:1088-91.

36. Coombs RW, Collier AC, Allain JP, et al. Plasma viremia in human immunodeficiency virus. N Engl J Med 1989; 321:1626-30.

37. Saag M, Crane MJ, Decker WD, et al. High level viremia in adults and children infected with human immunodeficiency virus: relation to disease stage and CD4+ lymphocyte levels. J Infect Dis 1991; 164:72-80.

38. Katzenstein DA, Holodniy M, Israelski DM, et al. Plasma viremia in human immunodeficiency virus infection: relationship to stage of disease and antiviral treatment. J AIDS 1992; 6:107-12.

39. Bourinbaiar AS. HIV and gag (letter). Nature 1991; 349:111.

40. Hendrix CW, Volberding PA, Chaisson RE. HIV antigen variability in ARC/AIDS. J AIDS 1991; 4:847-50.

41. Chaisson RE, Leuther MD, Allain JP, et al. Effect of zidovudine on serum human immunodeficiency virus core antigen levels. Results from a placebo-controlled trial. Arch Intern Med 1988; 148:2151-3.

42. Fischl MA, Richman DD, Greico MH, et al. The efficacy of azidothymidine (AZT) in the treatment of patients with AIDS and AIDS-related complex: a double-blind placebo-controlled trial. N Engl J Med 1987; 317:185-91.

43. Jackson GG, Paul DA, Falk LA, et al. Human immunodeficiency virus (HIV) antigenemia (p24) in the acquired immunodeficiency syndrome (AIDS) and effect of treatment with zidovudine (AZT). Ann Intern Med 1988; 108:175-80.

44. Yarchoan R, Mitsuya H, Thomas RV, et al. In vivo activity against HIV and favorable toxicity profile of 2'3'-dideoxyinosine. Science 1989; 245:245.

45. Lambert JS, Seidlin M, Reichman RC, et al. 2'-3' Dideoxyinosine (ddI) in patients with the acquired immunodeficiency syndrome or AIDS-related complex. N Engl J Med 1990; 322:1333-45.

46. Merigan TC, Skowron G, Bozzette SA, et al. Circulating p24 antigen levels and responses to dideoxycytidine in human immunodeficiency virus infection. Ann Intern Med 1989; 110:189-94.

47. Yarchoan R, Perno CF, Thomas RV, et al. Phase 1 studies of 2'-3' dideoxycytidine in severe human immunodeficiency virus infection as a single agent and alternating with zidovudine (AZT). Lancet 1988; 1:76-80.

48. Berglund O, Engman K, Ehrnst A, et al. Combined treatment of symptomatic human immunodeficiency virus type-1 infection with native interferon-alpha and zidovudine. J Infect Dis 1991; 163:710-5.

49. Kovacs JA, Deyton L, Davey R, et al. Combined zidovudine and interferon-alpha therapy in patients with Kaposi sarcoma and the acquired immunodeficiency syndrome. Ann Intern Med 1989; 111:280-7.

50. Krown SE, Gold JWM, Niedzwiecki D, et al. Interferon alpha with zidovudine: safety, tolerance, and clinical and virologic effects in patients with Kaposi sarcoma associated with the acquired immunodeficiency syndrome (AIDS). Ann Intern Med 1990; 112:812-21.

51. Jacobson MA, van der Horst C, Causey DM, et al. In vivo additive antiretroviral effect of combined zidovudine and foscarnet therapy for human immunodeficiency virus infection (ACTG Protocol 053). J Infect Dis 1991; 163:1219-2.

52. Collier AC, Bozzette S, Coombs RW, et al. A pilot study of low-dose zidovudine in human immunodeficiency virus infection. N Engl J Med 1990; 323: 1015-21.

53. Spector SA, Kennedy C, McCuthchan JA, et al. The antiviral effect of zidovudine and ribavirin in clinical trials and the use of p24 as a virologic marker. J Infect Dis 1989; 159:822-8.

54. Skowrin G, Merigan TC. Alternating and intermittent regimens of zidovudine and deoxycytidine in the treatment of patients with acquired immunodeficiency syndrome (AIDS) and AIDS-related complex. Am J Med 1990; 88:S5B-20S-5B-23S.

55. Schattenkerk JKME, Danner SAA, Lange JMA, et al. Persistence of human immunodeficiency virus antigenemia in patients with the acquired immunodeficiency syndrome treated with a reverse transcriptase inhibitor, suramin: ten patient case-control study. Arch Intern Med 1988; 209-11.

56. Abrams DI, Kuno S, Wong R, et al. Oral dextran sulfate in the treatment of acquired immunodeficiency syndrome (AIDS) and AIDS related complex. Ann Intern Med 1989; 110:183-8.

57. Torseth J, Bhatia G, Harkonen S, et al. Evaluation of the antiviral effect of rifabutin in AIDS-related complex. J Infect Dis 1989; 159:1115-8.

58. Schooley RT, Merigan TC, Gout P, et al. Recombinant soluble CD4 therapy with the acquired immunodeficiency syndrome (AIDS) and AIDS-related complex. Ann Intern Med 1990; 112:247-53.

59. Roberts RB, Jurica K, Meyer WA, et al. A phase 1 study of ribavirin in human immunodeficiency virus-infected patients. J Infect Dis 1990; 162:638-42.

60. Volberding PA, Lagakos SW, Koch MA, et al. Zidovudine in asymptomatic human immunodeficiency virus infection: a controlled trial in persons with

fewer than 500 CD4 positive cells per cubic milliliter. N Engl J Med 1990; 322:1340-5.

61. Fischl MA, Parker CB, Pettinelli C, et al. A randomized controlled trial of a reduced daily dose of zidovudine in patients with the acquired immunodeficiency syndrome. N Engl J Med; 323:1009-14.

62. Fischl MA, Richman DD, Hansen N, et al. The safety and efficacy of zidovudine (AZT) in the treatment of subjects with mildly symptomatic human immunodeficiency virus type 1 infection; a double-blind, placebo controlled trial. Ann Intern Med 1990; 112:727-37.

63. Jacobson MA, Bacchetti P, Kolokathin A, et al. Surrogate markers for survival in patients with AIDS and AIDS related complex treated with zidovudine. Brit Med J 1991; 302:73-8.

64. Zagury D, Fouchard M, Vol JC, et al. Detection of infectious HTLV-III/LAV virus in cell-free plasma from AIDS patients. Lancet 1989; 2:505-6.

65. Ehrnst A, Sonnerborg S, Bergdahl S, Strannegard. Efficient isolation of HIV from plasma during different stages of HIV infection. J Med Virol 1989; 26:23-32.

66. Groupe "Viremie Quantitative": A.C. 11-ANRS. Quantitative plasma viremia: comparison of two techniques. Abstract M.A. 1107. presented at the VII International Conference on AIDS, Florence Italy, June 16-21, 1991.

67. Escaich S, Ritter J, Rougier P, et al. Detection of HIV plasma viremia by culture and polymerase chain reaction (PCR) at different stages of HIV infection. Abstract M.A. 1109 presented at the VII International Conference on AIDS, Florence Italy, June 16-21, 1991.

68. Dewar RL, Sarmiento M, Lawton E, et al. Plasma viremia in a randomly selected group of HIV seropositive individuals. Abstract M.A. 1116. presented at the VII International Conference on AIDS, Florence Italy, June 16-21, 1991.

69. Cuneo P, Sigari G, Zemignan M, Arenare L, Bonafede L. Methodological aspects and clinical value of HIV recovery from peripheral-blood mononuclear cells, plasma, and whole-blood. (Abstract #1024) VIth International Conference on AIDS, San Francisco, California. June 20-24, 1990.

70. Venet A, Lu W, Beldjord K, Andrieu J-M. Correlation between CD4 cell counts and cellular and plasma viral load in HIV-1-seropositive individuals. AIDS 1991; 5:283-7.

71. Bayliss GJ, Jesson WJ, Mortimer PP, et al. Cultivation of human immunodeficiency virus from whole blood: effect of anti-coagulant and inoculum size on virus growth. J Med Virol 1990; 31:161-4.

72. Israel V, Srugo I, Chelyapox NV, Brunelle PA. Quantitation of HIV-1 in the blood of infected children. Clin Res 1991; 39:59A.

73. Schnittman SM, Greenhouse JJ, Lane HC, et al. Frequent detection of HIV-1 specific mRNAs in infected individuals suggests ongoing active viral expression in all stages of disease. AIDS Res Hum Retroviruses 1991; 7:361-7.

74. Shepp D, Ashareaf A. Effect of low-speed centrifugation on recovery of HIV from cell-free virus stocks and from serum. Abstr 1022. Presented at the VI International Conference on AIDS, June 22-24, 1990, San Francisco, CA.

75. Dimitrov DH, Melnick JL, Hollinger FB. Microculture assay for isolation of human immunodeficiency virus type 1 and for titration of infected peripheral blood cells. J Clin Microbiol 1990; 28:734-7.

76. Lane CH, Kovacs JA, Feinberg J, et al. Anti-retroviral effects of interferon-alpha in AIDS-associated Kaposi's sarcoma. Lancet 1988; ii:1218-22.

77. Lane CH, Davey V, Kovacs JA, et al. Interferon alpha in patients with asymptomatic human immunodeficiency virus (HIV) infection. A randomized placebo-controlled trial. Ann Intern Med 1990; 112:805-19.

78. Kwok S, Mack DH, Mullis KB, et al. Identification of human immunodeficiency virus sequences by using in vitro enzymatic amplification and oligomer cleavage detection. J Virol 1987; 61:1690-4.

79. Hewlett IK, Gregg RA, Ou CY, et al. Detection in plasma of HIV-1 specific DNA and RNA by polymerase chain reaction before and after seroconversion. J Clin Immunoassay 1988; 11:161-4.

80. Hart C, Schochetman G, Spira T, et al. Direct detection of HIV RNA expression in seropositive subjects. Lancet 1988; 2:596-9.

81. Goswami KK, Miller RF, Harrison MJ, et al. Expression of HIV-1 in the cerebrospinal fluid detected by the polymerase chain reaction and its correlation with central nervous system disease. AIDS 1991; 5:797-803.

82. Yolken RH, Shuojia L, Perman J, Viscidi R. Persistent diarrhea and fecal shedding of retroviral nucleic acids in children infected with human immunodeficiency virus. J Infect Dis 1991; 164:61-6.

83. Mermin JH, Holodniy M, Katzenstein DA, Merigan TC. Detection of human immunodeficiency virus DNA and RNA in semen by the polymerase chain reaction. J Infect Dis 1991; 164:769-72.

84. Bell J, Ratner L. Specificity of polymerase chain reactions for human immunodeficiency virus type 1 DNA sequences. AIDS Res Hum Retroviruses 1989; 5:87.

85. Lai-Goldman M, Lai E, Grody WW. Detection of human immunodeficiency virus (HIV) infection in formalin-fixed paraffin-embedded tissues by DNA amplification. Nucleic Acid Res 1988; 16:8191.

86. Varma V, Rimland D, Srinvasan A, Swan D. Diagnosis of HIV infection employing polymerase chain reaction (PCR) on paraffin embedded tissue. Lab Invest 1989; 60:101A.

87. Kwok S, Ehrlich G, Poiesz B, et al. Enzymatic amplification of HTLV I viral sequences from peripheral blood mononuclear cells and infected tissues. Blood 1988; 72:1117.

88. Openshaw H, H, Cantin E, Hinton D. HIV detection by polymerase chain reaction in AIDS brains. Neurology 1989; 39:379.

89. Jackson JB, Sannerud KJ, Hopsicker JS, et al. Hemophiliacs with HIV antibody are actively infected. JAMA 1988; 260:2236-9.

90. Horsburgh CR, Ou CY, Jason J, et al. Concordance of polymerase chain reaction with human immunodeficiency virus antibody detection. J Infect Dis 1990; 162:542-5.

91. Rogers MF, Ou CY, Rayfield M, et al. Use of the polymerase chain reaction for early detection of the proviral sequences of human immunodeficiency virus in infants born to seropositive mothers. N Engl J Med 1989; 320:1649-54.

92. Escaich S, Baginski WI, Ritter J, et al. Comparison of HIV detection by virus isolation in lymphocyte cultures and molecular amplification of HIV DNA and RNA by PCR in offspring of seropositive mothers. J Acq Immun Def Synd 1991; 4:130-5.

93. Wolinsky SM, Rinaldo CR, Kwok S, et al. Human immunodeficiency virus type 1 (HIV-1) infection a median of 18 months before a diagnostic Western blot. Ann Intern Med 1989; 111:961-72.

94. Imagawa DT, Lee MH, Wolinsky SM, et al. Human immunodeficiency virus type 1 infection in homosexual men who remain seronegative for prolonged periods of time. N Engl J Med 1989; 320:1458-62.

95. Jackson JB, MacDonald KL, Caldwell J, et al. Absence of HIV infection in blood donors with indeterminate Western blot tests for antibody to HIV-1. N Engl J Med 1989; 320:1458-62.

96. Dock NL, Kleinman SH, Rayfield MA, et al. Human immunodeficiency virus infection and indeterminate Western blot patterns. Prospective studies in a low prevalence population. Arch Intern Med 1991; 151:525-30.

97. Schnittman SM, Psallidopoulos MC, Lane HC, et al. The reservoir for HIV-1 in human peripheral blood is a T cell that maintains expression of CD4. Science 1989; 245:305-8.

98. Spear GT, Ou CY, Kessler HA, et al. Analysis of lymphocytes, monocytes and neutrophils from human immunodeficiency virus (HIV)-infected persons for HIV DNA. J Infect Dis 1990; 162:1239-44.

99. McElrath MJ, Steinman RM, Cohn ZA. Latent HIV-1 infection in enriched populations of blood monocytes and T cells from seropositive patients. J Clin Invest 1991; 87:27-30.

100. Dickover RE, Donovan RM, Goldstein E, et al. Quantitation of human immunodeficiency virus DNA by using the polymerase chain reaction. J Clin Micro 1990; 28:2130-3.

101. Coutlee F, Yang B, Bobo L, et al. Enzymatic immunoassay for detection of hybrids between PCR-amplified HIV-1 DNA and RNA probe: PCR-EIA. AIDS Res Hum Retroviruses 1990; 6:775-84.

102. Abbott MA, Poiesz BJ, Byrne BC, et al. Enzymatic gene amplification: qualitative and quantitative methods for detecting proviral DNA amplified in vitro. J Infect Dis 1988; 158:1158-64.

103. Simmonds P, Balfe P, Peutherer et al. Human immunodeficiency virus-infected individuals contain provirus in small numbers of peripheral mononuclear cells and at low copy number. J Virol 1990; 64:864-72.

104. Brinchman JE, Albert J, Vartdal F. Few infected CD4 + T cells but a high proportion of replication competent provirus copies in asymptomatic human immunodeficiency virus type 1 infection. J Virol 1991; 65:2019-23.

105. Lee TH, Sunzeri FJ, Tobler LH, et al. Quantitative assessment of HIV-1 DNA by coamplification of HIV-1 gag and HLA-DQ-a genes. AIDS 1991; 5:683-91.

106. Holodniy M, Katzenstein DA, Sengupta S, et al. Detection and quantification human immunodeficiency virus RNA in patient serum by the polymerase chain reaction. J Infect Dis 1991; 163:862-6.

107. Holodniy M, Katzenstein DA, Israelski DM, Merigan TC. Reduction in plasma human immunodeficiency virus ribonucleic acid following dideoxynucleoside therapy as determined by the polymerase chain reaction. J Clin Invest 1991; 88:1755-9.

108. Karpas A, Hewlett IK, Hill F, et al. Polymerase chain reaction evidence for human immunodeficiency virus 1 neutralization by passive immunization in patients with AIDS and AIDS-related complex. Proc Natl Acad Sci USA 1990; 87:7613-7.

109. Lefere JJ, Mariotte M, Poste Y, et al. Quantitation of viral copies through PCR in AIDS patients transfused with plasma rich in Anti-HIV antibodies. Program VII International Conference on AIDS, Florence Italy 1991 (Abstract W.B. 2132).

110. Ottman M, Innocenti P, Thanadey M, et al. The polymerase chain reaction for the detection of HIV-1 genomic RNA in plasma from infected individuals. J Virol Methods 1991; 31:273-84.

111. Bagnarelli P, Menzo S, Manzin A, et al. Detection of human immunodeficiency virus type 1 genomic RNA in plasma samples by reverse transcriptase polymerase chain reaction. J Med Virol 1991; 34:89-95.

112. Mitsuya H, Aoki-Sei S. Quantitative analysis of HIV-1 in clinical specimens from patients with HIV-1 infection by polymerase chain reaction (PCR). 1991 Workshop on Viral Quantitation in HIV Infection, Paris, France, June 13-14, 1991.

113. Aoki-Sei S, Yarchoan R, Kageyama S, et al. Quantitation of HIV-1 virus particles in plasma from patients with HIV-1 Infection by RNA polymerase

chain reaction: decrease in viral load in Plasma following treatment with 2', 3' dideoxyinosine (ddi). Program VII International Conference of AIDS, 1991, Florence, Italy (Abstract W.A. 79).

114. Genesca J, Wang RYH, Alter HJ, Smith JWK. Clinical correlation and genetic polymorphism of the human immunodeficiency virus proviral DNA obtained after polymerase chain reaction. J Infect 1990; 162:1025-30.

115. Oka S, Urayama K, Hirabayashi Y, et al. Quantitative estimation of human immunodeficiency virus type-1 provirus in CD4+ T lymphocytes using the polymerase chain reaction. Mol Cell Probes 1991; 5:137-42.

116. Pozansky MC, Walker B, Haseltine WA, et al. A rapid method for quantitating the frequency of peripheral blood cells containing HIV-1 DNA. J Acq Immun Def Synd 1991; 4:368-373.

117. Murphy R, Wolinsky S, Furtado MR. Enzymatic amplification of HIV-1 mRNA as a surrogate marker for anti-retroviral therapy. Program 31st Interscience Conference on Antimicrobial Agents and Chemotherapy. Chicago, IL, 1991, (Abstract 633).

118. Baxter JD, Byrne BC, HIV-1 Proviral is constant by quantitative polymerase chain reaction (PCR) over short time periods. Program 31st Interscience Conference on Antimicrobial Agents and Chemotherapy, Chicago, IL, 1991 (Abstract 635).

119. Donovan RM, Dickover RE, Goldstein E, et al. HIV-1 proviral number in blood mononuclear cells from AIDS patients on zidovudine therapy. J Acq Immun Def Synd 1991; 4:766-9.

120. Oka S, Urayama K, Hirabayshi Y, et al. Anti HIV activity of beta interferon (IFN) evaluated by changes of the number of HIV proviruses in blood. Program VII International Conference on AIDS, Florence, Italy, 1991 (Abstract W.B. 2149).

121. Aoki S, Yarchoan R, Thomas RV, et al. Quantitative analysis of HIV-1 proviral DNA in peripheral blood mononuclear cells from patients with AIDS or ARC: decrease of proviral DNA content following treatment with 2',3'-dideoxyinosine (ddI). AIDS Res Hum Retroviruses 1990; 6:1331-9.

122. Israel V, Chelyapov NV, Ho DD et al. Evaluation of efficacy of therapy and emergence of zidovudine (AZT) resistant HIV-1 by quantitative cultures and PCR. Program VII International Conference on AIDS, Florence, Italy, 1991 (Abstract Tu.B. 90).

123. Clark AGB, Holodniy M, Schwartz DH, et al. Decrease in HIV provirus in peripheral blood mononuclear cells during zidovudine and human rIL-2 administration. J AIDS 1992; 5:52-9.

124. Anderson RE, Lang W, Shiboski S, et al. Use of beta 2 microglobulin level and CD4 lymphocyte count to predict development of acquired immunodeficiency syndrome in persons with human immunodeficiency virus infection. Arch Intern Med 1990; 150:73-7.

125. Landay A, Ohlsson-Wilhelm B, Giorgi JV. Application of flow cytometry to the study of HIV infection. AIDS 1990; 4:479-97.

126. Ohlsson-Wilhelm BM, Eyster ME, Friedberg G, et al. Quantification of P24 + lymphocytes as a function of CD4 count. Program VII International Conference on AIDS, Florence, Italy, 1991 (Abstract Th.A. 71).

4

New Developments in Antiretroviral Drug Therapy for HIV Infection

Victoria A. Johnson
University of Alabama at Birmingham, Birmingham, Alabama

I. INTRODUCTION

Efforts are underway to further define the optimal therapy for human immunodeficiency virus type 1 (HIV-1) infection (1-3). Much attention has focused on HIV-1 reverse transcriptase (RT) inhibitors, including clinical studies of agents that may have enhanced therapeutic indices and/ or may act by different mechanisms than currently available drugs (1-3). There is also impressive progress in the development of agents that attack other virus-specific targets within the HIV-1 replicative cycle, such as inhibitors of HIV-1 protease or regulatory genes (e.g., *Tat*), which are undergoing clinical evaluation (1-3) (Fig. 1). Despite major advances in our understanding of the HIV-1 replicative cycle and potential chemotherapeutic interventions, the optimal determination of antiretroviral activity in patients during clinical trials remains unknown, although promising markers of viral load are under study (4-12) (see Chapter 3). The significance of the detection of drug-resistant virus variants from patients during prolonged monotherapy, both in regard to clinical disease progression and drug failure, as well as the permanence of the drug-resistant viral pheno-

Johnson

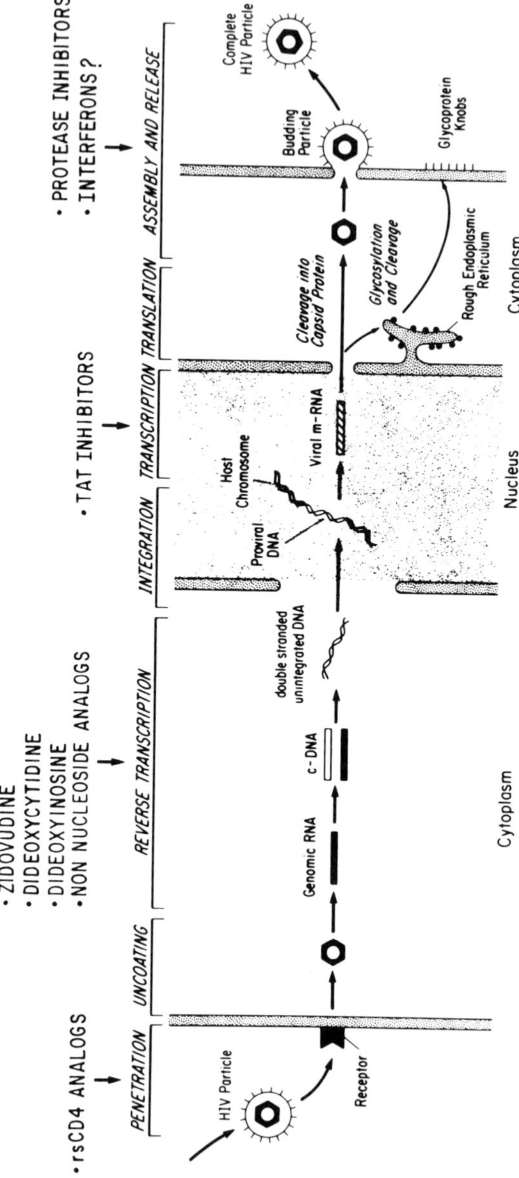

Figure 1 Schematic representation of the replication cycle of HIV-1 and the sites of action of antiretroviral agents.

Table 1 Targets for Anti-HIV Agents

Target in viral replicative cycle	Agents[a]
Viral adsorption or entry	Recombinant soluble CD4 analogs
	Neutralizing antibodies
	Inhibitors of viral uncoating
Reverse transcriptase inhibitors	Zidovudine
	Dideoxycytidine
	Dideoxyinosine
	Other nucleoside analogs
	Nonnucleoside analogs
	Inhibitors of RNase H activity
Integration of DNA into host genetic material	Inhibitors of integrase function
Viral gene expression	Anti-*Tat* or anti-*Rev* inhibitors
	Antisense oligodeoxynucleotides
	TAR decoys (to bind *Tat*)
	Ribozymes (to destroy HIV mRNA)
Posttranscriptional or posttranslational processing, assembly, or release	Glycoprotein processing inhibitors (e.g., castanospermine, deoxynojiri-mycin derivatives)
	Myristylation inhibitors
	Protease inhibitors
	Interferons

[a]The antiviral effect of some of these agents has not been firmly established; for some there may be more than one mode of action, and for others the mechanism is unclear. Some of these listings are theoretical interventions and not currently available for testing.

type and genotype, needs to be explored fully (13,14). As further information has accumulated regarding the natural history and pathogenesis of HIV-1 infection in infected humans, it is clear that progressive HIV-1 replication occurs resulting in increasing viral burden and immunological impairment (4-9, 15-18). As a result, there is increasing interest in antiviral intervention for asymptomative HIV-1-infected individuals (19,20). Based on clinical trials with available drugs, single-agent regimens will not be enough to provide long-term virus suppression in HIV-1-infected individuals. Therefore, combination therapy for HIV-1 infection will likely be required (21-25). A rapidly rising number of clinical trials involving combination antiviral therapies, both to potentially limit viral spread and/ or delay emergence of resistance to single agent regimens, attests to the growing support for this approach. This chapter will focus on progress in drug development for therapy of HIV-1 infection, review current knowledge regarding the development of drug-resistant HIV-1 during single-agent therapy, and discuss the role of combination therapy.

II. NUCLEOSIDE ANALOGS AND RESISTANCE

A. Zidovudine

The RT inhibitor zidovudine (also known as ZDV, 3'-azido-3'-deoxythymidine, azidothymidine, AZT, or Retrovir) is a pyrimidine nucleoside analog that inhibits HIV-1 replication in vitro and has demonstrated efficacy in vivo (26-44). Despite its proven benefit in patients with advanced HIV disease (28,30,31,37), long-term administration is often associated with drug-induced toxicities, which require dose modifications or withdrawals (29,32,37), particularly when higher doses ($\geqslant$1 g daily) are used.

To enhance the therapeutic index of zidovudine by limiting drug-induced toxicities, the safety and efficacy of a lower daily dose of zidovudine in patients with the acquired immunodeficiency syndrome (AIDS) was examined in a randomized, controlled trial (ACTG protocol 002) (35). Subjects with a history of a first episode of *Pneumocystis carinii* pneumonia (PCP) were assigned to receive either 1500 mg daily or 1200 mg daily for 4 weeks followed by 600 mg daily thereafter. After a median length of follow-up of 25.6 months, the reduced daily dose of zidovudine was found to be at least as effective as the standard 1500 mg daily dose, as measured by length of time to development of another opportunistic infection, changes in the CD4 + T-lymphocyte count, and declines in the serum level of HIV antigen (35). The lower-dose regimen resulted in less hematological toxicity than the higher-dose regimen. It was also associated with a better survival rate, which was attributed to the ability to maintain more continuous antiviral therapy using the less toxic lower-dose regimen than the higher-dose regimen (35).

A separate open-label, phase II pilot study examined lower-dose zidovudine therapy in patients with AIDS-related complex (ARC) with CD4 + T-lymphocyte counts of 200-500/mm^3 (36). Three daily doses of zidovudine were studied (300 mg, 600 mg, or 1500 mg). Very low-dose zidovudine therapy (300 mg daily) resulted in similar clinical and virological benefits as the higher daily dose regimens (600 and 1500 mg), although drug-related toxicities occurred most frequently at the 1500-mg dose (36). Based on the small numbers of patients evaluated, large-scale clinical studies will be required prior to recommending the use of zidovudine at these very low doses. Of note, one recent study documented that zidovudine at 150 mg/day in subjects with advanced HIV-1 infection produced suboptimal virological and immunological effects (45).

Several landmark randomized, double-blind, placebo-controlled clinical trials have evaluated the role of initiation of zidovudine therapy at early stages in HIV-1 infection. In one trial evaluating persons with mildly symptomatic HIV-1 infection and CD4 + T-lymphocyte counts of 200-500/mm³, zidovudine delayed progression of HIV disease and produced limited toxicity when compared to placebo (ACTG protocol 016) (33). A second trial evaluated asymptomatic HIV-1-infected individuals with CD4 + T-lymphocyte counts less than 500/mm³ treated with placebo, zidovudine 500 mg daily, or zidovudine 1500 mg daily, with a mean follow-up of 55 weeks (ACTG protocol 019) (34). The rates of progression to either AIDS or advanced ARC were 7.6, 3.6, and 4.3 per 100 person-years, respectively. Immunological and virological benefits were seen with both zidovudine doses when compared to the placebo-treated group. However, hematological toxicity was most frequent at the 1500-mg daily zidovudine-treated group. A minority subset data analysis of ACTG protocols 016 and 019 demonstrated beneficial effects of zidovudine on rates of progression to AIDS in subpopulations of blacks, Hispanics, women, and intravenous drug users (40).

In yet another placebo-controlled trial evaluating zidovudine in asymptomatic HIV-1-infected patients with hemophilia, similar observations regarding zidovudine benefit were seen in subjects over 30 years of age (NHF-ACTG protocol 036) (38) as in the larger study of its use in asymptomatic, nonhemophilic patients (ACTG protocol 019) (34). Based on all of these data, the current recommended dose of zidovudine is 100 mg every 4 hours (600 mg/day) for adult patients with symptomatic HIV infection and 100 mg every 4 hours while awake (500 mg/day) for adult patients with asymptomatic HIV infection (39). Alternatively, many clinicians are now giving zidovudine 200 mg every 8 hours orally due to ease of administration.

Favorable results of zidovudine therapy in children with HIV infection have also been reported (41-44). In a multicenter phase II study in children with advanced HIV disease, oral zidovudine was administered safely to children 4 months to 11 years of age (ACTG protocol 043) (44). Improvement in numerous clinical, immunological, and virological parameters during the course of zidovudine therapy in children have been reported, similar to those found in adults (41-44). A phase III randomized, placebo-controlled trial is underway to evaluate the efficacy, safety, and tolerance of oral zidovudine (ZDV) in pregnant HIV-infected women and their infants (ACTG protocol 076). The study will 1) evaluate the effect of zido-vudine on the incidence of HIV infection in infants by treating HIV-in-fected pregnant women and their infants; 2) evaluate the safety and toler-ance of zidovudine administered to HIV-1-infected women from 14-34 weeks of pregnancy until delivery; and 3) evaluate the safety and toler-ance of zidovudine administered to infants with perinatal HIV exposure from 0 to 6 weeks of age.

Despite the clear-cut benefits of zidovudine in multiple HIV-1-infected populations, prolonged single-agent treatment has been associated with observations that HIV-1 is incompletely suppressed during AZT therapy and that AZT activity may diminish after the first year (31,46,47). The potential etiologies for this phenomenon are multifactorial, including de-velopment of drug-resistant viruses, cellular toxicities or refractoriness to antivirals, and/or overwhelming viral burden. Although the clinical sig-nificance of the detection of zidovudine-resistant HIV-1 in vitro derived from drug-treated subjects is still being assessed, the clinical importance of drug resistance for other viruses (e.g., herpes simplex viruses, cyto-megaloviruses, varicella-zoster viruses, and influenza A viruses) has been described amply (13,14), particularly in the setting of prolonged exposure to drug, chronic viral infection, and underlying immunodeficiency (13, 14). It is clear that HIV-1 isolates exist in mixtures (48-51), and that mixed populations of zidovudine-sensitive and -resistant virus variants occur during therapy (52,53), which may have important implications for po-tential intervention using combined therapy regimens which still contain zidovudine (52).

Progress has been made in several areas of study of zidovudine-resis-tant HIV-1:

1. Multiple RT mutations have been shown to confer zidovudine resis-tance phenotypically (four have been described at RT codons 67, 70, 215, and 219, but more are likely to contribute) (13, 52-68) and occur in a stepwise fashion during prolonged zidovudine therapy (53).

2. Zidovudine-resistant HIV-1 has now been generated in vitro (69, 70), allowing better understanding of the activity of antiviral drugs at a molecular level and determination of the relative significance of sequential RT mutations that occur during therapy. This may then allow the design of anti-HIV-1 agents that are potentially more effective and safer.

3. A consensus protocol regarding standardized methodology for sur-veillance of drug-resistant HIV-1 during clinical antiretroviral trials

is now being developed by the NIAID AIDS Clinical Trials Group (ACTG) Virology Committee's Viral Resistance Working Group.

4. Several clinical trials aimed at determining the clinical significance of zidovudine resistance are being developed and sponsored, including collaborative efforts of the ACTG/NIAID/NIH, the FDA, and the military.

B. Dideoxyinosine

2',3'-Dideoxyinosine (ddI, dideoxyinosine, didanosine, Videx) is a purine nucleoside analog that inhibits HIV-1 reverse transcriptase in vitro (71). The potential advantages of ddI include 1) longer intracellular half-life of ddATP (the active form of ddI) than the triphosphates of zidovudine or ddC (72); 2) minimal bone marrow precursor toxicity when compared to zidovudine (73); and 3) zidovudine-resistant HIV-1 isolates have not been shown to be cross-resistant to ddI in vitro (72). Potential disadvantages of ddI include 1) acid lability, which may decrease oral bioavailability without concurrent antacid administration (citrate buffers used to increase gastric pH have been implicated for ddI-related diarrhea); 2) overlapping toxicity with 2',3'-dideoxycytidine (ddC) regarding reversible peripheral neuropathy (74), making combined ddI and ddC therapy administered simultaneously less desirable; 3) cases of severe pancreatitis and hepatitis have been reported, particularly at higher doses (72,75-86). ddI-related pancreatitis was noted most commonly in patients with advanced HIV disease, a previous history of pancreatitis, exposure to intravenous pentamidine, and concomitant disseminated cytomegalovirus (CMV) or *Mycobacterium avium-intracellulare* (MAI) infections (84).

In October 1991, ddI became the second RT inhibitor after zidovudine to be approved for therapy of HIV-1 infection. This agent was approved for the treatment of adult and pediatric patients (over 6 months of age) with advanced HIV-1 infection who are zidovudine-intolerant or who have demonstrated significant clinical or immunological deterioration during zidovudine therapy (87). Since initiation of clinical trials in August 1988, multiple centers have described benefits of ddI therapy in both HIV-1-infected adults and children, including increases in CD4+ T-lymphocyte counts, weight gains, and declines in levels of HIV-1 p24 antigens (72, 75-86). The effect of ddI on clinical progression of HIV infection or mortality rates, however, remains unknown, such that zidovudine should still be considered as initial therapy for advanced HIV infection. To address these questions, multiple ACTG phase II/III clinical trials are in progress to evaluate the role of ddI therapy. These studies include comparison of ddI and zidovudine with respect to efficacy and toxicity in patients with advanced HIV-1 infection before (ACTG protocol 116A) and after (ACTG protocol 116B/117) prolonged zidovudine therapy, as well as evaluation of ddI in zidovudine-intolerant patients (ACTG protocol 118). Phase I safety and pharmacokinetics studies of ddI administered daily to infants, children, and adolescents with AIDS or symptomatic HIV infection have been completed or are in progress (ACTG protocol 091) (81,85). A randomized, comparative trial of two doses of ddI is underway in children with HIV-1 infection unresponsive to zidovudine and/or who are intolerant to zidovudine (ACTG protocol 144). A comparative efficacy trial of zidovudine versus ddI in symptomatic HIV-1-infected pediatric subjects is also in progress at the NCI under the direction of Dr. Phillip Pizzo.

Despite multiple reports of clinical benefit with ddI therapy, several investigators have documented decreased ddI sensitivity of HIV-1 isolates in vitro obtained from recipients treated long-term with ddI (i.e., after at least 12 months of therapy) (88-91). In one study of persons switched from long-term zidovudine therapy to ddI, reversion of zidovudine-resistant to zidovudine-sensitive strains occurred, although ddI susceptibility declined during ddI therapy (89). The mechanism for this ddI-resistant phenotype appears to be a RT codon 74 mutation, which has been detected in HIV-1 isolates obtained from subjects after prolonged therapy (89).

C. Dideoxycytidine

With the advent of zidovudine and dideoxyinosine resistance, as well as the finding that long-term single-agent therapy may be associated with either drug failure and/or intolerance (31,46,47,83), increasing interest in alternative agents has emerged. The pyrimidine nucleoside analog 2′,3′-dideoxycytidine, also known as ddC or dideoxycytidine, also inhibits HIV-1 replication in vitro (71). In phase I clinical testing of ddC in patients with AIDS or ARC, declines in serum HIV p24 antigen and rises in CD4+ cell numbers were noted (1,24,92,93). Side effects included rashes, stomatitis, arthralgias, arthritis, fever, and dose-dependent late-onset painful peripheral neuropathy (1,24,92,93). Pancreatitis and esophageal ulcers during ddC therapy have also been described.

In 1990, in addition to ongoing efficacy trials, ddC was made available to patients with AIDS and ARC who were intolerant or did not respond to zidovudine or ddI through an open-label safety study by Hoffmann-LaRoche. In August 1991, these studies were switched by the FDA from open label to a treatment Investigational New Drug (IND) status. A phase II trial of two doses of ddC for treatment of children with symptomatic HIV infection who are zidovudine interolant and/or show signs of disease progression while receiving zidovudine therapy is in progress (ACTG protocol 138). To directly compare the efficacy and toxicity of ddI and ddC, a randomized open-label trial of ddI and ddC in HIV-1-infected patients who are intolerant or have failed zidovudine is also planned (NIAID's Community Programs for Clinical Research on AIDS [CPCRA] IND protocol 35,629).

Unfortunately, as with single-agent zidovudine or ddI therapy for HIV-1 infection, HIV-1 isolates resistant to ddC have now been reported (94). In patients receiving prolonged ddC therapy, an RT mutation at codon 69 was described which was associated with less ddC susceptibility phenotypically (94). One report suggested that HIV-1 may develop resistance to ddC and ddI less readily than to zidovudine in patients receiving antiviral therapy (95), although further studies are required to assess the relative rates of development of drug resistance among RT inhibitors during single-agent therapy.

III. NONNUCLEOSIDE ANALOGS AND RESISTANCE

A novel class of nonnucleoside RT inhibitors has received much attention as potential alternative anti-HIV-1 agents based on their excellent therapeutic ratio; namely, potent anti-HIV-1 activity in vitro with minimal cytotoxicity (96-108). These compounds include 1) TIBO derivatives (of the benzodiazepine class) (96-98); 2) BI-RG-587 (a dipyridodiazepinone, Nevirapine; Boehringer Ingelheim) (99-102); 3) pyridinone derivatives (L drugs, most potent derivatives named L697,639 and L697,661; Merck) (103-106); and 4) BHAPs (bis[heteroaryl]piperazines; Upjohn) (107,108). Albeit structurally diverse, these compounds probably inhibit HIV-1 RT (but not HIV-2) via a similar mechanism of action that is still being defined but appears to be distinct from that of 2',3'-dideoxynucleoside analogs (which compete with cellular nucleoside triphosphates and/or act as DNA chain terminators in the RT reaction).

Clinical phase I/II evaluation of a promising pyridinone RT inhibitor L697,661 was conducted at both the University of Alabama at Birmingham (UAB) and the NIAID/NIH. At UAB under the direction of Dr. Michael S. Saag, preliminary clinical results regarding safety and antiviral activity of L697,661 were: 1) L697,661 is an active antiretroviral compound in vivo; 2) the drug is well tolerated by most individuals with few serious side effects; 3) the most serious side effect noted was asymptomatic liver function test elevations in a few subjects, which resolved when drug was temporarily discontinued, and did not recur in two participants rechallenged with drug; 4) there was no clear-cut difference between L697,661 and zidovudine regarding antiviral activity short-term in vivo, in contrast to previous in vitro studies which demonstrated a 10- to 1000-fold increased activity of L697,661 over zidovudine (103); and 5) the apparent development of viral strains resistant to L697,661 amont patients taking the drug. Although only limited data exist regarding seven L-drug-treated subjects, all seven had viruses sensitive to L697,661 before receiving treatment, which became resistant to drug within 6-12 weeks after initiation of L697, 661 therapy. In contrast, two control patients (assigned to zidovudine therapy) showed no development of resistance to L697,661 while receiving zidovudine (as expected). The development of viral strains resistant to L697,661 was anticipated as a potential problem for this drug based on in vitro studies (conducted in parallel with the in vivo trials) that selected L-drug-resistant HIV-1 during drug pressure (106), as well as on the observation that this class of compounds (i.e., nonnucleoside RT inhibitors) demonstrated highly selective activity against HIV-1 but not HIV-2 (96-108). However, the rapid development of resistance in an apparently substantial number of individuals was quite surprising and unanticipated, although the clinical significance of this finding remains unclear. Because of intensive laboratory evaluations of viral markers performed in collaboration with Dr. George M. Shaw (at UAB), the investigators were able to detect, at least in a few patients, rising HIV-1 p24 antigen levels which were associated with the development of resistant viral isolates. This finding prompted discontinuation of the clinical trial of L697,661 as a single agent (M. Saag, personal communication), although the role of L drugs in combination with zidovudine is still being evaluated in clinical trials (E. Emini, personal communication).

One study of drug resistance to this class of compounds has documented changes at RT codons 103 and 181 in drug-resistant HIV-1 which display phenotypic resistance (106). These viruses were generated during drug treatment in vitro. Cross-resistance of HIV-1 to other nonnucleoside analogs supports a similar mechanism of action (106). Despite their high potency, the long-term role of this class of compounds as single agents for HIV-1 infection is unclear given the rapid emergence of resistance during drug therapy.

IV. ALTERNATIVE ANTIRETROVIRAL AGENTS

A. *Tat* Inhibitors

A better understanding of complex regulatory gene functions that are essential for HIV-1 replication has led to the development of novel compounds for HIV-1 intervention, including agents that interrupt HIV-1 regulatory gene products such as *Tat* (109). The HIV-encoded Tat protein increases gene expression directed by the HIV-1 long terminal repeat (LTR) promoter and is critical for elongation of transcription and may also increase transcription initiation (109) (see Fig. 1). Through a screening program at Hoffmann-LaRoche, one promising compound, Ro 5-3335, demonstrated inhibition of HIV-1 LTR promoter activity in cloned cell lines that contained integrated *Tat* and indicator genes (under the control of the HIV-1 LTR promoter). The inhibition of gene expression by Ro 5-3335 was due to interruption of *Tat* transactivation of the HIV-1 LTR promoter (109). In addition to efficacy of Ro 5-3335 in cells acutely HIV-1-infected, the compound also inhibits HIV-1 replication in chronically infected cells due to its mechanism of action (109). This finding, as well the ability to inhibit replication of both HIV-1 and HIV-2, makes Ro 5-3335 an attractive agent for drug development (109). Phase I/II clinical trials evaluating *Tat* inhibitors are now in progress.

B. Protease Inhibitors

Due to intense interest in the ability to attack HIV-1-specific genes other than RT therapeutically, efforts have lead to the identification of HIV-1 protease inhibitors (110-120). For mature infectious virions to be formed, the viral precursor polyproteins $Pr55^{gag}$ and $Pr160^{gag-pol}$ must undergo a posttranslational cleavage reaction which requires HIV-1 protease in order to form the virion core structural proteins of *gag* (p17,p24,p15,p9,p6) and the essential enzymes of *pol* (reverse transcriptase, ribonuclease H, integrase). This occurs only after the HIV-1 protease has autocatalytically cleaved itself from the $Pr160^{gag-pol}$ precursor polyprotein (2). The HIV-1 protease is enzymatically active when it self-assembles monomers into a dimeric form, which may occur very late in the HIV-1 replicative cycle, even after virions have been released from cells (2,3) (see Fig. 1). Mutations of either the HIV-1 protease or the *gag* or *pol* cleavage sites result in virus particles that are noninfectious and immature (120). Substrate-based inhibitors of HIV-1 protease that compete with natural substrate have been developed, including 1) C_2 symmetric inhibitors, which correspond to the

C_2 symmetric active site of the HIV-1 protease homodimer, and 2) "transition-state mimetic" peptide analogs that mimic the natural transition state intermediate achieved during normal peptide bond cleavage of substrate by HIV-1 protease yet contain a noncleavable peptide bond (110-120). These compounds demonstrate low cytotoxicity and high antiviral potency in vitro against both acute and chronic infected cells including activity against HIV-1 (including AZT-resistant viruses) and HIV-2 (110-120). Initially, clinical development of this class of agents was limited by high lipophilicity, poor aqueous solubility, rapid metabolism, and limited oral bioavailability (110-120). However, several lead compounds are now undergoing evaluation in phase I/II clinical trials.

V. COMBINATION THERAPY FOR HIV INFECTION

A. Background

Combination chemotherapeutic agent regimens have been used successfully in treating a variety of bacterial and fungal diseases, as well as in cancer chemotherapy. Single-agent therapy has been associated with the emergence of drug resistance and the development of drug-related toxicities (particularly at higher doses) and/or drug failure over time (31,46,47, 83). Based on these findings, there is now tremendous interest in the combined agent therapeutic approach to HIV-1 infection. Due to some confusion regarding terminology, several definitions are worth reviewing:

1. *Combination therapy*: Multiple drugs used in combination against a specific pathogen (e.g., HIV-1).
2. *Concomitant therapy*: Multiple drugs used in combination against HIV-1 infection *plus* HIV-1-associated opportunistic infections.

This discussion will focus on anti-HIV combined regimens. When two agents are combined, they may have one of three types of interactions (21,22,121):

1. Additive effect: Two drugs are said to be additive when the activity of the drugs in combination is equal to the sum (or a partial sum) of their independent activities when studied separately.
2. Synergism: The combined effect of a synergistic pair of agents is greater than the sum of their independent activities when measured separately (i.e., greater than the expected additive effect).
3. Antagonism: If two drugs are antagonistic, the activity of the combination is less than the sum of their independent effects when measured alone (i.e., less than the expected additive effect).

It is difficult to ascertain the nature of drug interactions in complex biological assays, leading to general agreement that we should attempt to apply mathematical/statistical methods to yield determinations of additive effects, synergism, or antagonism. Unfortunately, there is as yet no consensus regarding methodology for the mathematical/statistical assessments of either in vitro or in vivo drug interactions, although a Contractors' Workshop on Combination Therapies, sponsored by the Division of AIDS/NIAID/NIH and held in September 1991, has initiated discussions to achieve this goal. In collaboration with Dr. Martin S. Hirsch (Massachusetts General Hospital and Harvard Medical School, Boston), we have evaluated drug interactions by the median-effect principle and the isobologram technique (122-124). Full discussions of the methods available and their limitations are described elsewhere (122-128).

There are many potential advantages of anti-HIV combined-agent regimens over single-agent therapy, particularly if antiviral additive or synergistic interactions occur, which may lead to more complete virus suppression. This strategy may also allow the use of individual agents below their toxic concentrations and may prevent the emergence of drug-resistant HIV mutants. Ideally, these combination regimens should affect viral replication in a broad range of cell types, provide activity against heterogeneous viral populations, and should not display additional toxicity in combination or share cross-resistance. The overall goal for anti-HIV combination therapy is to achieve increased efficacy and/or decreased toxicity when treating patients. However, drugs should generally not be used in combination in patients until they have been evaluated thoroughly as single agents, in order to avoid incorrect conclusions regarding combined efficacies and/or toxicities.

B. Drug Combinations Tested Against HIV Replication In Vitro

Many combination therapies (Table 2) have been studied in vitro under the direction of Dr. Martin S. Hirsch, (Massachusetts General Hospital and Harvard Medical School, Boston). Several promising in vitro combined anti-HIV-1 strategies will be reviewed:

1. Two-Drug Combinations of Zidovudine, ddl, and Recombinant Interferon-α A (rIFN-αA) Against Zidovudine-Resistant HIV-1 In Vitro

Zidovudine-sensitive and -resistant isolate pairs derived from two individuals before and after extended zidovudine therapy were evaluated (52).

Table 2 In Vitro Interactions of Drug Combinations for HIV Infection Studied in the Laboratory of Dr. Martin S. Hirsch, Massachusetts General Hospital and Harvard Medical School, Boston

Virus	Combination	Interaction	Ref.
AZT-sensitive:			
HTLV-IIIB	Foscarnet + IFN-alpha	Synergism	129
HTLV-IIIB	AZT + IFN-alpha	Synergism	130
HTLV-IIIB	AZT + Ribavirin	Antagonism	131
HTLV-IIIB	ddC + IFN-alpha	Synergism	132
HTLV-IIIB or HIV-2/ROD	AZT + Castanospermine	Synergism	133
HTLV-IIIB	AZT + recombinant soluble CD4 (rsCD4)	Synergism	134
HTLV-IIIB	AZT + N-butyl 1-deoxynojirimycin (N-butyl DNJ)	Synergism	135
HTLV-IIIB	AZT + rsCD4 + rIFN-α-A	Synergism	136
HTLV-IIIB	ddI + either AZT, rsCD4, or IFN-alpha	Synergism	137
HTLV-IIIB	AZT + ddC	Synergism	138
Clinical HIV-1	AZT + ddC	Synergism	139
Clinical HIV-1	Protease inhibitor + AZT, ddC, or IFN-alpha	Additive/ Synergism	140
AZT-resistant:			
Clinical HIV-1	AZT + either ddI or IFN-alpha; ddI + IFN-alpha	Synergism	52
Clinical HIV-1	AZT + ddC	Synergism	139
Clinical HIV-1	Protease inhibitor + AZT, ddC, or IFN-alpha	Additive/ Synergism	140

Using the zidovudine-resistant isolate from each individual, zidovudine, ddI, and recombinant interferon-α A were evaluated in acutely HIV-1-infected peripheral blood mononuclear cells (PBMC). The compounds were tested as single agents and in the following drug regimens: zidovudine combined with ddI (i.e., the addition of another anti-HIV-1 agent that inhibits RT); zidovudine combined with rIFN-αA (i.e., the addition of an anti-HIV-1 agent acting by a different mechanism) (see Fig. 1); and ddI combined with rIFN-αA (i.e., use of a regimen that did not include zidovudine). Synergistic interactions (as determined mathematically) were seen among zidovudine, ddI, and rIFN-αA in 2-drug regimens against zidovudine-resistant HIV-1 in vitro, even when zidovudine was included in the treatment regimen (52). The concentrations of agents tested (0.125-1.0 μM zidovudine, 0.625-5.0 μM ddI, and 4-32 U/ml rIFN-αA) are easily achievable in vivo (52). Mixtures of genomes encoding both wild-type and mutant RT codons 67 and 70 were found in one of the late-zidovudine therapy isolates, suggesting that the mechanism of synergy of zidovudine-containing regimens may involve inhibition of zidovudine-sensitive viruses in the viral pool (52). However, alternative mechanisms for synergistic inhibition of phenotypically zidovudine-resistant viruses by zidovudine-containing two-drug regimens should also be considered. Synergy may still occur when one combines partly effective agents that act at different viral targets (e.g., zidovudine plus rIFN-αA). Another possible mechanism is that one chain-terminating nucleoside analog may potentiate the effect of another (e.g., zidovudine plus ddI) by stereochemically altering the agent's RT binding. With either mechanism, more complete viral inhibition may occur within infected cell. These studies suggest that zidovudine may still be useful in drug combination regimens, even when zidovudine-resistant viruses are isolated in vitro (52).

2. Zidovudine Plus 2',3'-Dideoxycytidine (ddC)

In work conducted in collaboration with Dr. Joseph Eron, synergistic interactions were seen using the combination of zidovudine and ddC against HIV-1 replication in acutely infected PBMC or T-cell lines (139,140). The viruses tested included HIV-1$_{IIIB}$, as well as zidovudine-sensitive and -resistant HIV-1 isolates derived from a clinical source (139,140).

3. Protease Inhibitor Ro 31-8959 plus Either Zidovudine, ddC, or rIFN-αA

We assessed in vitro the interactions of two-drug combined regimens including a potent protease inhibitor Ro 31-8959 against HIV-1 replication using acutely infected PBMC (114,119,140). Both zidovudine-sensitive and -resistant HIV-1 isolates (52) were used. Ro 31-8959, also called Compound XVII, was developed by Roche Products Limited (Welwyn Garden City, England) using the transition state mimetic approach. Concentrations tested were 7.5-30 nM Ro 31-8959, 0.005-0.02 μM zidovudine for zidovudine-sensitive HIV-1, 0.25-1.0 μM zidovudine for zidovudine-resistant HIV-1, 0.025-0.1 μM ddC, and 8-32 U/ml rIFN-αA. When Ro 31-8959 was combined with each of these agents in two-drug regimens, additive to synergistic anti-HIV-1 interactions were seen, without additive toxicity (140).

Many other promising combination therapies for HIV-1 infection tested in vitro in other laboratories are presented in Table 3.

C. Clinical Trials of Combination Therapy

The many potential benefits and problems conducting clinical trials using combination regimens are reviewed elsewhere (21-25,173). Given the exponential number of potential combined regimens that may be considered for anti-HIV-1 therapy in the future, the ACTG is developing a "master protocol" (under the direction of Drs. Martin Hirsch [Harvard], Thomas Merigan [Stanford], and David Schoenfeld [Harvard]) for screening and identifying those combined drug regimens that are most promising for further large-scale phase II/III clinical trials in HIV-1-infected patients with CD4+ lymphocyte cell numbers $\leqslant 500/mm^3$. Numerous clinical trials already in progress are outlined in Table 4. One strategy includes alternating antiretroviral therapies to attempt to diminish cumulative toxicities of individual agents (e.g., AZT alternating with ddC) (1,3,24,25). Another strategy includes combinations of antiretrovirals, as well as combining antiretrovirals with biologic response modifiers and/or immunomodulators (174-178).

Results of several promising clinical trials of anti-HIV-1 combined regimens will be highlighted. The combination of zidovudine plus interferon-α has been examined in humans and animal models at multiple centers, resulting in the largest number of publications (24,179-192). Several studies have reported combined benefits for HIV-1-infected individuals (24, 179-185), including those with Kaposi's sarcoma (KS). Both tumor responses and anti-HIV-1 effects (sustained CD4+ T-lymphocyte count increases and declines in HIV-1 p24 antigen) were described, although these benefits were detected more frequently at the highest tolerated doses of the combination (179-185). In one study, tumor regression was seen in responders receiving combined therapy, even in those subjects with pretreatment CD4+ T-lymphocyte counts $\leqslant 200$ cells/mm^3 (184). Of note, several patients with sustained suppression of HIV-1 p24 antigen levels later developed breakthrough of detectable levels of antigen following 31-55 weeks of therapy (184). Preliminary analysis of their HIV-1 isolates following 1 year of therapy did not demonstrate changes in zidovudine susceptibility (184), suggesting alternative mechanisms for breakthrough (e.g., overwhelming viral load due to disease progression and/or loss of drug efficacy). These data present a glimmer of hope that combined therapy will provide more complete virus suppression and may possibly delay

Table 3 Antiretroviral Combinations Tested In Vitro Elsewhere

Combination	Ref.
Zidovudine and acyclovir	141,142
Zidovudine and GM-CSF	143,144
Zidovudine and dextran sulfate	145-147
Zidovudine and ampligen	148
Zidovudine and amphotericin B	149
Zidovudine and dipyridamole	150
Ribavarin and dideoxycytidine	151
Purine nucleoside analogue NSC-614846 and either ribavarin or zidovudine	152
Zidovudine and an acyclic adenosine analogue (PMEA)	153
Zidovudine and foscarnet	154,155
Zidovudine and interferon-beta	156
Zidovudine and isoprinosine	157
Zidovudine alternating with dideoxycytidine	158
Dideoxyinosine and ribavirin	151,159
2',3'-Dideoxy-2,6-diaminopurine riboside and ribavarin	160
Recombinant soluble CD4 and either zidovudine, dideoxyinosine, and dideoxycytidine	161
Dextran sulfate and either zidovudine, dideoxyinosine, and dideoxycytidine	161
Sulfated sugar alpha-cyclodextrin sulfate and zidovudine	162
Sodium pentosan polysulfate and zidovudine	163
Dideoxyinosine and GM-CSF	164
Dideoxycytidine and GM-CSF	164
Zidovudine and 3'-fluoro-3'-deoxythymidine	165
Phosphorothioate oligonucleotide S-dC28 and either zidovudine, interferon-alpha, or dextran sulfate	166
1-[(2-Hydroxyethoxy)methyl]-6-phenylthiothymine (HEPT) and recombinant alpha interferon	167
Inhibitors of IMP dehydrogenase and either 2',3'-dideoxyadenosine or 2',3'-dideoxyinosine	168
Zidovudine and dideoxyinosine	169
5-Ethyl-1-ethoxymethyl-6-(phenylthio)uracil (E-EPU) and zidovudine	170
Pyridinone RT inhibitors and nucleoside analogs	106,171
BI-RG-587 (Nevaripine) and zidovudine	100
C_2 symmetric HIV protease inhibitors and AZT or ddI	172

Table 4 Clinical Trials of Combination Therapies for HIV Infection in Progress or Planned

Zidovudine (AZT) plus:
acyclovir
BI-RG-587
CD4-IgG
ddI
ddI versus AZT versus ddI
ddI versus AZT plus ddC
ddI versus ddI versus AZT plus ddC versus AZT
ddC
erythropoietin
foscarnet
GM-CSF
GM-CSF plus EPO
interferon-alpha
interferon-alpha plus GM-CSF
IL-2
IL-2 (PEG) or ddI plus IL-2 (PEG)
L-697,661
N-butyl DNJ
AZT alternating with ddC
AZT alternating with GM-CSF
Weekly alternating regimens of:
AZT and acyclovir (week 1)
ddI (week 2)
ddC (week 3)
IFN-α + IL-2

the emergence of resistance when compared to single agent regimens. The major toxicities of the combination included bone marrow suppression (both anemia and neutropenia) and hepatotoxicity (24,179-185). Other investigators have demonstrated that low-dose GM-CSF may ameliorate neutropenia associated with combined zidovudine and interferon-α without affecting antiretroviral benefits (191,192).

The preliminary results of clinical trials employing zidovudine with other nucleoside analogs are also encouraging (24,25). Zidovudine in combination with ddI is being evaluated in HIV-1-infected adults and children in multiple centers, and appears to be well-tolerated (24,193,194). Zidovudine combined with foscarnet, another RT inhibitor with anti-HIV-1 effects, resulted in an additive (albeit transient) in vivo effect (195), as predicted from previous in vitro studies (154,155). Zidovudine in combination with ddC was well tolerated in other studies (24,25), and sustained elevations in CD4+ T-lymphocyte numbers were seen with the combination when compared to those studies reported previously for either agent alone (45). A randomized, double-blind phase II/III trial of monotherapy versus combination therapy with nucleoside analogs is in development for HIV-1-infected persons with CD4+ T-lymphocyte cell numbers $\geq$ 200 and $\leq$ 500/mm^3 (ACTG protocol 175). The relative efficacy of zidovudine versus either ddI, ddI combined with zidovudine, or ddC combined with zidovudine will be evaluated with respect to change in CD4+ T-lymphocyte cell numbers below 50% of baseline level, to the development of AIDS-defining events, to survival, and to serious toxicities.

VI. CONCLUSIONS

Ongoing research efforts should still focus on the development of novel, effective, nontoxic anti-HIV-1 agents. However, it is unlikely that any single agent regimen will be sufficient to control chronic HIV-1 infection based on clinical trials with available drugs to date. The final results of the numerous combination anti-IIIV therapy trials currently in progress are awaited eagerly, including assessment of the development of drug resistance when compared to single agent regimens. The ultimate test will be whether they provide more complete virus suppression and prolongation of therapeutic benefits in HIV-1-infected persons. Efforts to halt progressive immunological deterioration, including evaluation of combined strategies involving antiretrovirals with either immunomodulators, biological response modifiers, or HIV-1-specific cytotoxic T lymphocytes, should be pursued to enhance host factors that limit viral spread and emergence of drug resistance. Further efforts to identify better virological markers will also help define the role of antiretroviral therapy for intervention at even earlier stages of HIV-1 disease.

ACKNOWLEDGMENTS

The author thanks Dr. Michael S. Saag for review of the manuscript and helpful comments.

REFERENCES

1. Yarchoan R, Pluda JM, Perno C-F, et al. Anti-retroviral therapy of human immunodeficiency virus infection: current strategies and challenges for the future. Blood 1991; 78:859-84.

2. De Clercq E. Basic approaches to anti-retroviral treatment. J AIDS 1991; 4:207-18.

3. Mitsuya H, Yarchoan R, Kageyama S, Broder S. Targeted therapy of human immunodeficiency virus-related disease. FASEB J 1991; 5:2369-81.

4. Ho DD, Moudgil T, Alam M. Quantitation of human immunodeficiency virus type 1 in the blood of infected persons. N Engl J Med 1989; 321:1621-5.

5. Coombs RW, Collier AC, Allain JP, et al. Plasma viremia in human immunodeficiency virus infection. N Engl J Med 1989; 321:1626-31.

6. Ratner L. Measurement of human immunodeficiency virus load and its relation to disease progression. AIDS Res Hum Retro 1989; 5:115-9.

7. Schnittman SM, Greenhouse JJ, Psallidopoulos MC, et al. Increasing viral burden in CD4 + T cells from patients with human immunodeficiency virus (HIV) infection reflects rapidly progressive immunosuppression and clinical disease. Ann Intern Med 1990; 113:438-43.

8. Clark SJ, Saag MS, Decker WD, et al. High titers of cytopathic virus in plasma of patients with symptomatic primary HIV-1 infection. N Engl J Med 1991; 324:954-60.

9. Daar ES, Moudgil T, Meyer RD, et al. Transient high levels of viremia in patients with primary human immunodeficiency virus type 1 infection. N Engl J Med 1991; 324:961-4.

10. Aoki S, Yarchoan R, Thomas RV, et al. Quantitative analysis of HIV-1 proviral DNA in peripheral blood mononuclear cells from patients with AIDS or ARC: decrease of proviral DNA content following treatment with 2',3'-dideoxyinosine (ddI). AIDS Res Hum Retro 1990; 6:1331-9.

11. Clark AGB, Holodniy M, Schwartz DH, et al. Decrease in HIV provirus in peripheral blood mononuclear cells during zidovudine and human rIL-2 administration. J AIDS 1992; 5:52-9.

12. Dickover RE, Donovan RM, Goldstein E, et al. Decreases in unintegrated HIV DNA are associated with antiretroviral therapy in AIDS patients. J AIDS 1992; 5:31-6.

13. Richman DD. Zidovudine resistance of human immunodeficiency virus. Rev Infect Dis 1990; 12:S507-12.

14. Laughlin CA, Black RJ, Feinberg J, et al. Resistance to antiviral drugs: although relatively new and poorly understood, viral resistance to drugs is an increasingly significant clinical issue. ASM News 1991; 57:514-7.

15. Levy JA. Changing concepts in HIV infection: challenges for the 1990s. AIDS 1990; 4:1051-8.

16. Fauci AS, Schnittman SM, Poli G, et al. Immunopathogenic mechanisms in human immunodeficiency virus (HIV) infection. Ann Intern Med 1991; 114: 678-93.

17. Pantaleo G, Graziosi C, Butini L, et al. Lymphoid organs function as major reservoirs for human immunodeficiency virus. Proc Natl Acad Sci USA 1991; 88:9838-42.

18. Michael NL, Vahey M, Burke DS, et al. Viral DNA and mRNA expression correlate with the stage of human immunodeficiency virus (HIV) type 1 infection in humans: evidence for viral replication in all stages of HIV disease. J Virol 1992; 66:310-6.

19. Friedland GH. Early treatment for HIV: the time has come. N Engl J Med 1990; 322:1000-2.

20. National Institute of Allergy and Infectious Diseases, National Institutes of Health, U.S. Public Health Service. State-of-the-art conference on azidothymidine therapy for early HIV infection. Am J Med 1990; 89:335-44.

21. Johnson VA, Hirsch MS. Combination therapy for HIV infection. In: Mills J, Corey L, eds. Antiviral chemotherapy: new directions for clinical application and research. Vol. 2. New York: Elsevier, 1989:275-302.

22. Johnson VA, Hirsch MS. New developments in combination chemotherapy of anti-human immunodeficiency virus drugs. In: Georgiev VS, McGowan JJ, eds. AIDS: anti-HIV agents, therapies, and vaccines. Vol. 616. New York: Annals of the New York Academy of Sciences, 1990:318-55.

23. Hoth D. Rationale for development of multidrug therapy. J AIDS 1990; 3(suppl 2):S95-S96.

24. Merigan TC. Treatment of AIDS with combinations of antiretroviral agents. Am J Med 1991; 90(suppl 4A):8S-17S.

25. Yarchoan R, Pluda JM, Perno CF, et al. Initial clinical experience with dideoxynucleosides as single agents and in combination therapy. In: Georgiev VS, McGowan JJ, eds. AIDS: anti-HIV agents, therapies, and vaccines. Vol. 616. New York: Annals of the New York Academy of Sciences, 1990:328-43.

26. Mitsuya H, Weinhold KJ, Furman PA, et al. 3'-Azido-3'-deoxythymidine (BW A509U): an antiviral agent that inhibits the infectivity and cytopathic effect of human T-lymphotropic virus type III/lymphadenopathy-associated virus in vitro. Proc Natl Acad Sci USA 1985; 82:7096-100.

27. Yarchoan R, Klecher RW, Weinhold KJ, et al. Administration of 3'-azido-3'-deoxythymidine, an inhibitor of HTLV-III/LAV replication, to patients with AIDS or AIDS-related complex. Lancet 1986; 1:575-80.

28. Fischl MA, Richman DD, Grieco MH, et al. The efficacy of azidothymidine (AZT) in the treatment of patients with AIDS and AIDS-related complex: a double-blind, placebo-controlled trial. N Engl J Med 1987; 317:185-91.

29. Richman DD, Fischl MA, Grieco MH, et al. The toxicity of azidothymidine (AZT) in the treatment of patients with AIDS and AIDS-related complex: a

double-blind, placebo-controlled trial. N Engl J Med 1987; 317:192-7.

30. Creagh-Kirk T, Doi P, Andrews E, et al. Survival experience among patients with AIDS receiving zidovudine: follow-up of patients in a compassionate plea program. JAMA 1988; 260:3009-15.

31. Fischl MA, Richman DD, Causey DM, et al. Prolonged zidovudine therapy in patients with AIDS and advanced AIDS-related complex. JAMA 1989; 262:2405-10.

32. Groopman JE. Zidovudine intolerance. Rev Infect Dis 1990; 12:S500-6.

33. Fischl MA, Richman DD, Hansen N, et al. The safety and efficacy of zidovudine (AZT) in the treatment of subjects with mildly symptomatic human immunodeficiency virus type 1 (HIV) infection: a double-blind, placebo-controlled trial. Ann Intern Med 1990; 112:727-37.

34. Volberding PA, Lagakos SW, Koch MA, et al. Zidovudine in asymptomatic human immunodeficiency virus infection: a controlled trial in persons with fewer than 500 CD4-positive cells per cubic millimeter. N Engl J Med 1990; 322:941-9.

35. Fischl MA, Parker CB, Pettinelli C, et al. A randomized controlled trial of a reduced daily dose of zidovudine in patients with the acquired immunodeficiency syndrome. N Engl J Med 1990; 323:1009-14.

36. Collier AC, Bozzette S, Coombs RW, et al. A pilot study of low-dose zidovudine in human immunodeficiency virus infection. N Engl J Med 1990; 323:1015-21.

37. Moore RD, Creagh-Kirk T, Keruly J, et al. Long-term safety and efficacy of zidovudine in patients with advanced human immunodeficiency virus disease. Arch Intern Med 1991; 151:981-6.

38. Merigan TC, Amato DA, Balsley J, et al. Placebo-controlled trials to evaluate zidovudine in treatment of human immunodeficiency virus infection in asymptomatic patients with hemophilia. Blood 1991; 78:900-6.

39. Fischl MA. New developments in dideoxynucleoside antiretroviral therapy for HIV infection. In: Volberding P, Jacobson MA, eds. AIDS Clinical Review 1991. New York: Marcel Dekker, Inc., 1991:197-214.

40. Lagakos S, Fischl MA, Stein DS, et al. Effects of zidovudine therapy in minority and other subpopulations with early HIV infection. JAMA 1991; 266:2709-12.

41. Pizzo PA, Eddy J, Falloon J, et al. Effect of continuous intravenous infusion of zidovudine (AZT) in children with symptomatic HIV infection. N Engl J Med 1988; 319:889-96.

42. Balis FM, Pizzo PA, Murphy RF, et al. The pharmacokinetics of zidovudine administered by continuous infusion in children. Ann Intern Med 1989; 110:279-85.

43. DeCarli C, Fugate L, Falloon J, et al. Brain growth and cognitive improve-

ment in children with human immunodeficiency virus-induced encephalopathy after 6 months of continuous infusion zidovudine therapy. J AIDS 1991; 4:585-92.

44. McKinney RE, Maha MA, Connor EM, et al. A multicenter trial of oral zidovudine in children with advanced human immunodeficiency virus disease. N Engl J Med 1991; 324:1018-25.

45. Meng T-C, Fischl MA, Boota AM, et al. Combination therapy with zidovudine and dideoxycytidine in patients with advanced human immunodeficiency virus infection: a phase I/II study. Ann Intern Med 1992; 116:13-20.

46. Dournon E, Matheron S, Rozenbaum W, et al. Effects of zidovudine in 365 consecutive patients with AIDS or AIDS-related complex. Lancet 1988; 2: 1297-302.

47. Reiss P, Lange JMA, Boucher CA, et al. Resumption of HIV antigen production during continuous zidovudine treatment. Lancet 1988; 1:421.

48. Saag MS, Hahn BH, Gibbons J, et al. Extensive variation of human immunodeficiency virus type 1 in vivo. Nature 1988; 334:440-4.

49. Fischer AG, Ensoli B, Looney D, et al. Biologically diverse molecular variants within a single HIV-1 isolate. Nature 1988; 334:444-7.

50. Meyerhans A, Cheynier R, Albert J, et al. Temporal fluctuations in HIV quasispecies in vivo are not reflected by sequential HIV isolations. Cell 1989; 58:901-10.

51. Goodenow M, Huet T, Saurin W, et al. HIV-1 isolates are rapidly evolving quasispecies: evidence for viral mixtures and preferred nucleotide substitutions. J AIDS 1989; 2:344-52.

52. Johnson VA, Merrill DP, Videler JA, et al. Two-drug combinations of zidovudine, didanosine, and recombinant interferon-α A inhibit replication of zidovudine-resistant human immunodeficiency virus type 1 synergistically in vitro. J Infect Dis 1991; 164:646-55.

53. Boucher CAB, O'Sullivan E, Mulder JW, et al. Ordered appearance of zidovudine resistance mutations during treatment of 18 human immunodeficiency virus-positive subjects. J Infect Dis 1992; 165:105-10.

54. Larder BA, Darby G, Richman DD. HIV with reduced sensitivity to zidovudine (AZT) isolated during prolonged therapy. Science 1989; 243:1731-4.

55. Larder BA, Kemp SD. Multiple mutations in HIV-1 reverse transcriptase confer high-level resistance to zidovudine (AZT). Science 1989; 246:1155-8.

56. Rooke R, Tremblay M, Soudeyns H, et al. Isolation of drug-resistant variants of HIV-1 from patients on long-term zidovudine therapy. AIDS 1989; 3: 411-5.

57. Richman DD, Grimes JM, Lagakos SW. Effect of stage of disease and drug dose on zidovudine susceptibilities of isolates of human immunodeficiency virus. J AIDS 1990; 3:743-6.

58. Larder BA, Chesebro B, Richman DD. Susceptibilities of zidovudine-susceptible and -resistant human immunodeficiency virus isolates to antiviral agents determined by using a quantitative plaque reduction assay. Antimicrob Agents Chemother 1990; 34:436-41.

59. Land S, Treloar T, McPhee D, et al. Decreased in vitro susceptibility to zidovudine of HIV isolates obtained from patients with AIDS. J Infect Dis 1990; 161:326-9.

60. Boucher CAB, Tersmette M, Lange JMA, et al. Zidovudine sensitivity of human immunodeficiency viruses from high-risk, symptom-free individuals during therapy. Lancet 1990; 336:585-90.

61. Richman DD. Susceptibility to nucleoside analogues of zidovudine-resistant isolates of human immunodeficiency virus. Am J Med 1990; 88(Suppl 5B): 8S-10S.

62. Lopéz-Galíndez C, Rojas JM, Nájera R, et al. Characterization of genetic variation and 3′-azido-3′-deoxythymidine-resistance mutations of human immunodeficiency virus by the RNAse A mismatch cleavage method. Proc Natl Acad Sci USA 1991; 88:4280-4.

63. Larder BA, Kellman P, Kemp SD. Zidovudine resistance predicted by direct detection of mutations in DNA from HIV-infected lymphocytes. AIDS 1991; 5:137-44.

64. Mayers D*, McCutchan FE, Sanders-Buell E, et al. Molecular characterization of HIV-1 variants arising after prolonged zidovudine (AZT) therapy. J AIDS 1991; 4:343.

65. Boucher C, Larder B, Tijnagel J, et al. Proviruses with mutation causing zidovudine resistance can persist after discontinuation of therapy. J AIDS 1991; 4:346.

66. D'Aquila RT, Videler JA, Bechtel LB, et al. Specific PCR detection and DNA sequence analysis of the AZT-resistant RT genotype of HIV-1. J AIDS 1991; 4:346-7.

67. D'Aquila RT, Videler JA, Eron J, et al. Plasma and PBMC derived HIV-1 isolates differ in RT genotype and AZT susceptibility. Seventh International Conference on AIDS, Florence, Italy, 1991; Abstract W.B. 2084.

68. Fitzgibbon JE, Howell RM, Schwartzer TA, et al. In vivo prevalence of azidothymidine (AZT) resistance mutations in an AIDS patient before and after AZT therapy. AIDS Res Hum Retro 1991; 7:265-9.

69. Larder BA, Coates KE, Kemp SD. Zidovudine-resistant human immunodeficiency virus selected by passage in cell culture. J Virol 1991; 65:5232-6.

70. Gao Q, Gu Z, Parniak MA, et al. In vitro selection of variants of human immunodeficiency virus type 1 resistant to 3′-azido-3′-deoxythymidine and 2′, 3′-dideoxyinosine. J Virol 1992; 66:12-9.

71. Mitsuya H, Broder S. Inhibition of the in vitro infectivity and cytopathic effect of human T-lymphotrophic virus type III/lymphadenopathy-associated

virus (HTLV-III/LAV) by 2′,3′-dideoxynucleosides. Proc Natl Acad Sci USA 1986; 83:1911-5.

72. Yarchoan R, Mitsuya H, Thomas RV, et al. In vivo activity against HIV and favorable toxicity profile of 2′,3′-dideoxyinosine. Science 1989; 245:412-5.

73. Molina JM, Groopman JE. Bone marrow toxicity of dideoxyinosine. N Engl J Med 1989; 321:1478.

74. LeLacheur SF, Simon GL. Exacerbation of dideoxycytidine-induced neuropathy with dideoxyinosine. J AIDS 1991; 4:538-9.

75. Lambert JS, Seidlin M, Reichman RC, et al. 2′,3′-Dideoxyinosine (ddI) in patients with the acquired immunodeficiency syndrome or AIDS-related complex. A phase I trial. N Engl J Med 1990; 322:1333-40.

76. Cooley TP, Kunches LM, Saunders CA, et al. Once-daily administration of 2′,3′-dideoxyinosine (ddI) in patients with the acquired immunodeficiency syndrome or AIDS-related complex. Results of a phase I trial. N Engl J Med 1990; 322:1340-5.

77. Yarchoan R, Mitsuya H, Pluda JM, et al. The National Cancer Institute phase I study of 2′,3′-dideoxyinosine administration in adults with AIDS or AIDS-related complex: analysis of activity and toxicity profiles. Rev Infect Dis 1990; 12:S522-33.

78. Valentine FT, Seidlin M, Hochster H, et al. Phase I study of 2′,3′-dideoxyinosine: experience with 19 patients at New York University Medical Center. Rev Infect Dis 1990; 12:S534-9.

79. Dolin R, Lambert JS, Morse GD, et al. 2′,3′-Dideoxyinosine in patients with AIDS or AIDS-related complex. Rev Infect Dis 1990; 12:S540-51.

80. Cooley TP, Kunches LM, Saunders CA, et al. Treatment of AIDS and AIDS-related complex with 2′,3′-dideoxyinosine given once daily. Rev Infect Dis 1990; 12:S552-60.

81. Pizzo PA. Considerations for the evaluation of antiretroviral agents in infants and children infected with human immunodeficiency virus: a perspective from the National Cancer Institute. Rev Infect Dis 1990; 12:S561-9.

82. Rozencweig M, McLaren C, Beltangady M, et al. Overview of phase I trials of 2′,3′-dideoxyinosine (ddI) conducted on adult patients. Rev Infect Dis 1990; 12:5570-5.

83. Yarchoan R, Pluda JM, Thomas RV, et al. Long-term toxicity/activity profile of 2′,3′-dideoxyinosine in AIDS or AIDS-related complex. Lancet 1990; 336:526-9.

84. Lai KK, Gang DL, Zawacki JK, et al. Fulminant hepatic failure associated with 2′,3′-dideoxyinosine (ddI). Ann Intern Med 1991; 115:283-4.

85. Butler KM, Husson RN, Balis FM, et al. Dideoxyinosine in children with symptomatic human immunodeficiency virus infection. N Engl J Med 1991; 324:137-44.

86. Connolly KJ, Allen JD, Fitch H, et al. Phase I study of 2'-3'-dideoxyinosine administered orally twice daily to patients with AIDS or AIDS-related complex and hematologic intolerance to zidovudine. Am J Med 1991; 91:471-8.

87. Dobkin JF. ddI Approved for HIV infection. Infections in Medicine 1991: 12.

88. Japour AJ, Chatis PA, Eigenrauch HA, et al. Detection of human immunodeficiency virus type 1 clinical isolates with reduced sensitivity to zidovudine and dideoxyinosine by RNA·RNA hydridization. Proc Natl Acad Sci USA 1991; 88:3092-6.

89. St. Clair MH, Martin JL, Tudor-Williams G, et al. Resistance to ddI and sensitivity to AZT induced by a mutation in HIV-1 reverse transcriptase. Science 1991; 253:1557-9.

90. Reichman R, Lambert J, Strussenberg J, et al. Decreased dideoxyinosine (ddI) sensitivity of HIV isolates obtained from long term recipients of ddI. Seventh International Conference on AIDS, Florence, Italy, 1991; Abstract TU.B. 92.

91. McLeod GX, McGrath JM, Connolly KJ, et al. Dideoxyinosine (DDI) and zidovudine (AZT) resistance patterns in clinical isolates of HIV-1. 31st Interscience Conference on Antimicrobial Agents and Chemotherapy, Chicago, IL, 1991; Abstract 1355.

92. Yarchoan R, Perno CF, Thomas RV, et al. Phase I studies of 2',3'-dideoxycytidine in severe human immunodeficiency virus infection as a single agent and alternating with zidovudine (AZT). Lancet 1988; 1:76-81.

93. Merigan TC, Skowron G, Bozzette SA, et al. Circulating p24 antigen levels and responses to dideoxycytidine in human immunodeficiency virus (HIV) infections: a phase I and II study. Ann Intern Med 1989; 110:189-94.

94. Fitzgibbon JE, Howell RM, Haberzettl CA, et al. Human immunodeficiency virus type 1 *pol* gene mutations which cause decreased susceptibility to 2',3'-dideoxycytidine. Antimicrob Agents Chemother 1992; 36:153-7.

95. Shirasaka T, Yarchoan R, Husson R, et al. HIV may develop resistance preferentially to azidothymidine (AZT) as compared to dideoxycytidine (ddC) and dideoxyinosine (ddI) in patients receiving antiviral therapy. Seventh International Conference on AIDS, Florence, Italy, 1991; Abstract W.A. 9.

96. Pauwels R, Andries K, Desmyter J, et al. Potent and selective inhibition of HIV-1 replication in vitro by a novel series of TIBO derivatives. Nature 1990; 343:470-4.

97. Debyser Z, Pauwels R, Andries K, et al. An antiviral target on reverse transcriptase of human immunodeficiency virus type 1 revealed by tetrahydroimidazo-[4,5,1-*jk*][1,4]benzodiazepin-2(1*H*)-one and -thione derivatives. Proc Natl Acad Sci USA 1991; 88:1451-5.

98. White EL, Buckheit RW, Ross LJ, et al. A TIBO derivative, R82913, is a potent inhibitor of HIV-1 reverse transcriptase with heteropolymer templates. Antiviral Res 1991; 16:257-66.

99. Merluzzi VJ, Hargrave KD, Labadia M, et al. Inhibition of HIV-1 replication by a nonnucleoside reverse transcriptase inhibitor. Science 1990; 250: 1411-3.

100. Richman D, Rosenthal AS, Skoog M, et al. BI-RG-587 is active against zidovudine-resistant human immunodeficiency virus type 1 and synergistic with zidovudine. Antimicrob Agents Chemother 1991; 35:305-8.

101. Koup RA, Merluzzi VJ, Hargrave KD, et al. Inhibition of human immunodeficiency virus type 1 (HIV-1) replication by the dipyridodiazepinone BI-RG-587. J Infect Dis 1991; 163:966-70.

102. Shih CK, Rose JM, Hansen GL, et al. Chimeric human immunodeficiency virus type 1/type 2 reverse transcriptases display reverse sensitivity to nonnucleoside analog inhibitors. Proc Natl Acad Sci USA 1991; 88:9878-82.

103. Goldman ME, Nunberg JH, O'Brien JA, et al. Pyridinone derivatives: specific human immunodeficiency virus type 1 reverse transcriptase inhibitors with antiviral activity. Proc Natl Acad Sci USA 1991; 88:6863-7.

104. Davey R, Laskin O, Decker M, et al. L-697,639 and L-697,661, novel agents for treatment of HIV-1 infection. 31st Interscience Conference on Antimicrobial Agents and Chemotherapy, Chicago, IL, 1991; Abstract 697.

105. Laskin OL, Dupont AG, Buntinx A, et al. Human pharmacokinetics and tolerability of L-697,661 and L-697,639; non-nucleoside HIV-1 reverse transcriptase inhibitors. 31st Interscience Conference on Antimicrobial Agents and Chemotherapy; September 29 - October 2, 1991, Chicago; Abstract 698.

106. Nunberg JH, Schleif WA, Boots EJ, et al. Viral resistance to human immunodeficiency virus type 1-specific pyridinone reverse transcriptase inhibitors. J Virol 1991; 65:4887-92.

107. Romero DL, Busso M, Tan C-K, et al. Nonnucleoside reverse transcriptase inhibitors that potently and specifically block human immunodeficiency virus type 1 replication. Proc Natl Acad Sci USA 1991; 88:8806-10.

108. Dueweke TJ, Kezdy FJ, Waszak GA, et al. The binding of a novel bisheteroarylpiperazine mediates inhibition of human immunodeficiency virus type 1 reverse transcriptase. J Biol Chem 1992 (in press).

109. Hsu MC, Schutt AD, Holly M, et al. Inhibition of HIV replication in acute and chronic infections in vitro by a Tat antagonist. Science 1991; 254:1799-802.

110. Seelmeier S, Schmidt H, Turk V, von der Helm K. Human immunodeficiency virus has an aspartic-type protease that can be inhibited by pepstatin A. Proc Natl Acad Sci USA 1988; 85:6612-6.

111. Dreyer GB, Metcalf BW, Tomaszek TA, et al. Inhibition of human immunodeficiency virus 1 protease in vitro: rational design of substrate analogue inhibitors. Proc Natl Acad Sci USA 1989; 86:9752-6.

112. Meek TD, Lambert DM, Dreyer GB, et al. Inhibition of HIV-1 protease in infected T-lymphocytes by synthetic peptide analogues. Nature 1990; 343: 90-2.

113. McQuade TJ, Tomasselli AG, Liu L, et al. A synthetic HIV-1 protease inhibitor with antiviral activity arrests HIV-like particle maturation. Science 1990; 247:454-6.

114. Roberts NA, Martin JA, Kinchington D, et al. Rational design of peptide-based HIV proteinase inhibitors. Science 1990; 248:358-61.

115. DesJarlais RL, Seibel GL, Kuntz ID, et al. Structure-based design of nonpeptide inhibitors specific for the human immunodeficiency virus 1 protease. Proc Natl Acad Sci USA 1990; 87:6644-8.

116. Ashorn P, McQuade TJ, Thaisrivongs S, et al. An inhibitor of the protease blocks maturation of human and simian immunodeficiency viruses and spread of infection. Proc Natl Acad Sci USA 1990; 87:7472-6.

117. Swain AL, Miller MM, Green J, et al. X-ray crystallographic structure of a complex between a synthetic protease of human immunodeficiency virus 1 and a substrate-based hydroxyethylamine inhibitor. Proc Natl Acad Sci USA 1990; 87:8805-9.

118. Sham HL, Betebenner DA, Wideburg NE, et al. Potent HIV-1 protease inhibitors with antiviral activities in vitro. Biochem Biophys Res Commun 1991; 175:914-9.

119. Craig JC, Duncan IB, Hockley D, et al. Antiviral properties of Ro 31-8959, an inhibitor of human immunodeficiency virus (HIV) proteinase. Antiviral Res 1991; 16:295-305.

120. Kempf DJ, Marsh KC, Paul DA, et al. Antiviral and pharmacokinetic properties of C_2 symmetric inhibitors of the human immunodeficiency virus type 1 protease. Antimicrob Agents Chemother 1991; 35:2209-14.

121. Moellering RC. Principles of anti-infective therapy. In: Mandell GL, Douglas RG, Bennett JE, eds. Principles and practice of infectious diseases. 3rd ed. New York: Churchill Livingstone Inc, 1990:212-3.

122. Chou T-C, Talalay P. Applications of the median-effect principle for the assessment of low-dose risk of carcinogens and for the quantitation of synergism and antagonism of chemotherapeutic agents. In: Harrap KR, Connors TA, eds. New avenues in developmental cancer chemotherapy. Bristol-Myers Cancer Symposia Series. Orlando, FL: Academic Press, 1987:37-64.

123. Chou T-C, Talalay P. Quantitative analysis of dose-effect relationships: the combined effects of multiple drugs or enzyme inhibitors. Adv Enzyme Regul 1984; 22:27-55.

124. Chou J, Chou T-C. Dose-effect analysis with microcomputers: quantitation of ED_{50}, LD_{50}, synergism, antagonism, low-dose risk, receptor-ligand binding and enzyme kinetics. In: A computer software for IBM-PC and

manual. Cambridge, UK: Elsevier-Biosoft, 1987.

125. Greco WR, Park HS, Rustum YM. Application of a new approach for the quantitation of drug synergism to the combination of *cis*-diamminedichloroplatinum and 1- -D-arabinofuranosylcytosine. Cancer Res 1990; 50:5318-27.

126. Prichard MN, Shipman C Jr. MacSynergy. A three-dimensional model to analyze drug-drug interactions. Antiviral Res 1990; 14:181-206.

127. Bunow B, Weinstein JN. Combo: a new approach to the analysis of drug combinations in vitro. Vol. 616. New York: Annals of the New York Academy of Sciences, 1990:490-4.

128. Weinstein JN, Bunow B, Weislow OS, et al. Synergistic drug combinations in AIDS therapy: Dipyridamole/3'-azido-3'-deoxythymidine in particular and principles of analysis in general. Vol. 616. New York: Annals of the New York Academy of Sciences, 1990:367-84.

129. Hartshorn KL, Sandstrom EG, Neumeyer D, et al. Synergistic inhibition of human T-cell lymphotropic virus type III replication in vitro by phosphonoformate and recombinant alpha-A interferon. Antimicrob Agents Chemother 1986; 30:189-91.

130. Hartshorn KL, Vogt MW, Chou T-C, et al. Synergistic inhibition of human immunodeficiency virus in vitro by azidothymidine and recombinant alpha A interferon. Antimicro Agents Chemother 1987; 31:168-72.

131. Vogt MW, Hartshorn KL, Furman PA, et al. Ribavirin antagonizes the effect of azidothymidine on HIV replication. Science 1987; 235:1376-9.

132. Vogt MW, Durno AG, Chou T-C, et al. Synergistic interaction of 2',3'-dideoxycytidine and recombinant interferon-α-A on replication of human immunodeficiency virus type 1. J Infect Dis 1988; 158:378-85.

133. Johnson VA, Walker BD, Barlow MA, et al. Synergistic inhibition of human immunodeficiency virus type 1 and type 2 replication in vitro by castanospermine and 3'-azido-3'-deoxythymidine. Antimicrob Agents Chemother 1989; 33:53-7.

134. Johnson VA, Barlow MA, Chou T-C, et al. Synergistic inhibition of human immunodeficiency virus type 1 (HIV-1) replication in vitro by recombinant soluble CD4 and 3'-azido-3'-deoxythymidine. J Infect Dis 1989; 159:837-44.

135. Johnson VA, Merrill DP, Chou T-C, et al. Synergistic inhibition of HIV-1 replication by N-butyl-deoxynojirimycin (N-butyl-DNJ) and zidovudine (AZT). Twenty-ninth Interscience Conference on Antimicrobial Agents and Chemotherapy, Houston, Texas, 1989; Abstract 504.

136. Johnson VA, Barlow MA, Merrill DP, et al. Three-drug synergistic inhibition of HIV-1 replication in vitro by zidovudine, recombinant soluble CD4, and recombinant interferon-alpha A. J Infect Dis 1990; 161:1059-67.

137. Johnson VA, Merrill DP, Chou T-C, et al. HIV-1 inhibitory interactions between 2',3'-dideoxyinosine (ddI) and either zidovudine (AZT), recombi-

nant soluble CD4 (rsCD4), or recombinant interferon-alpha-A. Sixth International Conference on AIDS, San Francisco, California, 1990; Abstract F.A. 66.

138. Eron JJ, Hirsch MS, Merrill DP, et al. Synergistic inhibition of HIV-1 by the combination of zidovudine (AZT) and 2′,3′-dideoxycytidine (ddC) in vitro. Seventh International Conference on AIDS, Florence, Italy, 1991; Abstract W.B. 2110.

139. Eron JJ, Johnson VA, Merrill DP, et al. Synergistic inhibition of replication of HIV-1, including a zidovudine resistant isolate, by the combination of zidovudine and 2′,3′-dideoxycytidine (ddC) in vitro (submitted).

140. Johnson VA, Merrill DP, Chou TC, et al. Human immunodeficiency virus type 1 (HIV-1) inhibitory interactions between HIV-1 protease inhibitor (Ro 31-8959, Compound XVII) and either zidovudine (AZT), 2′,3′-dideoxycytidine (ddC) or recombinant interferon-alpha-A (rIFN-α-A) using either AZT-sensitive or AZT-resistant HIV-1 in vitro. Fourth Conference of the NIH National Cooperative Drug Discovery Groups for the Treatment of HIV Infection, San Diego, California, November 3-7, 1991; Abstract 38.

141. Mitsuya H, Broder S. Strategies for antiviral therapy in AIDS. Nature 1987; 325:773-8.

142. Yarchoan R, Mitsuya H, Myers CE, et al. Clinical pharmacology of 3′-azido-2′,3′-dideoxythymidine (zidovudine) and related dideoxynucleosides. N Engl J Med 1989; 321:726-38.

143. Hammer SM, Gillis JM. Synergistic activity of granulocyte-macrophage colony-stimulating factor and 3′-azido-3′-deoxythymidine against human immunodeficiency virus in vitro. Antimicrob Agents Chemother 1987; 31:1046-50.

144. Perno C-F, Yarchoan R, Cooney DA, et al. Replication of human immunodeficiency virus in monocytes. Granulocyte/macrophage colony-stimulating factor (GM-CSF) potentiates viral production yet enhances the antiviral effect mediated by 3′-azido-2′3′-dideoxythymidine (AZT) and other dideoxynucleoside congeners of thymidine. J Exp Med 1989; 169:933-51.

145. Ueno R, Kuno S. Dextran sulphate, a potent anti-HIV agent in vitro having synergism with zidovudine. Lancet 1987; 1:1379.

146. Ueno R, Kuno S. Anti-HIV synergism between dextran sulphate and zidovudine. Lancet 1987; 2:796-7.

147. Mitsuya H, Looney DJ, Kuno S, et al. Dextran sulfate suppression of viruses in the HIV family: inhibition of virion binding to CD4 + cells. Science 1988; 240:646-9.

148. Mitchell WM, Montefiori DC, Robinson WE. Mismatched double-stranded RNA (ampligen) reduces concentration of zidovudine (azidothymidine) re-

quired for in-vitro inhibition of human immunodeficiency virus. Lancet 1987; 1:890-2.

149. Pontani D, Sun D, Brown J, et al. Synergistic activity of amphotericin B methyl ester and azidothymidine. Fourth International Conference on AIDS, Stockholm, Sweden, 1988; Abstract 3128.

150. Szebeni J, Wahl SM, Popovic M, et al. Dipyridamole potentiates the inhibition by 3'-azido-3'-deoxythymidine and other dideoxynucleosides of human immunodeficiency virus replication in monocyte-macrophages. Proc Natl Acad Sci USA 1989; 86:3842-6.

151. Baba M, Pauwels R, Balzarini J, et al. Ribavirin antagonizes inhibitory effects of pyrimidine 2'-3'-dideoxynucleosides but enhances inhibitory effects of purine 2',3'-dideoxynucleosides on replication of human immunodeficiency virus in vitro. Antimicrob Agents Chemother 1987; 31:1613-7.

152. Shannon WM, Lavelle GC, Qualls KJ, Hua M, et al. Enhancement of the antiviral efficacy of a new purine nucleoside analog (NSC-614846) against human immunodeficiency virus (HIV) by combination with ribavarin or with other anti-HIV compounds in vitro. Fourth International Conference on AIDS, Stockholm, Sweden, 1988; Abstract 3019.

153. Smith MS, Brain EL, De Clercq E, et al. Susceptibility of human immunodeficiency virus type 1 replication in vitro to acyclic adenosine analogs and synergy of the analogs with 3'-azido-3'-deoxythymidine. Antimicrob Agents Chemother 1989; 33:1482-6.

154. Eriksson BFH, Schinazi RF. Combinations of 3'-azido-3'-deoxythymidine (zidovudine) and phosphonoformate (foscarnet) against human immunodeficiency virus type 1 and cytomegalovirus replication in vitro. Antimicrob Agents Chemother 1989; 33:663-9.

155. Koshida R, Vrang L, Gilljam G, Harmenberg J, et al. Inhibition of human immunodeficiency virus in vitro by combinations of 3'-azido-3'-deoxythymidine and foscarnet. Antimicrob Agents Chemother 1989; 33:778-80.

156. Carron WC, Colby CB, Ho DD. Anti-HIV activity of beta-interferon in combination with zidovudine. Fourth International Conference on AIDS, Stockholm, Sweden, 1988; Abstract 3633.

157. Schinazi RF, Cannon DL, Arnold BH, et al. Combinations of isoprinosine and 3'-azido-3'-deoxythymidine in lymphocytes infected with human immunodeficiency virus type 1. Antimicrob Agents Chemother 1988; 32:1784-7.

158. Spector SA, Ripley D, Hsia K. Human immunodeficiency virus inhibition is prolonged by 3'-azido-3'-deoxythymidine alternating with 2',3'-dideoxycytidine compared with 3'-azido-3'-deoxythymidine alone. Antimicrob Agents Chemother 1989; 33:920-3.

159. Balzarini J, Lee CK, Schols D, et al. 1-beta-D-ribofuranosyl-1,2,4-triazole-3-carboxamide (ribavirin) and 5-ethynyl-1-beta-D-ribofuranosylimidazole-4-carboxamide (EICAR) markedly potentiate the inhibitory effect of 2',3'-

dideoxyinosine on human immunodeficiency virus in peripheral blood lymphocytes. Biochem Biophys Res Commun 1991; 178:563-9.

160. Balzarini J, Naesens L, Robins MJ, et al. Potentiating effect of ribavirin on the in vitro and in vivo antiretrovirus activities of 2′,3′-dideoxyinosine and 2′,3′-dideoxy-2,6-diaminopurine riboside. J AIDS 1990; 3:1140-7.

161. Hayashi S, Fine RL, Chou T-C, et al. In vitro inhibition of the infectivity and replication of human immunodeficiency virus type 1 by combination of antiretroviral 2′,3′-dideoxynucleosides and virus-binding inhibitors. Antimicrob Agents Chemother 1990; 34:82-8.

162. Anand R, Nayyar S, Pitha J, et al. Sulphated sugar alpha-cyclodextrin sulphate, a uniquely potent anti-HIV agent, also exhibits marked synergism with AZT, and lymphoproliferative activity. Antiviral Chemistry Chemother 1990; 1:41-6.

163. Anand R, Nayyar S, Galvin TA, et al. Sodium pentosan polysulfate (PPS), an anti-HIV agent also exhibits synergism with AZT, lymphoproliferative activity, and virus enhancement. AIDS Res Hum Retro 1990; 6:679-89.

164. Perno CF, Cooney DA, Currens MJ, et al. Ability of anti-HIV agents to inhibit HIV replication in monocyte/macrophages or U937 monocytoid cells under conditions of enhancement by GM-CSF or anti-HIV antibody. AIDS Res Hum Retro 1990; 6:1051-5.

165. Harmenberg J, Akesson-Johansson A, Vrang L, et al. Synergistic inhibition of human immunodeficiency virus replication in vitro by combinations of 3′-azido-3′-deoxythymidine and 3′-fluoro-3′-deoxythymidine. AIDS Res Hum Retro 1990; 6:1197-1202.

166. Chou T-C, Zhu Q-Y, Stein CA. Differential alteration of the anti-HIV-1 effect of phosphorothioate oligonucleotide S-dC28 by AZT, interferon-alpha, and dextran sulfate. AIDS Res Hum Retro 1991; 7:943-51.

167. Ito M, Baba M, Shigeta S, et al. Synergistic inhibition of human immunodeficiency virus type 1 (HIV-1) replication in vitro by 1-[(2-hydroxyethoxy) methyl]-6-phenylthiothymine (HEPT) and recombinant alpha interferon. Antiviral Res 1991; 15:323-30.

168. Hartman NR, Ahluwalia GS, Cooney DA, et al. Inhibitors of IMP dehydrogenase stimulate the phosphorylation of the anti-human immunodeficiency virus nucleosides 2′,3′-dideoxyadenosine and 2′,3′-dideoxyinosine. Mol Pharmacol 1991; 40:118-124.

169. Dornsife RE, St. Clair MH, Huang AT, et al. Anti-human immunodeficiency virus synergism by zidovudine (3′-azidothymidine) and didanosine (dideoxyinosine) contrasts with their additive inhibition of normal human marrow progenitor cells. Antimicrob Agents Chemother 1991; 35:322-8.

170. Baba M, Ito M, Shigeta S, et al. Synergistic inhibition of human immunodeficiency virus type 1 replication by 5-ethyl-1-ethoxymethyl-6-(phenylthio)

uracil (E-EPU) and azidothymidine in vitro. Antimicrob Agents Chemother 1991; 35:1430-3.

171. Nunberg JH, Quintero JC, Schleif WA, et al. HIV-1 specific pyridinone reverse transcriptase inhibitors: 111. Synergism in the combined in vitro use with nucleoside analogs. Seventh International Conference on AIDS, Florence, Italy, 1991; Abstract W.A. 1012.

172. Kageyama S, Erickson J, Weinstein J, et al. In vitro inhibtion of HIV-1 replication by C_2 symmetric HIV protease inhibitors as single agents or in combinations with azidothymidine (AZT) or dideoxyinosine (ddI). Seventh International Conference on AIDS, Florence, Italy, 1991; abstract W.A. 1054.

173. Schoenfeld DA. Issues in the testing of drug combinations. J AIDS 1990; 3:S104-7.

174. Groopman JE. Antiretroviral therapy of immunomodulators in patients with AIDS. Am J Med 1991; 90(suppl 4A):18S-21S.

175. Fischl MA, Galpin JE, Levine JC, et al. Recombinant human erythropoietin for patients with AIDS treated with zidovudine. N Engl J Med 1990; 322:1488-93.

176. Pluda JM, Yarchoan R, Smith PD, et al. Subcutaneous recombinant granulocyte-macrophage colony-stimulating factor used as a single agent and in an alternating regimen with azidothymidine in leukopcnic patients with severe human immunodeficiency virus infection. Blood 1990; 76:463-72.

177. Miles SA, Mitsuyasu RT, Moreno J, et al. Combined therapy with recombinant granulocyte colony-stimulating factor and erythropoletin decreases hematologic toxicity from zidovudine. Blood 1991; 77:2109-17.

178. Schwartz DH, Skowron G, Merigan TC. Safety and effects of interleukin-2 plus zidovudine in asymptomatic individuals infected with human immunodeficiency virus. J AIDS 1991; 4:11-23.

179. Kovacs JA, Deyton L, Davey R, et al. Combined zidovudine and interferon-α therapy in patients with Kaposi sarcoma and the acquired immunodeficiency syndrome (AIDS). Ann Intern Med 1989; 111:280-7.

180. Orholm M, Pedersen C, Mathiesen L, et al. Suppression of p24 antigen in sera from HIV-infected individuals with low-dose α-interferon and zidovudine: a pilot study. AIDS 1989; 3:97-100.

181. Krown SE, Gold JWM, Niedzwiecki D, et al. Interferon-α with zidovudine: safety, tolerance, and clinical and virological effects in patients with Kaposi sarcoma associated with the acquired immunodeficiency syndrome (AIDS). Ann Intern Med 1990; 112:812-21.

182. Mildvan D, Ruprecht R, Krown S, et al. Application of the combination index method in the design of a clinical antiretroviral trial: ACTG 068. J AIDS 1990; 3:S111-3.

183. Fischl MA. Antiretroviral therapy in combination with interferon for AIDS-

related Kaposi's sarcoma. Am J Med 1991; 90(suppl 4A):2S-7S.

184. Fischl MA, Uttamchandani RB, Resnick L, et al. A phase 1 study of recombinant human interferon-$_{2a}$ or human lymphoblastoid interferon-α_{n1} and concomitant zidovudine in patients with AIDS-related Kaposi's sarcoma. J AIDS 1991; 4:1-10.

185. Berglund O, Engman K, Ehrnst A, et al. Combined treatment of symptomatic human immunodeficiency virus type 1 infection with native interferon-α and zidovudine. J Infect Dis 1991; 163:710-5.

186. Zeidner NS, Myles MH, Mathiason-DuBard CK, et al. Alpha interferon (2b) in combination with zidovudine for the treatment of presymptomatic feline leukemia virus-induced immunodeficiency syndrome. Antimicrob Agents Chemother 1990; 34:1749-56.

187. Hom RC, Finberg RW, Mullaney S, et al. Protective cellular retroviral immunity requires both CD4 + and CD8 + immune T cells. J Virol 1991; 65:220-4.

188. Ruprecht RM, Mullaney S, Bernard LD, et al. Vaccination with a live retrovirus: the nature of the protective immune response. Proc Natl Acad Sci 1990; 87:5558-62.

189. Ruprecht RM, Chou T-C, Chipty F, et al. Interferon- and 3'-azido-3'-deoxythymidine are highly synergistic in mice and prevent viremia after acute retrovirus exposure. J AIDS 1990; 3:591-600.

190. Ruprecht RM, Gama-Sosa MA, Rosas HD. Combination therapy after retroviral inoculation. Lancet 1988; i:239-40.

191. Davey RT, Davey VJ, Metcalf JA, et al. A phase I/II trial of zidovudine, interferon- , and granulocyte-macrophage colony-stimulating factor in the treatment of human immunodeficiency virus type 1 infection. J Infect Dis 1991; 164:43-52.

192. Scadden DT, Bering HA, Levine JD, et al. GM-CSF as an alternative to dose modification of the combination zidovudine and interferon-alpha in the treatment of AIDS-associated Kaposi's sarcoma. Am J Clin Oncol 1991; 14(suppl 1):S40-4.

193. Collier AC, Fischl MA, Kaplan LD, et al. Effect of combination therapy with zidovudine (ZDV) and didanosine (ddI) on surrogate markers. Seventh International Conference on AIDS, Florence, Italy, 1991; Abstract TU.B. 2.

194. Husson R, Tishler D, Kovacs A, et al. A phase I study of zidovudine (AZT) and dideoxyinosine (ddI) in children with HIV infection. 31st Interscience Conference on Antimicrobial Agents and Chemotherapy, Chicago, IL, 1991; Abstract 474.

195. Jacobson MA, van der Horst C, Causey DM, et al. In vivo additive antiretroviral effect of combined zidovudine and foscarnet therapy for human immunodeficiency virus infection (ACTG protocol 053). J Infect Dis 1991; 163:1219-22.

Toxoplasmic Encephalitis

Peter R. Mariuz and Benjamin J. Luft
State University of New York at Stony Brook,
Stony Brook, New York

I. INTRODUCTION

Toxoplasmosis is a ubiquitous protozoal infection found throughout the world. In the immunocompetent host, upon acquisition of the infection, most individuals remain asymptomatic or develop mild localized lymphadenopathy (1,2). There have been relatively few cases reported of severe disease due to toxoplasma in the immunocompetent patient (3); however, toxoplasmosis is a significant opportunistic infection in the severely immunocompromised host, usually occurring as a result of a recrudescence of a latent infection (3). With the advent of the acquired immunodeficiency syndrome (AIDS) due to infection with either HIV-1 or HIV-2, toxoplasmic encephalitis has become recognized as the most prominent cause of encaphalitis and focal intracerebral lesions in this patient population (4–9). In order to appreciate the diagnostic and therapeutic challenges posed by toxoplasma in the AIDS patient, it is essential to have an appreciation of the biology of the organism and the host-parasite immunological interaction.

II. EPIDEMIOLOGY

Toxoplasma gondii is found throughout the world. The organism infects all mammals and some birds and it usually acquired by eating foods contaminated with the oocyst or meat from animals previously infected with *T. gondii*. Raw milk, in particular goats milk, has also been implicated as a source for infection (10). Knowing the epidemiological pattern of acquisition of infection, it is not surprising that common source outbreaks within families (11) and groups eating together (12–14) are common. The prevalence of infection is generally higher in warm, humid climates. In the United States, between 10 and 60% of adults are seropositive for toxoplasma depending on the geographical location (15). In France 80% of adults are seropositive for toxoplasma (15). This geographical difference in the seroprevalence of toxoplasma infection may also reflect a difference in culinary habits. The incidence of toxoplasmic encephalitis, which results from a recrudescence of latent infection, is directly related to the seroprevalence rate in a given risk group. Thus, depending on the risk associated with the development of AIDS and geographical variations in the seroprevalence of toxoplasmic infections, toxoplasmic encephalitis has been reported in 5–40% of patients with AIDS (9,16–24). In the United States, toxoplasmic encephalitis appears to occur most frequently in Florida, in both Haitian and nonHaitian patients (23). There is a suggestion that toxoplasmic encephalitis may occur more frequently in intravenous drug abusers (24). It has been calculated that approximately 30% of AIDS patients who are seropositive for toxoplasma will ultimately develop toxoplasmic encephalitis (22). In a recent study from Austria, 47.4% of seropositive patients developed toxoplasmic encephalitis (25).

Therefore, it is no surprise that in areas of the world where the seroprevalence of toxoplasma is high (e.g., France, equatorial Africa, Haiti) the incidence of toxoplasmic encephalitis is also high. In the review of clinical experience of neurological disease in AIDS patients, it has been shown that toxoplasma accounts for approximately 40% of known central nervous system infections and one third of intracerebral lesions (26–30). It has been estimated that in the United States toxoplasmic encephalitis may eventually afflict between 10 and 20% of AIDS patients, thereby causing severe disease in 20,000–40,000 AIDS patients by 1991 (4). These studies emphasize the pervasiveness of toxoplasma infection as a significant cause of morbidity and mortality in AIDS patients.

III. PATHOGENESIS

In order to understand the pathogenesis, the clinical manifestations, the response to therapy, and the prevention of toxoplasmic encephalitis, it is important to appreciate the life cycle of this organism (31). The cat is the definitive host for toxoplasma. In the cat the organism undergoes its complete life cycle including both an enteroepithelial cycle and extraintestinal cycle. After the cat becomes infected with the organism by ingesting food which contains toxoplasma (the cyst or oocyst form), the organism is released and invades the epithelial cells of the small intestine. Within the intestinal lumen, *T. gondii* undergoes sequential stages of development and multiplication, resulting in the formation of the oocyst. Millions of oocysts are excreted in the stool approximately 3-24 days after infection. In the environment the oocyst undergoes sporogony resulting in the formation of the infectious oocysts. Under favorable conditions such as warm climate and moist soil, the oocyst may remain infectious for as long as a year.

In all infected mammals, including cats, ingestion of food contaminated with viable toxoplasma results in an extraintestinal form of infection. After ingestion of food containing the organism, the tachyzoite form can be found in the lamina propria, mesenteric nodes, and distant organs. The tachyzoite is an obligate intracellular parasite that can infect every cell and can be found in every tissue or organ. The tachyzoites proliferate within vacuoles in the host cell until 8–16 organisms accumulate, at which time the cell lyses. Tachyzoites may also form pseudocysts, which are present in host cells for prolonged periods of time without forming a true tissue cyst.

The tissue cyst varies in size and may contain up to 3,000 bradyzoites. The cyst is characteristic of chronic infection. It is most commonly found in the heart, striated muscle, and brain. However, any organ can be chronically infected. The mechanism involved in the transformation of actively dividing tachyzoites to the cyst form of infection has not been delineated. The wall of the mature tissue cyst is believed to represent a combination of host and parasitic components (32). Although the cyst form of the organism is the predominant form during chronic infection, there is evidence from animal experimentation to suggest that the cyst periodically ruptures, releasing the organism, which then goes on to develop daughter cysts (33, 34). These recurrent episodes of subclinical active infection may be responsible for the lifelong persistence of antibodies and cell-mediated immunity to toxoplasma. Furthermore the spontaneous rupture of the cyst may be the initial event in the development of encephalitis in patients whose immune system has been so compromised so as not to be able to contain the infectious process. In the patient with AIDS and toxoplasmic encephalitis, the tachyzoite is the form of the organism responsible for the destructive, necrotizing process (31). However, even within these lesions the tissue cyst can be found. The tissue cyst is associated with transmission because it persists in tissues of chronically infected animals, which may be ingested by carnivores, including humans. Undercooked meat has been implicated as the source of several outbreaks of toxoplasmosis. In particular, meats such as mutton and pork are commonly contaminated with toxoplasma.

The pathological findings found in toxoplasmic encephalitis and AIDS are consistent with the hypothesis that the encephalitis results from the local recrudescence of a latent infection. Although widely diffuse necrotizing encephalitis has been reported (35), focal areas of encephalitis separated by normal brain tissue is far more common. The histopathological appearance of the focal encephalitis also suggests that the primary event is the recrudescence of infection from a single or group of closely related cysts. Post et al. (36) noted the lesions to have three distinct zones. The central zone contains necrotic amorphous material and few if any identifiable organisms. In the intermediate zone there is spotty necrosis and numerous extracellular and intracellular tachyzoites, and in the outer zone, necrosis was rare and the cyst form of the organism is most prominent. The cellular infiltrate consists of acute and chronic inflammatory cells, reactive astrocytes, macrophages, and a mixture of B and T lymphocytes (32). Prominent vascular proliferation, endothelial hyperplasia, and frank vasculitis may be present, resulting in further necrosis due to infarction (27,37–38). Acute infection can also occur. Partisani et al. (39) reported a 5.5% seroconversion rate in 72 HIV-infected patients followed prospectively for a median of 28 months.

IV. CLINICAL MANIFESTATIONS

Although *T. gondii* can infect all cells and organ systems, the predominant manifestation of infection in the immunocompromised host is encephalitis. The clinical symptoms at time of presentation can vary between focal and nonfocal symptoms of central nervous system dysfunction (3). Systemic symptoms of infection such as fever and malaise are variable, although patients can have a diffuse encephalitic process that can be rapidly fatal (35). In general, patients who present with nonfocal abnormalities usually develop signs of focal neurological disease as the infection progresses. The focal neurological abnormalities that develop are a function of the multifocal nature of this necrotizing encephalitis as well as the association of edema, vasculitis, and hemorrhage (36–38), which occur concomitantly with active infection. The clinical presentation varies between an insidious process evolving over weeks to an acute confusional state with or without focal neurological deficits. Focal abnormalities include hemiparesis, hemiplegia, hemisensory loss, cerebellar tremor, visual field defects, cranial nerve palsies, aphasia, severe localized headache, and focal seizures. The focal neurological problems may at first be subtle and transient, and with time evolve to persistent focal neurological deficits (40). Nonfocal symptoms and signs of neurological dysfunction can predominate and include weakness, disorientation, frank psychosis, lethargy, confusion, or coma. There may be difficulty differentiating cerebral toxoplasmosis from herpes encephalitis (41). Panhypopituitarism (42) and hyponatremia resulting from inappropriate antidiuretic hormone secretion (21) can complicate the neurological symptoms. Patients with global cognitive impairment associated with attention deficits, impaired recent memory, and slowness of global and motor responses may be haid to differentiate from the AIDS-related dementia syndrome. Furthermore, after successful treatment for toxoplasmosis, patients may continue to have generalized cognitive impairment, which progressively deteriorates. In these cases there has been a failure to identify *T. gondii* after repeat brain biopsy. This pattern of neurological dysfunction may occur in the majority of patients witrh AIDS and toxoplasmic encephalitis, and it is not clear whether this is a result of the acute encephalitis.

Recently a diffuse encephalitis has been described (35), manifested by rapidly progressive fatal global cerebral dysfunction without focal neurological deficits. Focal lesions are absent on neuroradiographic studies. Macroscopically the brain was normal in 3 of 4 cases (35), while numerous microglial nodules mainly involving the grey matter, most with central toxoplasma cysts or free tachyzoites, were noted upon microscopic examination. This appears to be a form of toxoplasmic encephalitis unique to AIDS patients (35).

An autopsy study of 55 cases of cerebral toxoplasmosis revealed diffuse toxoplasmic encephalitis without focal lesions as the sole manifestation in 7 patients (43). CT scans are frequently unremarkable, underestimating the true incidence of this infection (44). Toxoplasmic myelitis has been described involving the cervical spine in a patient presenting with weakness and numbness of the left arm (45). Corpus medullaris syndrome has also been described.

Although *T. gondii* can infect any cell in the brain, specific focal neurological symptoms vary depending on the area of brain affected. There is a tendency for *T. gondii* to cause localized disease in the brain stem, basal ganglia, the pituitary, and the white matter-cortex junction (30,36,47). With brain stem involvement, neurological symptoms such as ataxia, cranial palsies (48), and dysmetria are not uncommon (49,50). Choreiform movements and choreoathetosis have been found in patients with basal ganglia infection. Acquired hydrocephalus may also develop (51). Because *T. gondii* infection causes predominantly an encephalitis with little to no meningeal involvement, meningismus is rare and the cerebrospinal fluid may be normal or have a mild pleocytosis and elevated protein level with no depression of the glucose concentration. Autopsy studies of patients infected with *T. gondii* have demonstrated multiple organ system involvement (52). However, clinical manifestations of severe organ involvement have been infrequently mentioned in case reports or series of cases. It is important to be aware that infections in the skin, lung, heart, eye, and liver can occur independently of central nervous system involvement (32,36,52–54). Concomitant systemic and/or cerebral infections with *Pneumocystis carinii*, cytomegalovirus, *Mycobacterium tuberculosis, Mycobacterium avium-intracellulare,* and *Candida albicans* have been reported to occur with toxoplasmic encephalitis (3,32).

In most reported cases of toxoplasmic pneumonia (55–60) the clinical manifestations are nonspecific, similar to those seen with *P. carinii* pneumonia (PCP). Patients may have fever, dyspnea, and a nonproductive cough. Hemoptysis has occasionally been described (60). The onset of disease tends to be more rapid than PCP, and patients can present with acute respiratory failure in a setting similar to septic shock with hypotension, metabolic acidosis, and disseminated intravascular coagulation (60,55). Chest x-rays usually demonstrate bilateral interstitial infiltrates, while single nodules, nodular infiltrates, and hilar adenopathy may occur (55–60). Pathologically, *T. gondii* in tissue is associated most often with necrosis and mixed inflammation. Intracellular and free tachyzoites, bradyzoites, and cysts in healthy tissue can be found (55,61–63). Diagnosis can be made using Giemsa or eosin methylene blue fast stains of bronchoalveolar lavage fluid or lung biopsy specimens. False-negative biopsy results have occurred and can be overcome using the peroxidase-antiperoxidase method (55). *T. gondii* pneumonia usually represents activation of latent infection, but knowledge of the pathogenesis of pulmonary disease is incomplete.

Primary toxoplasma myocarditis manifested by cardiac tamponade or biventricular failure has been reported (64–66), but cardiac infection is usually asymptomatic and is diagnosed in the setting of disseminated disease in which central nervous system infection predominates (67). Definitive diagnosis is extremely difficult as it requires an endomyocardial biopsy and the small amounts of tissue obtained coupled with the patchy tissue involvement decrease the sensitivity of this procedure.

Retinochoroiditis can occur with or without concomitant encephalitis. At times, the development of toxoplasmic retinochoroiditis is a harbinger for toxoplasmic encephalitis (68–70). Orchitis and peritonitis due to *T. gondii* have occasionally been reported in AIDS patients (71–73).

V. DIAGNOSIS

Currently, treatment for toxoplasmic encephalitis is usually initiated upon presumptive diagnosis. This clinical practice has evolved with the advent of AIDS since the attendant morbidity associated with brain biopsy, as well as the inability to biopsy all the numerous and inaccessible lesions, often preclude brain biopsy. In addition, since *T. gondii* is the most common opportunistic pathogen of the central nervous system in AIDS patients, the practice of presumptive therapy for patients fulfilling the following criteria is almost universally practiced: 1) a characteristic finding on computerized axial tomography (CAT) scan or magnetic resonance imaging (MRI) study (3,4,21,30,32); 2) a serological test positive for antitoxoplasma antibody. Using these criteria, the predictive value has been estimated to be as great as 80% (74). However, in patient populations such as intravenous drug abusers in whom other central nervous processes are more prevalent, the predictive value of a positive toxoplasma serology may be diminished (75). In patients who are empirically started on therapy, a clear clinical response to therapy should be evident within 14 days of therapy, and there should be a clear radiographic response in all lesions within 3 weeks (32). In patients who fail to respond, brain biopsy with or without alteration of therapy should be sought.

VI. ISOLATION AND DETECTION OF ORGANISMS

The definitive diagnosis of toxoplasmic infection is made by the demonstration of toxoplasma tachyzoites in clinical specimens. In patients with toxoplasmic encephalitis and pneumonitis, detection of the pathogen from the cerebrospinal fluid (76) and bronchoalveolar lavage (55,77), respectively, has been found to be useful in the diagnosis of central nervous system and pulmonary involvement. Previously, isolation of *T. gondii* from clinical specimens required inoculation of the specimen into a laboratory animal, most commonly a mouse (78). Using this technique, as much time as 6 weeks may be necessary to demonstrate the organism by direct observation of the tissue cyst in the brain of these animals or by seroconversion. Recently, isolation in tissue culture systems, commonly used for viral isolation, has been shown to be useful for the isolation of *T. gondii* from clinical specimens (78). This technique may offer a more practical and expedient methodology for the microbiological demonstration of this pathogen. Another diagnostic methodology that is still being evaluated is the usefulness of selective amplification of DNA products specific to *T. gondii* by the polymerase chain reaction. This latter work holds great promise as a sensitive and specific assay for the direct identification of a product of *T. gondii* in amniotic fluid, however, its utility for the detection of specific nucleic acid sequences in CSF remains to be determined.

The utility of brain biopsy for the diagnosis of toxoplasmic encephalitis in AIDS patients has been a source of controversy. Although other infectious and noninfectious processes can cause a focal abnormality indistinguishable on CAT scan or MRI from *T. gondii*, the predictive value of a positive antitoxoplasma antibody in most patient populations with a characteristic contrast-enhancing lesion on CAT scan appears to be very good (79,80) in predicting the presence of toxoplasma encephalitis. In contrast, biopsy has proved diagnostic by histopathological examination in only 50% of reported cases of toxoplasmic encephalitis (74). Intraoperative sonography and needle biopsy with a sterotactic device have proved useful for the diagnosis of deep intracerebral lesions; however, significant morbidity continues to be associated with brain biopsy. Utilizing these new techniques, morbidity and mortality due to biopsy has been decreased; however, the size of the biopsy is small, which limits the extent of immunohistological examination that can be performed. Given that the histological changes associated with toxoplasma may closely resemble those of viral encephalitis and that tachyzoites may be difficult to distinguish from nuclear debris, the diagnosis of toxoplasma may be difficult (5). Specialized immunohistochemical techniques are also necessary to detect the organism or its antigens. The reactive round cell infiltrates found in toxoplasmic encephalitis may be difficult to differentiate from an intracerebral lymphoma (32). In our experience, similarities of morphological appearance of the reactive lymphocytes and monocytes may be indistinguishable from the malignant B cell found in a lymphoma. Usually, if the entire pathological specimen is reviewed from wide excisional biopsy or autopsy, the distribution and composition of cells are reactive, but in isolated areas the infiltrate is highly atypical and not vasocentric (32). It is therefore obvious that a needle biopsy, which is a small sampling by virtue of the technology, may be misleading. In these cases, immunohistological strains of the atypical cells found in toxoplasma lesions consist predominantly of T cells and histiocytes (32). Thus, it is recommended that if the needle biopsy does not definitively diagnose a *T. gondii* infection or a lymphoma, immunohistological studies with pathogen (e.g., peroxidase antiperoxidase staining) and cell-specific antibodies be performed. Thus, brain biopsy is generally reserved for those patients who present with a diagnostic dilemma or do not fulfill the criteria for presumptive treatment or who have not responded to appropriate antitoxoplasmic chemotherapy.

VII. NEURORADIOLOGICAL STUDIES

Characteristically, patients with toxoplasmic encephalitis will have focal or multifocal abnormalities demonstrable on MRI or CAT scan. These focal areas of encephalitis may be single or multiple, bilateral, isodense or hypodense, contrast-enhancing lesions. These findings are not specific for toxoplasmic encephalitis. In a recent review, 40% of CNS lymphomas were multifocal, and almost 50% had ring enhancement (81). In 70-80% of patients, the lesions of toxoplasmic encephalitis on CAT scan are multiple, and the contrast-enhancing lesions are located in both cerebral hemispheres (26–28,30,36,81). The basal ganglia and corticomedullary junction are most commonly involved. The lesions are frequently associated with edema. It has been suggested that a delayed double-dose contrast CAT scan study may be a more sensitive means of diagnosis of toxoplasmic encephalitis (30,80). Although the CAT scan seems to be a sensitive diagnostic modality in patients with focal neurological symptoms, it may underestimate the minimal inflammatory response seen during early disease (32,82–84). It is believed that, given the increased sensitivity of the MRI scan (82), the demonstration of a single lesion with this diagnostic modality strongly suggests etiologies other than toxoplasmosis (e.g., lymphoma) (83,84). Therefore, it is recommended that an MRI be performed in patients with neurological symptoms and antibody to toxoplasma whose CAT scans show no abnormality.

The MRI or CAT scan is useful for assessment of response to empirical treatment. The radiographic response to therapy may lag behind the clinical response. Complete resolution of abnormalities on CAT scan may vary between 3 weeks and 6 months, although patients who respond to therapy will usually have radiographic evidence of improvement within 3 weeks of initiation of therapy. The time to resolution of the lesions may depend on the area of the brain involved. Peripheral lesions seem to respond more quickly than deeper lesions. As a rule, patients with encephalitis should have evidence of either clinical or radiographic improvement within 2 weks of initiation of empirical therapy.

VIII. SEROLOGY

Toxoplasmic encephalitis occurs most often as a result of recrudescence of a latent infection. Therefore, serological evidence of toxoplasmic infection is seen in virtually all patients prior to the development of encephalitis (22). Upon the development of encephalitis, significant rises in antibody titers are found in only a minority of AIDS patients with toxoplasmic encephalitis (22,29). The level of antibody titer does not seem to be predictive for the presence of toxoplasmic encephalitis (5,29). The Sabin-Feldman dye test titers vary between negative and 1:1024 in patients with AIDS and toxoplasmic encephalitis. Approximately one fifth of patients have antibody titers of 1:1024 and <3% have no demonstrable antitoxoplasmic antibody at the time of their toxoplasmic encephalitis. The toxoplasma agglutination test may be a more sensitive indicator of active disease (5,85). Antitoxoplasma IgM antibody is rarely found in AIDS patients with toxoplasmic encephalitis.

Determination of antitoxoplasma antibodies in the spinal fluid may be a useful adjunct in the diagnosis of toxoplasmic encephalitis (86). In using this technique, it is important to determine whether there is intrathecal production of antitoxoplasma antibody. This can be determined by the following formula: CSF dye test titer (reciprocal)/total CSF globulin × total serum globulin/serum dye test titer (reciprocal). Using this formula, a value greater than 1 is indicative of the intrathecal production of antitoxoplasma antibody.

IX. GENERAL THERAPY

Toxoplasmic encephalitis is suspected in patients with AIDS who are both seropositive for *T. gondii* and who have CAT scans or MRI studies indicative of a focal or multifocal encephalitis. Characteristically, the CAT scan may show one or more lesions, whereas the MRI with its increased sensitivity almost invariably reveals multiple lesions. Although multiple infectious and noninfectious etiologies including cerebral lymphoma and *Mycobacterium tuberculosis* may cause abnormalities on imaging studies that are distinguishable from toxoplasmic encephalitis, patients are presumptively started on specific antitoxoplasma chemotherapy if they fulfill these two diagnostic criteria. Patients treated for toxoplasmic encephalitis should be carefully monitored for evidence of clinical deterioration during the early course of therapy, and significant clinical improvement should be sought within 10–14 days after the initiation of therapy as a confirmation of the original diagnosis. Concomitant with clinical improvement, neuroradiographic studies performed within 3 weeks after initiation of therapy should reveal improvement. Because corticosteroids stabilize the blood-brain barrier and have a dramatic antiinflammatory effect, clinical or radiographic improvement while on corticosteroids must be interpreted with caution. Furthermore, after discontinuation of steroids, repeat radiographic studies should be performed to determine whether there is any exacerbation of disease. In view of the fact that other infectious and noninfectious entities may be indistinguishable from toxoplasmic encephalitis and that toxoplasmic encephalitis has been reported to occur in association with other infectious diseases such as tuberculosis and cryptococcosis, patients with poor clinical response or who continue to have focal abnormalities that do not change during the course of therapy should be strongly considered for a brain biopsy.

X. SPECIFIC THERAPY

The mainstay of therapy for toxoplasmic encephalitis is the combination of pyrimethamine, a dihydrofoliate reductase inhibitor, and sulfadiazine, a dihydrofolate synthetase inhibitor, which sequentially block folic acid metabolism and thereby act synergistically against *T. gondii*. Folinic acid (leucovorin), which is preferentially transported across mammalian cell membranes and not across *T. gondii* cell membranes, is a useful adjunct to prevent the bone marrow toxicity of pyrimethamine. Both pyrimethamine and sulfadiazine are well absorbed from the gut, cross the blood-brain barrier, and possess activity only against the tachyzoite. Unfortunately, this combination is plagued with toxicity rates that may preclude its use in up to 40% of patients (53,54). Drug rash is the most frequent dose-limiting toxicity during the early phase of acute therapy, occurring in up to 20% of patients. The rash, however, does not preclude the subsequent use of pyrimethamine and sulfadiazine for maintenance treatment. Hematological toxicities manifested as cytopenias may occur at any time during therapy (88). The concomitant use of antiretroviral agents may potentiate these toxicities (89). Nephrotoxicity, including crystaluria, hematuria, radiolucent stones, and renal failure, are well-known adverse effects of sulfonamides (90,91). Treatment includes hydration, alkalinization of urine, and dose reduction. The treatment of toxoplasma encephalitis is further complicated by the erratic levels of pyrimethamine found in the serum of patients with AIDS and toxoplasmic encephalitis (92). Recently we examined the pharmacokinetics of pyrimethamine (in collaboration with Louis Weiss, Einstein College of Medicine, New York) in five consecutive patients with toxoplasmic encephalitis treated with 75 mg of pyrimethamine per day. The half-life of pyrimethamine varied between 26 and 90 hours in these patients, and concomitant mean serum levels obtained over 24 hours after 3 weeks of therapy varied between 500 and 2000 ng/ml. It therefore becomes apparent that, given our limited knowledge of the erratic serum pyrimethamine levels achieved with oral therapy and the distribution of the drug in the brain or in the cerebral spinal fluid, synergistic combination therapy should be used for initial treatment. Further studies are needed to correlate the levels of antitoxoplasmic chemotherapeutic agents found in the serum to the therapeutic response as well as to hematological toxicity. Currently pyrimethamine is given as a 200-mg loading dose and then 50–75 mg/day by mouth. Sulfadiazine is given 4–6 g/day in four divided doses by mouth. Folinic acid is commonly given at a dose of 10 mg/day for 6 weeks followed by chronic suppressive therapy. The precise dosing and amount of folinic acid needed to circumvent the hematological toxicity of pyrimethamine has not been established. Reversal of the antitoxoplasma effect of sulfadiazine by exogeneously administered folic or folinic acid in murine toxoplasmosis has been reported (87). Studies are needed to determine the dosing necessary to optimize delivery of folinic acid.

As stated above, pyrimethamine and sulfadiazine are active only against the tachyzoite, not against the cyst form of *T. gondii*. Since both forms are present in patients with active encephalitis, discontinuation of specific chemotherapy almost invariably results in recrudescence of the encephalitis (74). Thus, after an initial 6 weeks of therapy for toxoplasmic encephalitis, patients are maintained on 25–50 mg pyrimethamine with 2–4 g sulfadiazine daily. In instances when sulfonamides cannot be continued, pyrimethamine 75 mg/day in combination with clindamycin (450 mg every 8 hours) can be used. There has been anecdotal evidence to indicate that pyrimethamine when given at sufficient dose (≥75 mg/day) may be adequate as chronic suppressive therapy.

Trimetrexate, a potent inhibitor of *T. gondii* dihydrofolate reductase, has also been shown to have both in vitro and in vivo (murine toxoplasmosis) activity against *T. gondii* (93,94). Unfortunately, in AIDS patients with biopsy-proven toxoplasmic encephalitis, a recrudescence of toxoplasmic encephalitis was noted while on therapy with this drug (95). Piritrexin, another lipid-soluble antifolate (96), has not been studied in humans.

Dapsone (diaminodiphenyl sulfone) is the most potent sulfone against *T. gondii* in experimental murine infection (97). Dapsone inhibits *T. gondii* dihydropteroate synthase (98). Dapsone is well absorbed from the gut and possesses a longer serum half-life than sulfadiazine. In vitro synergism with pyrimethamine has been demonstrated (99). Dapsone alone or in combination with pyrimethamine has no effect on the tissue cyst. Dapsone is an attractive alternative agent for maintenance therapy given its longer serum half-life and better toxicity profile over sulfadiazine (100), however, it does not cross the blood-brain barrier effectively.

Spiramycin, a macrolide antibiotic, is commonly used in Europe for the treatment of toxoplasmosis during pregnancy. However, this agent has been ineffective for prophylaxis or treatment of a small number (four patients) of patients with toxoplasmic encephalitis (101).

Clindamycin has been recognized to be an effective drug for treatment of murine toxoplasmosis, although it lacks in vitro activity against *T. gondii* (102,103). In bacteria, clindamycin inhibits protein synthesis by acting on the 50S ribosome. The mechanism of action of this drug against *T. gondii* is not known. Clindamycin is well absorbed from the gastrointestinal tract, and peak serum levels occur 1–2 hours after administration. Although clindamycin has excellent tissue penetration, the concentrations reached in the CSF and brain tissue are erratic and have precluded its use in bacterial meningitis in humans (104,105). It is not known whether the drug may accumulate in necrotic areas of the brain or as a consequence of local destruction of the blood brain barrier (106). Although these reports suggest a role for clindamycin in the treatment of toxoplasmosis, further studies are necessary to determine the relative role of this combination chemotherapy and whether oral therapy with clindamycin is useful in the initial treatment of toxoplasmic encephalitis.

There have been several reports of patients with AIDS and toxoplasmic encephalitis for whom therapy with pyrimethamine (25–75 mg/day) and oral or intravenous clindamycin (1200–4800 mg/day) yielded apparent improvement (43,44,74,110,111). Recently a prospective study by the California Universitywide Task Force on AIDS—California Collaborative Treatment Group reported that clindamycin (1200 mg IV every 6 hours) combined with pyrimethamine (75 mg/day) was efficacious in the initial treatment of toxoplasmic encephalitis (44). Unfortunately, the size of the study did not allow determination of whether this combination therapy was as efficacious as pyrimethamine and sulfadiazine. Both regimens appear to have similar frequencies of toxicity. The preliminary findings of a large prospective trial in Europe using pyrimethamine (50 mg/day) and oral clindamycin (2.4 g/day orally) vs. pyrimethamine 50 mg/day and sulfadiazine (4 g/day orally) have confirmed these results (113). In a nonrandomized prospective study performed by the AIDS Clinical Trial Group, pyrimethamine (75 mg/day) and clindamycin (2.4 g/day) had a greater than 80% efficacy rate in patients who could tolerate therapy (B. J. Luft, unpublished data). The toxicities of clindamycin are well known and include nausea, vomiting, diarrhea, neutropenia, rash, and pseudomembranous colitis (114). Myopathy with typical electromyographic findings and elevated creatine phosphokinase levels, which reversed upon discontinuation of clindamycin, has also been reported (115). Although these reports suggest a role for clindamycin in the treatment of toxoplasmosis, further studies are necessary to determine the relative role of this combination chemotherapy and whether oral therapy with clindamycin is useful in the initial treatment of toxoplasmic encephalitis.

Recently, roxithromycin, clarithromycin, and azithromycin, three new macrolide antibiotics, have been found to be highly active in treating murine toxoplasmosis (45,46,116,117). These agents possess both improved pharmacokinetic properties (greater bioavailability, higher and more persistent serum and tissue levels) and potent antimicrobial activity (118,119). Azithromycin possesses in vivo activity against the cyst form (120). In human toxoplasmic encephalitis, the combination of pyrimethamine and clarithromycin seemed effective in a prospective pilot study of 13 AIDS patients (121). Hearing loss and increased transminase levels were noted. Further studies are necessary to determine whether these agents may have a role in the acute treatment or chronic suppression of this disease. Other agents such as arprinocid, a purine analog (122), and the hydroxynaphtoquinone BW566C80 may prove to be useful for the treatment of toxoplasmic encephalitis (123). BW566C80 was shown to be very effective in experimental (murine) toxoplasmosis, possessing activity against the tissue cyst (123). This drug was also shown to be effective in a rat model of PCP (124).

The optimal agents and dosing schedule for chronic maintenance therapy and chemoprophylaxis have yet to be determined. Combinations of oral pyrimethamine 25–50 mg, plus sulfadiazine 2–4 g daily or bi- or triweekly have been used (4,32,125,126). Folinic acid at a dose of 5–15 mg daily is added to this regimen. As stated earlier, clindamycin can be substituted for sulfadiazine in the sulfa-allergic patient. The efficacy of a biweekly oral regimen using either pyrimethamine 25 mg/day and sulfadiazine 4 g/day or clindamycin 600 mg every 6 hours in the sulfa-allergic patient was recently reported by Pedrol et al. (126). The efficacy of pyrimethamine and clindamycin for chronic maintenance therapy has been reported by others (127,128), while relapses of toxoplasmic encephalitis using this regimen have also been noted (107,112).

Prophylactic therapy is particularly appealing given the ease with which patients at risk of developing toxoplasmic encephalitis (those seropositive for *T. gondii*) can be identified. Small studies reported that pyrimethamine alone or with dapsone or trimethoprim-sulfamethoxazole as primary prophylaxis were ineffective (129,130), while others have reported these agents to be promising for primary prophylaxis (131). Large comparative trials of various agent doses and drug combinations will be needed to determine maintenance regimens of choice. Such studies are currently underway.

REFERENCES

1. Remington JS. Toxoplasmosis in the adult. Bull NY Acad Med 1974; 50:211.

2. Faruqi A, Frank MA, Rosvali M, et al. Acute acquired toxoplasmosis. South Med J 1976; 69:1234.

3. Luft BJ, Remington JS. Toxoplasmosis of the central nervous system. In: Remington JS, Swartz MN, eds. Current topics in infectious disease, Vol. 6. New York: McGraw-Hill, 1985.

4. Luft BJ, Remington JS. Toxoplasmic encephalitis. J Infect Dis 1988; 157:1–6.

5. Luft BJ, Brooks RC, Conley FK et al. Toxoplasmic encephalitis in patients with AIDS. JAMA 1984; 252:913.

6. Luft BJ, Conley FK, Remington JS. Outbreak of central-nervous system toxoplasmosis in Western Europe and North America. Lancet 1983; 1:781–4.

7. Kloser PC, Mangia AJ, Leonard J, Lombardo JM, Michaels J, Denny TN, Shaer L, Sathe S, Weiss SH, Schable C, et al. HIV-2-associated AIDS in the United States. The first case. Arch Intern Med 1989; 149:1875–7.

8. Ruef C, Dickey P, Schable CA, Griffith B, Williams AE, D'Aquila RT. A second case of the acquired immunodeficiency syndrome due to hyman immunodeficiency virus type 2 in the United States: the clinical implications. Am J Med 1989; 86:709–12.

9. Levy RM, Bredesen DE, Rosenblum ML. Neurological manifestations of the acquired immunodeficiency syndrome (AIDS). Experience of UCSF and review of the literature. J Neurosurg 1985; 62:475.

10. Sacks JJ, Roberto RR, Brooks WF. Toxoplasmosis infection associated with goat's milk. JAMA 1982; 248:1728.

11. Luft BJ, Remington JS. Acute toxoplasma infection among family members of patients with acute lymphadenopathic toxoplasmosis. Arch Intern Med 1984; 144:53.

12. Teutsch SM, Juranek DD, Sulzer A, et al. Epidemic toxoplasmosis associated with infected cats. N Engl J Med 1979; 300:695.

13. Benson MW, Takafuji Et, Lemon SM, et al. Oocyst transmitted toxoplasmosis associated with the ingestion of contaminated water. N Engl J Med 1982; 307:666.

14. Weinman D, Chandler AH. Toxoplasmosis in men and swine: an investigation of the possible relationship. JAMA 1956; 161:229.

15. Remington JS, Desmonts G. Toxoplasmosis. In: Remington JS, Klein JO, eds. Infectious diseases of the fetus and newborn infant. Philadelphia: WB Saunders Company, 1983:

16. Viera J, et al. Acquired immune deficiency in Haitians: opportunistic infections in previously healthy Haitian immigrants. N Engl J Med 1983; 308:125.

17. Moskowitz LB, et al. Unusual causes of death in Haitians residing in Miami. High prevalence of opportunistic infections. JAMA 1983; 250:1187.

18. Clumeck N, et al. Acquired immunodeficiency syndrome in African patients. N Engl J Med 1984; 310:492.

19. Snider WD, et al. Neurological complications of acquired immuno-deficiency syndrome. Analysis of 50 patients. Ann Neurol 1983; 14:403.

20. Chan JC, et al. Toxoplasma encephalitis om recent Haitian entrants. South Med J 1983; 76:211.

21. Navia BA, Petito CK, Gold JW, Cho E, Jordan BD, Price RW. Cerebral toxoplasmosis complicating the acquired immune deficiency syndrome: clinical and neuropathological findings in 27 patients. Ann Neurol 1986; 224:38.

22. Carme B, M'Pele P, Mbitsi A, Kissila AM, Aya GM, Mouanga-Vidika G, Mboussa J, Itoua-Ngaporo A. Opportunistic parasitic diseases and mycoses in AIDS. Their frequencies in Brazzaville (Congo). Bull Soc Pathol Exot Filiales 1988; 81:311–6.

23. Levy RM, Janssen RS, Bush TJ, Rosenblum ML. Neuroepidemiology of acquired immunodeficiency syndrome. In: Rosenblum ML, et al. eds. AIDS and the nervous system. New York: Raven Press, 1988:13–27.

24. Ambros Ra, Lee EY, Sharer LR, Khan MY, Robboy SJ. The acquired immunodeficiency syndrome in intravenous drug abusers and patients with a sexual risk: clinical and postmortem comparisons. Human Pathol 1987; 18: 1109–14.

25. Zangerle R, Allenberger F, Pohl, et al. High risk of developing toxoplasmic encephalitis in AIDS patients seropositive for *Toxoplasma gondii*. Med Microbiol Immunol 1991; 180:59–66.

26. Levy RM, Bredesen DE, Rosenblum ML. Neurological manifestations of the acquired immunodeficiency syndrome (AIDS): experience at UCSF and review of the literature. J Neurosurg 1985; 62:475–95.

27. Levy RM, Rosenbloom S, Perrett LV. Neuroradiological findings in the acquired immunodeficiency syndrome (AIDS): a review of 200 cases. AJNR 1986; 7:833–9.

28. Post MJD, Kursunoglu SJ, Hensley CT, et al. Cranial CT in acquired immunodeficiency syndrome: spectrum of diseases and optimal contrast enhancement technique. AJR 1985; 145:929–40.

29. Wong B, Gold JWM, Brown AE, et al. Central-nervous-system toxoplasmosis in homosexual men and parenteral drug abusers. Ann Intern Med 1984; 100:36–42.

30. Whelan MA, Krichoff II, Handler M, et al: A.I.D.S.: Cerebral computed tomographic manifestations. Radiology 1983; 149:477.

31. Frenkel JK. Toxoplasmosis: parasite life cycle, pathology and immunology. In: D. M. Hammond, ed., The coccidia. Baltimore University Park Press, 1973:343.

32. Luft BJ. *Toxoplasma gondii*. In: Walzer PD, Gertz RM, eds. Parasitic infection in the compromised host. New York: Marcel Dekker, 1989:

33. Lainson R. Observations on the development and nature of pseudocysts and cysts of *Toxoplasma gondii*. Trans R Soc Trop Med Hyg 1958; 12:221.

34. Van der Waaj D. Formation, growth and multiplication of *Toxoplasma gondii* cysts in mouse brains. Trop Georg Med 1959; 11:345.

35. Gray F, Gherardi R, Wingate E, Wingate J, Fenelon G, Gaston A, Sobel A, Poirier J. Diffuse encephalitic cerebral toxoplasmosis in AIDS. Report of four cases. J Neurol 1989; 236:273–7.

36. Post MJD, Chan JC, Hensley GT, et al. Toxoplasma encephalitis in Haitian adults with acquired immunodeficiency syndrome: a clinical-pathologic-CT correlation. AJR 1983; 140:861-8.

37. Chaudhari AB, Singh A, Jindal S, Poon TP. Hemorrhage in cerebral toxoplasmosis: a report on a patient with the acquired immunodeficiency syndrome. S Afr Med J 1989; 76:272-4.

38. Casado-Naranjo I, Lopez-Trigo J, Ferrandiz A, Cervello A, Navarro V. Hemorrhagic abscess in a patient with the acquired immunodeficiency syndrome. Neuroradiology 1989; 31:289.

39. Partisani M, Candolfi H, De Mautort E, et al. Seroprevalence of latent *Toxoplasma gondii* infection in HIV-infected individuals and long-term follow up of toxoplasma seronegative subjects. [Abstract] W.B. 2294 from the VII International Conference on AIDS, Florence, Italy, 1991.

40. Engstrom JW, Lowenstein DH, Bredesen DE. Cerebral infarctions and transient neurologic deficits associated with acquired immunodeficiency syndrome. Am J Med 1989; 86:528-32.

41. Carrazana EJ, Rossitch E, Jr., Schachter S. Cerebral toxoplasmosis masquerading as herpes encephalitis in a patient with the acquired immunodeficiency syndrome. Am J Med 1989; 86:730-2.

42. Milligan SA, Katz MS, Craven PC. Toxoplasmosis presenting as panhypopituitarism in a patient with the acquired immune deficiency syndrome. Am J Med 1984; 77:760-4.

43. Rolston KV. Clindamycin in cerebral toxoplasmosis (letter). Am J Med 1988; 85:285.

44. Danneman BR, Israelski DM, McCutchan JA, et al. Treatment of toxoplasma encephalitis in AIDS: Primary report of the California Collaborative Treatment Group randomized trial of pyrimethamine plus sulfadiazine versus pyrimethamine plus clindamycin. Los Angeles, 28th ICAAC, 1988.

45. Araujo FG, Guptill DR, Remington JS. Azithromycin, a macrolide antibiotic with potent activity against *Toxoplasma gondii*. Antimicrob Agents Chemother 1988; 32:755-7.

46. Luft BJ. In vivo and in vitro activity of roxithromycin against *Toxoplasma gondii* in mice. Eur J Clin Microbiol 1987; 6:479-81.

47. Farkash AE, Maccabbee PJ, Sher JH. CNS toxoplasmosis in acquired immune deficiency syndrome: A clinical-pathological-radiological review of 12 cases. J Neurol Neurosurg Psychiatry 1986; 49:744-8.

48. Hamed LM, Schatz NJ, Galetta SL. Brainstem ocular motility defects and AIDS. Am J Opthalmol 1988; 106:437-42.

49. Sanchez-Ramos JR, Factor SA, Weiner WJ, Marquez J. Hemichorea-hemiballismus associated with acquired immune deficiency syndrome and cerebral toxoplasmosis. Mov Discord 1989; 4:266-73.

50. Helweg-Larsen S, Jakobsen J, Boeser F, Artier-Siberg P. Neurological complications and concomitants of AIDS. Act Neurol Scand 1986; 74:467–744.

51. Nolla-Sallas J, Ricart C, D'Ohlaberringue L, Gali F, Lamorca J. Hydrocephalus: an unusual CT presentation of cerebral toxoplasmosis in a patient with acquired immunodeficiency syndrome. Eur Neurol 1987; 27:130.

52. Tschirhart D, Klatt EC. Disseminated toxoplasmosis in the acquired immunodeficiency syndrome. Arch Pathol Lab Med 1988; 112:1237–41.

53. Haverkos HW. Assessment of therapy of toxoplasma encephalitis. The TE Study Group. Am J Med 1987; 82:907.

54. Leport C, Raffi F, Matheron S, et al. Treatment of central nervous system toxoplasmosis with pyrimethamine-sulfadiazine combination in 35 AIDS patients: efficacy of long term continuous therapy. Am J Med (in press).

55. Catterall JR, Hofflin JM, Remington JS. Pulmonary toxoplasmosis. Am Rev Respir Dis 1986; 133:704–11.

56. Couvreur J, Lepoumon, et al. Toxoplasmosis. Rev Fr Mal Resp 1975; 3: 525.

57. Tourani JM, Israe-Biet D, Veret A, Andriew JM. Unusual pulmonary infection in a puzzling presentation of AIDS. Lancet 1985; 1:989.

58. Mendelson MH, Finkel LJ, Meyers BR, et al. Pulmonary toxoplasmosis in AIDS. Scand J Infect Dis 1987; 19:703–6.

59. Tawney S, Masci J, Berger HW, et al. Pulmonary toxoplasmosis: an unusual nodular radiographic pattern in a patient with AIDS. Mt. Sinai J Med 1986; 53:683–5.

60. Oskenhendler E, Cadranel J, Sarfati C, et al. *Toxoplasma gondii* pneumonia in patients with the acquired immunodeficiency syndrome. Am J Med 1989; 88(5M):18–21.

61. Maguire GP, Tatz J, Giose R, Ahmed T. Diagnosis of pulmonary toxoplasmosis by bronchoalveolar lavage. NY Stat J Med 1986; 78:204–50.

62. Tschirhart D, Klatt E. Disseminated toxoplasmosis in the acquired immunodeficiency syndrome. Arch Pathol Lab Med 1988; 112:1237–41.

63. Marche C, Mayorga R, Trophilme D, et al. Pathological study of extraneurological toxoplasmosis in AIDS. IV International Conference on AIDS, Stockholm, Sweden, 1988.

64. Wertlake PT, Winter TS. Fatal toxoplasma myocarditis in an adult patient with acute lymphocyte leukemia. N Engl J Med 1965; 237:438–40.

65. Adair OV, Randive N, Krasnow N. Isolated toxoplasma myocarditis in acquired immunodeficiency syndrome. Am Heart J 1989; 118(4):856–7.

66. Moskowitz L, Hemsley GT, Chan JC, et al. Immediate causes of death in acquired immunodeficiency syndrome. Arch Pathol Lab Med 1985; 109:735–8.

67. Roldan EO, Moskowitz L, Hemsley GT. Pathology of the heart in acquired immunodeficiency syndrome. Arch Pathol Lab Med 1987; 111:943–6.

68. Perke DW. Diffuse toxoplasmic retinochoroiditis in a patient with AIDS. 1986; 104:571.

69. Weiss A, Margo EC, Ledford DK, Lockey RF, Brinser JH. Toxoplasmic retinochoroiditis as an initial manifestation of the acquired immunodeficiency syndrome. Am J Ophthalmol 1986; 101:248.

70. Friedman AH. The retinal lesions of the acquired immunodeficiency syndrome Trans Am Ophthalmol Soc 1984; 82:447.

71. Crider SR, Horstman WG, Massey GS. Toxoplasma orchitis: report of a case and a review of the literature. Am J Med 1988; 95:421–4.

72. Nistral M, Santana A, Paniaqua R, et al. Testicular toxoplasmosis in two men with the acquired immunodeficiency syndrome (AIDS). Arch Pathol Lab Med 1986; 110:744–6.

73. Israelski DM, et al. Toxoplasma peritonitis in a patient with AIDS. Arch Int Med (submitted for publication).

74. Cohn JA, McMeeking A, Cohen W, Jacobs J, Holzman RS. Evaluation of the policy of empiric treatment of suspected Toxoplasma encephalitis in patients with the acquired immunodeficiency syndrome. Am J Med 1989; 86: 521–7.

75. Bishburg E, Eng RH, Slim J, Perez G, Johnson E. Brain lesions in patients with acquired immunodeficiency syndrome. Arch Intern Med 1989; 149:941–3.

76. DeMent Sh, Cox MC, Gupta PK. Diagnosis of central nervous system Toxoplasma gondii from the cerebrospinal fluid in a patient with acquired immunodeficiency syndrome. Diagn Cytopathol 1987; 3:148–51.

77. Derouin F, Sarfati C, Beauvais B, et al. Laboratory diagnosis of pulmonary toxoplasmosis in patients with AIDS. J Clin Microbiol 1989; 27:1661–3.

78. Derouin F, Mazeron MC, Garin YJF. Comparative study of tissue culture and mouse inoculation methods for demonstration of *Toxoplasma gondii*. J Clin Microbiol 1987; 25:1597–1600.

79. Wanke CH, Tuazon CU, Kovaks A, et al. Toxoplasma encephalitis in patients with acquired immunodeficiency syndrome. Am J Trop Med Hyg 1987; 36:509–16.

80. Post MJ, Kursonoglu SJ, Hensley GT, Chan JC, Moskowitz LB, Hoffman TA. Cranial CT in acquired immunodeficiency syndrome: spectrum of diseases and optimal contrast enhancement technique. Am J Roentgenol 1985; 145:929.

81. Weisberg LA, Greenberg J, Stazio A. Computed tomographic findings in cerebral toxoplasmosis in adults. Comput Med Imaging Graph 1988; 12:379–83.

82. Jarvik JG, Hesselink JR, Kennedy C, Teschke R, Wiley C, Spector S, Richman D, McCutchan JA. Acquired immunodeficiency syndrome. Magnetic resonance patterns of brain involvement with pathologic correlation. Arch Neurol 1988; 45:731-6.

83. Ostertun B, Dewes W, Suss H, Steudel A, Brassel H, Harder T. MR tomography of non-tumor diseases of the brain and cervical cord. ROFO 1988; 148: 408-14.

84. Gill PS, Graham RA, Boswell W, Meyer P, Krailo M, Levine A. A comparison of imaging, clinical, and pathologic aspects of space-occupying lesions within the brain in patients with acquired immunedeficiency syndrome. Am J Physiol Imaging 1986; 1:134-41.

85. Suzuki Y, Israelski DM, Dannemann BR, Stepick-Biek P, Thulliez P, Remington JS. Diagnosis of toxoplasmic encephalitis in patients with acquired immunodeficiency syndrome by using a new serologic method. J Clin Microbiol 1988; 26:2541-3.

86. Potsman I, Resnick L, Luft BJ, Remington JS. Intrathecal production of antibodies against *Toxoplasma gondii* in patients with toxoplasmic encephalitis and the acquired immunodeficiency syndrome (AIDS). Ann Intern Med 1988; 108:49-51.

87. Luft BJ, Steinberg S, Frankel R. The effect of folic and folinic acid on the anti-toxoplasma activity of pyrimethamine and sulfadiazine. [Abstract] 1238 ICAAC, Houston, 1988.

88. Torroba Alvarez L, Hermida Donate JM, Ezpeleta Baquedano C, Munoz Zato E. Methemoglobinemia secondary to the treatment of opportunistic infections in patients with AIDS (letter). Rev Clin Esp 1988; 182:289-90.

89. Leport C, Chakroun M, Matheron S, Rozenbaum W, Dournon E, Regnier B. Zidovudine efficacy and tolerance in 32 patients with cerebral toxoplasmosis in the acquired immunodeficiency syndrome (letter). Presse Med 1988; 17:1813-4.

90. Carbone LG, Bendixen B, Appel GB. Sulfadiazine-associated obstructive nephropathy occurring in a patient with the acquired immunodeficiency syndrome. Am J Kidney Dis 1988; 12:72-5.

91. Sahai J, Heimberger T, Collins K, Kaplowitz L, Polk R. Sulfadiazine-induced crystalluria in a patient with the acquired immunodeficiency syndrome: a reminder. Am J Med 1988; 84:791-2.

92. Weiss LM, Harris C, Berger M, Tanowitz HB, Wittner M. Pyrimethamine concentrations in serum and cerebrospinal fluid during treatment of acute toxoplasma encephalitis in patients with AIDS. J Infect Dis 1988; 157:580-3.

93. Kovacs JA, Altegra JC, Chabner BA, et al. Potent in vitro and in vivo antitoxoplasma activity of the new lipid soluble antifolate trimetrexate [Abstract]. Clin Res 1986; 34:522A.

94. Kovacs JA, Allegra JC, Chabner BA, et al. Potent effect of trimetrexate, a lipid-soluble antifolate on *Toxoplasma gondii*. J Inf Dis 1987; 155:627–1032.

95. Polis MA, Masur H, Tuazon C, et al. Salvage trial of trimetrexate-leukovorin for treatment of cerebral toxoplasmosis in AIDS patients [Abstract]. Clin Res 1989; 37:437A.

96. Kovacs JA, Allegra CJ, Swan JC, et al. Potent antipneumocystis and antitoxoplasma activities of piritrexin. Antimicrob Agents Chemother 1988; 32:430–3.

97. Eyles DE, Coleman M. An evaluation of the effect of sulfones on experimental toxoplasmosis in the mouse. Antibiot Chemother (Basel) 1957; 7:577–85.

98. Allegra CJ, Boarman D, Kovacs JA, et al. Interaction of sulfonamide and sulfone compounds with *Toxoplasma gondii* dihydropteroate synthase. J Clin Invest 1989; 85:371–79.

99. Derouin F, Piketty C, Chastang C, et al. Antitoxoplasma effects of dapsone alone and combined with pyrimethamine. Antimicrob Agents Chemother 1991; 35:252–5.

100. Lee BL, Medina I, Berowitz NL, et al. Dapsone, trimethoprim, and sulfamethoxazole plasma levels during treatment of pneumocystis pneumonia in patients with the acquired immunodeficiency syndrome (AIDS). Ann Int Med 1989; 110:606–11.

101. Leport C, Vilde JL, Katlama C, et al. Failure of spiramycin to prevent neurotoxoplasmosis in immunosuppressed patients. JAMA 1986; 255:2290.

102. Mack DG, McLeod R. New micromethod to study the effect of antimicrobial agents on *Toxoplasma gondii*: comparisons of sulfadoxine and sulfadiazine individually and in combination with pyrimethamine and study of clindamycin, metronidazole and cyclosporin A. Antimicrob Agents Chemother 1983; 26:26–30.

103. Harris C, Salgo MP, Tanowitz HB, Wittner M. In vitro assessment of antimicrobial agents against *Toxoplasma gondii*. J Inf Dis 1988; 157:14–17.

104. Picardi JL, Lewis HD, Tan JS, Phair JP. Clindamycin concentrations in the central nervous system of primates before and after head trauma. J Neurosurg 1975; 42:717–20.

105. Danneman BR, Israelski DM, Remington JS. Treatment of toxoplasmic encephalitis with intravenous clindamycin. Arch Intern Med 1988; 148:2477–82.

106. Hofflin J, Remington JS. Clindamycin in a murine model of toxoplasmic encephalitis. Antimicrob Agents Chemother 1987; 31:492–6.

107. Leport C, Bastuji-Garin S, Perronne C, Salmon D, Marche C, Bricaire F, Vilde JL. An open study of the pyrimethamine-clindamycin combination in AIDS patients with brain toxoplasmosis (letter). J Infect Dis 1989; 160: 557-8.

108. Hofflin JM, Remington JS. Clindamycin in a murine model of toxoplasmic encephalitis. Antimicrob Agents Chemother 1986; 31:492-6.

109. Santos Gil I, Noguerado Asensio A, Del Arco Galan C, Garcia Polo I. Clindamycin in the treatment of cerebral toxoplasmosis in a patient with AIDS (letter). Rev Clin Esp 1989; 185:47.

110. Dannemann BR, Israelski DM, Remington JS. Treatment of toxoplasmic encephalitis with intravenous clindamycin. Arch Intern Med 1988; 148: 2477-82.

111. Podzamczer D, Gudiol F. Clindamycin in cerebral toxoplasmosis (letter). Am J Med 1988; 84:136-9.

112. Rolston KV, Hoy J. Role of clindamycin in the treatment of central nervous system toxoplasmosis. Am J Med 1987; 83:551-4.

113. Katlama C. Evaluation of the efficacy and safety of clindamycin plus pyrimethamine for induction and maintenance therapy of toxoplasmic encephalitis in AIDS. Eur J Clin Microb Inf Dis 1991; 10:189-91.

114. Tedesco FJ. Clindamycin and colitis: a review. J Inf Dis 1977; 135:S95-98.

115. Coppola S, Angarano G, Monno L, et al. Adverse effects of clindamycin in the treatment of cerebral toxoplasmosis in AIDS patients. [Abstract] W. B.2333 VII International Conference on AIDS, Florence, Italy, 1991.

116. Chan J, Luft BJ. RU28965: An effective drug in the treatment of murine toxoplasmosis. Antimicrob Ag Chemother 1986; 30:323-7.

117. Chang HR, Rudareang FC, Pechere JC. Activity of 56268 (TE-031) a new macrolide against *Toxoplasma gondii*. Antimicrob Agents Chemother 1988; 32:755-7.

118. Kirst HA, Sides GD. New direction for macrolide antibiotics, pharmacokinetics and clinical efficacy. Antimicrob Agents Chemother 1989; 33:1419-22.

119. Kirst HA, Sides GD. New directions for macrolide antibiotics: structural modifications and in vitro activity. Antimicrob Agents Chemother 1989; 33:1413-18.

120. Huskinson-Mark J, Araujo F, Remington JS. Evaluation of the effect of drugs on the cyst form of *Toxoplasma gondii*. J Inf Dis 1991; 164:170-7.

121. Leport C, Fdez-Maartin J, Morlat P, et al. Combination of pyrimethamine-clarithromycin for acute therapy of toxoplasmic encephalitis. A pilot study. Abstracts from 29th ICAAC, Atlanta, 1990.

122. Luft BJ. Potent in vivo activity of arprinocid, a purine analog, against murine toxoplasmosis. J Infect Dis 1986; 154:692–5.

123. Araujo FG, Huskinson J, Remington JS. Remarkable in vitro and in vivo activities of the hydroxynaph to quinone 566C80 against tachyzoites and tissue cysts of *Toxoplasma gonii*. Antimicrob Agents Chemother 1991; 35: 293–9.

124. Hughes WT, Gray VL, Gutteridge WE, et al. Efficacy of a hydroxynaphthoquinone, 566C80 in experimental *Pneumocystis carinii* pneumonitis. Antimicrob Agents Chemother 1990; 34:225–8.

125. Luft BJ, Hafner R. Toxoplasmic encephalitis. AIDS 1990; 4:593–7.

126. Pedrol E, Gonzalez Clemente JM, Gatell J, et al. Central nervous system toxoplasmosis in AIDS patients: efficacy of an intermittent maintenance therapy. AIDS 1990; 4:511–17.

127. Rolston K. V.I. Treatment of acute toxoplasmosis with oral clindamycin. Eur J Clin Microbiol Infect Dis 1991; 10:181–3.

128. Uberti Foppa C, Bini T, Gregis G, et al. A retrospective study of primary and maintenance therapy of toxoplasmic encephalitis with oral clindamycin and pyrimethamine. Eur J Clin Microbiol Infect Dis 1991; 10:187–9.

129. Clotet B, Sirera G, Romen J, et al. Twice-weekly dapsone-pyrimethamine for preventing PCP and cerebral toxoplasmosis. AIDS 1991; 5:601–2.

130. Zamora L, Mallolas J, Gatell J, et al. Primary prophylaxis for CNS toxoplasmosis (TX) in HIV infected patients. [Abstract] W.B. 2342 VII International Conference on AIDS, Florence, Italy, 1991.

131. Nicholas P, Pierone G, Lin J, Gertman A, Schechter C, Masci J. Trimethoprim-sulfamethoxazole in the prevention of cerebral toxoplasmosis (abstract). Th.B.482, VII International Conference on AIDS, Florence, Italy, 1991.

6

Disseminated *Mycobacterium avium* Complex Infection

Clark B. Inderlied
Children's Hospital Los Angeles and University of Southern California School of Medicine, Los Angeles, California

Carol A. Kemper
Stanford University School of Medicine, Stanford, and Santa Clara Valley Medical Center, San Jose, California

I. INTRODUCTION

Disseminated *Mycobacterium avium* complex (MAC) disease has emerged as perhaps the most debilitating and relentlessly progressive infection in patients with AIDS, limiting both the survival and the quality of life. In the past year, advances in our understanding of this infection and the results of several encouraging clinical treatment trials have challenged the previously held tenet that treatment of this opportunistic infection was both futile and potentially harmful. Recent case-controlled studies indicate that survival is decreased in patients with disseminated MAC compared with noninfected controls and that treatment may enhance survival. A series of clinical trials using various combinations of traditional and investigational antimycobacterial agents demonstrate both modest clinical and microbiological success. The results of these trials suggest there is a correlation between quantitatively determined mycobacteremia and clinical response, providing a microbiological marker of clinical efficacy. Preliminary results from single agent trials of new macrolides, clarithromycin and azithromycin, are very encouraging and await confirmation.

Also, the efficacy of these agents in combination with other active drugs is of great interest. Additional data from several ongoing and recently completed controlled trials, including several single agent studies, will soon be available.

Nevertheless, the incidence of disseminated MAC disease in AIDS patients appears to be increasing, and this disease continues to challenge our clinical acumen and therapeutics. Our knowledge of the epidemiology and pathogenesis of disseminated MAC disease is incomplete; this information is necessary to provide a rational basis for earlier and more effective therapeutic intervention. Unraveling the complex interactions of mycobacteria with the host immune system may lead to exciting breakthroughs in adjunctive immunotherapy. In addition, the discovery of even more effective antimicrobial agents and the correlation of in vitro activity of these agents with clinical effectiveness will lead to the design of optimal combination regimens for the treatment of this infection.

II. MICROBIOLOGY OF THE *MYCOBACTERIUM AVIUM* COMPLEX

A. Classification

Mycobacteria are classified into broad taxonomic groups by general criteria such as pathogenicity, rate of growth at optimum temperatures, and the effect of visible light on pigment production (62,143,158). Accordingly, the *Mycobacterium avium* complex (MAC) is classified as acid-fast, slowly growing bacilli that may produce a yellow pigment in the absence of light (exposure to light often intensifies pigment production).

MAC is a serological complex of 28 serovars of two species, *M. avium* and *M. intracellulare*, which is sometimes extended to included three additional serovars of a third species, *M. scrofulaceum* (160). Serovar distinctions are based on a seroagglutination procedure originally described by Schaefer et al. (148). Later, Brennan (20,21) showed that the serovar specificity was conferred by specific oligosaccharide residues linked to the cell wall glycopeptidolipid. Although most of our knowledge about the epidemiology of MAC disease is based on serovar analysis, the process of serotyping is complex and at times imprecise. Several efforts have been made to clarify the taxonomy of the complex and provide a basis for more precise epidemiological studies. Recently, Wasem et al. (168) examined 35 strains of MAC and other mycobacteria by multilocus enzyme electrophoretic typing. Two distinct clusters were apparent in the resulting dendogram: an *M. intracellulare* cluster and an *M. avium* cluster. When compared with serovar identities, all but one serovar separated into these two clusters.

Three DNA homology groups comprise the *M. avium* complex of mycobacteria (140). DNA homology studies, first performed by Baess (4) and later confirmed by Yoshimura and Graham (179), showed that serovars 1-6 and 8-11 were *M. avium*, whereas serovars 7 and 12-28 were *M. intracellulare*. More recently, Saito et al. (144a), using a DNA-rRNA hybridization system to analyze the species distribution of serovars, concluded that serovar 21 is most likely *M. avium* and that serovars 7, 12-20, and 25 are *M. intracellulare*. However, he also concluded that serovars 22-24 and 26-28 were too disordered to assign a species epithet. Although the results of these studies are partially conflicting, thus making the clinical relevance unclear, these techniques are useful epidemiological tools (see Sections II.B and IV.A).

An important but incompletely understood microbiological feature of MAC is the occurrence of colony type variations. Three colony variants have been described: (1) a smooth, opaque, and domed type; (2) a smooth, translucent, and flat type; and (3) a rough type, only seen in laboratory studies. Clinical isolates of MAC usually appear as smooth translucent or smooth opaque types or as a mixture of these two types. In primary blood cultures, MAC colonies are frequently only of the smooth translucent type, which may not be apparent unless the blood sample has been diluted prior to plating onto Middlebrook 7H11 agar (colony-type variations are not apparent when the organism is grown on egg-based media such as Lowenstein-Jensen). The translucent colony variants are reported to be more resistant to antimicrobial agents (118,139,146), and there is evidence that this variant more readily infects macrophages (9) and is more virulent in animal models of infection (16,148). Stormer and Falkinham (154) isolated nonpigmented colony variants from both environmental sources and clinical material from AIDS patients and showed these variants were significantly more resistant to antimicrobial agents than pigmented segregants of the same strains.

B. Natural Habitat and Environmental Epidemiology

Organisms of the MAC are ubiquitous in nature and are commonly isolated from dust, soil, sediments, water, and aerosols (52,88,165). For humans, the most likely source of exposure to *M. avium* appears to be contaminated water (24,27,40,41,45,63,115,132,152,172). Indeed, mycobacteria have been isolated from the water supplies of some of the largest metropolitan areas in the United States, including the water supply systems of hospitals (24,27,40). Whether all strains of MAC found in the environment are capable of causing disease in patients with AIDS is unclear (see Section IV.A).

Comparisons of MAC isolates revealed that clinical isolates were more likely to contain plasmids than environmental isolates (95), to possess certain growth characteristics, or to display unusual resistance markers (resistance to streptomycin and cadmium) (52). However, of the various environmental sources, only the isolates from aerosols above natural bodies of water frequently possess features common to the clinical isolates (116). Various recent studies indicate that MAC isolates from AIDS patients are no more likely to carry plasmids than MAC isolates from non-AIDS patients. However, MAC serovars 4 and 8 commonly carry small plasmids or sections of plasmids (75,96,121). Environmental isolates of serovars 4 and 8 also carry these distinct plasmids (96). The presence of plasmids may have important clinical significance, since virulence factors have been associated with the presence of plasmids (30,54). In addition, one study suggests that differences in susceptibility to antimicrobial agents may be attributable to plasmids (117). Kunze et al. (107) recently described the presence of an insertion sequence (IS901) in certain strains of MAC which were more virulent in an animal model of infection than other closely related strains; however, this sequence was not present in MAC strains isolated from AIDS patients. Nevertheless, the association of such a genetic element with virulence is an intriguing observation which hopefully will be pursued.

III. LABORATORY DIAGNOSIS

A. Strategy and Alternatives

The laboratory diagnosis of MAC infection in AIDS patients should be directed primarily at identifying those patients with disseminated infection. The detection or isolation of MAC from stools, duodenal biopsy or other gastrointestinal tract specimens, and bronchial washings or other respiratory tract specimens should be interpreted with a certain amount of caution. The finding of MAC in such specimens clearly may be antecedent to the isolation of organisms from blood or other evidence of dissemination (34,39,51,137). However, the presence of MAC isolates in these sites may indicate colonization rather than infection (see Section V.A) (157). Repeated isolation from such potentially colonized sites should facilitate assessment of the clinical significance of such isolates. Neither skin test sensitivity (PPD-B or Battey antigen) nor serological assessment of anti-MAC antibodies by enzyme immunoassay (which is not readily available) are of clinical use (108,170,171,174).

MAC may be cultured from a variety of sterile sites, including bone marrow, liver, spleen, and lymph nodes, and cultures should be done if these tissues are available. However, with recent improvements in techniques, blood culture is an easy, relatively noninvasive, and highly sensitive procedure and, in most circumstances, the procedure of choice for the detection of disseminated disease (47,48,76,101,137). Bacteremia can be detected in 86-98% of patients with disseminated disease, and high grades of bacteremia with 10^4-10^6 colony forming units (cfu) per ml of blood have been commonly reported (68,119,164,175). In one study, colony counts ranged from one to a few hundred to greater than 20,000 cfu/ml of blood, but in tissues such as liver and spleen, the cfu/ml may be a millionfold or higher than in blood (175). Yagupsky and Menegus (176) using the Isolator™ system, concluded that two blood cultures are sufficient to detect MAC bacteremia. In their experience, nearly 20% of these cultures contained only 1 cfu/ml. However, in at least one report bone marrow culture was more sensitive than blood culture for detecting disseminated MAC infection (127a).

Our recent experience suggests that we may be identifying patients earlier in the course of their infection while bacteremia is still low grade (approximately 1-100 cfu/ml). In addition, 6 of 60 (10%) patients enrolled in our recent trial exhibited bacteremias that spontaneously resolved without treatment (C. A. Kemper, unpublished data). These findings may reflect the enhanced sensitivity of blood culture techniques and the use of more aggressive screening protocols for MAC.

The direct examination of blood lymphocytes (buffy coat blood film) may reveal mycobacteria when stained with an acid-fast stain, or when negatively stained with Wright's or Romanovsky's stain (43,60,128). Auramine-rhodamine staining with fluorescent microscopy of bone marrow aspirations also may be of value (162). However, in our experience we have not found these techniques to be clinically useful. They are cumbersome to perform, the positive predictive value is variable (35-86%), and one cannot exclude *M. tuberculosis* bacteremia (43,60,128). Mixed infections can occur, and clinicians and laboratorians should be alert to the possibility that the presence of MAC on the culture plate may obscure the detection of *M. tuberculosis* (43).

Alternate diagnostic procedures may be helpful in certain situations including: 1) the appearance of negative images of bacilli in Romanovsky-stained material from fine needle biopsies of lymph nodes, liver, bone marrow, and bronchoalveolar lavage (153); 2) disseminated MAC infection revealed by cutaneous gallium uptake with whole body imaging (2); 3) endoscopy with biopsy in the diagnosis of upper GI tract MAC disease (120); and 4) abdominal CT scans, which may reveal radiological features of disseminated MAC disease (138).

B. Culture and Identification

Several methods can be used to culture MAC from blood, bone marrow, or other specimens (57,101,147). In general, contaminated specimens, such as respiratory and stool specimens, are processed to eliminate rapidly growing bacteria and yeasts prior to culture. With the radiometric Bactec™ method, a sterile tissue specimen, blood (concentrated or unconcentrated), or decontaminated specimen is inoculated into a liquid medium containing radioactively labeled palmitic acid (Bactec™ TB System, Becton-Dickinson Diagnostic Instrument Systems, Sparks, MD) (76,101,104). The presence of mycobacteria is indicated by the production of ^{14}C-labeled carbon dioxide in 7-14 days. Alternatively a larger volume ($\leqslant$5 ml) of unconcentrated blood is inoculated directly into Bactec™ 13A medium (102,155), a medium developed specifically for detecting mycobacteremia. There is one report that MAC grows in the Bactec™ 6A medium, which is used with the nonradioactive Bactec™ 660 blood culture system (122). However, this requires performing an AFB smear, and *M. tuberculosis* does not grow in this medium.

In addition, specimens can be inoculated onto an agar-based medium such as Middlebrook 7H11 and/or an egg-based medium such as Lowenstein-Jensen using either a conventional plate method (101) or using a new biphasic Septi-Chek™ AFB system developed by Roche Diagnostic Systems, Nutley, NJ. In two reports, the Septi-Chek™ AFB system proved as sensitive or more sensitive than either conventional culture or the Bactec™ radiometric system (33,92).

M. avium, like *M. tuberculosis*, is an intracellular pathogen, and organisms found in blood are most likely to be present in the circulating monocytes. Therefore, lysis of the blood cells using a commercial lysis-centrifugation method (Isolator™, Wampole Laboratories, Cranbury, NJ) appears to significantly improve detection by blood culture (57,101,182). Using blood inoculated with known concentrations of mycobacteria, von Reyn et al. (163) recently demonstrated that MAC isolates remain viable in Isolator™ tubes for at least 7 days. Furthermore, lysis-centrifugation may be used to quantitate the mycobacteremia in terms of cfu/ml. Although this technique is laborious (the high level of the mycobacteremia requires serial dilution of the blood), monitoring the cfu/ml during the course of therapy may provide useful information regarding efficacy in clinical trails. However, the Bactec™ system may provide a convenient and reliable approximation of the level of bacteremia, since there appears to be a good correlation between the rate of growth (days to positive blood culture) in the Bactec™ 13A system and the degree of bacteremia as determined by lysis-centrifugation (67). Bactec™ blood cultures that were positive in less than 7 days had greater than 400 cfu/ml, whereas those that were positive at ≥12 days had low levels of bacteremia (<9 cfu/ml).

MAC colonies tend to be visible sooner and colony morphology is more apparent on agar-based media, while the egg-based media promotes pigment production. In general positive cultures are detected within 7-14 days using the radiometric method, 21-28 days (or longer) by the conventional method (104), and approximately 20 days using the SeptiChek™ AFB system (92). None of the culture methods has proven to be 100% sensitive; therefore, a common strategy is to use a combination of methods. At present the most sensitive system would be a combination of the Bactec™ radiometric system using either 12B or 13A media and the Roche SeptiChek™ AFB system. Positive cultures are routinely confirmed by performing an acid-fast stain on the broth culture or isolated organism. At that point, an experienced mycobacteriologist may be willing to report a presumptive identification based on the growth characteristics and microscopic morphology.

The identification of clinically significant mycobacteria can be achieved within a few hours, once sufficient growth is available, using nonradioactively labeled DNA probes (38,61,110,134,149). Positive broth cultures can be concentrated by centrifugation and directly tested with the probes; some investigators believe the results should be confirmed by testing organisms isolated on solid media (42,133). The DNA probe tests are considered highly specific and sensitive. In a typical evaluation of the probe identification method, 114 MAC isolates were tested with the three available probes and compared with conventional identification (124). Initial results yielded a sensitivity of 93% and a specificity of 97%, but on repeat testing the sensitivity and specificity increased to 97% and 100%, respectively. Lim and co-workers (110) found that the SNAP™ oligonucleotide probes (Syngene, San Diego, CA) were more sensitive than the GenProbe™ probes primarily because 7 isolates that were negative by GenProbe™ assay were positive using the Syngene X-probe. The X-probe detects MAC isolates that do not react with the species-specific probes. By first testing isolates from AIDS patients with the MAC probe or highly characteristic colonies with the *M. tuberculosis* probe, the high cost of these probes can be controlled (38,61). If it is not possible to use DNA probes for identification, conventional methods can be improved by using a strategy that limits the number of biochemical tests (169).

By combining the radiometric method of detection and the DNA probe method of identification, a definitive laboratory diagnosis of disseminated MAC infection should take no longer than 4 weeks. It is not unreasonable for a clinician to expect a reliable detection and presumptive identification of disseminated MAC infection within 7-10 days. The results of studies that have evaluated polymerase chain reaction (PCR) for the direct detection and identification of mycobacteria (to genus and species) should be available soon.

C. Susceptibility Testing

In general, MAC are predictably resistant to isoniazid and only variably susceptible to rifampin and ethambutol (89). The susceptibility profiles of MAC are considerably less uniform than those of *M. tuberculosis*, therefore, it seems warranted to perform in vitro susceptibility tests (Fig. 1) (69,70,74,91,159). However, there are no standardized methods for testing MAC, and there is only limited evidence that in vitro results with MAC isolates correlate with clinical efficacy (82,83).

Most clinical laboratories (in the United States), as a matter of routine, test the MAC against primary and secondary antituberculosis agents by the proportion method. The "critical concentrations" of drugs tested by the proportion method relate to clinical efficacy with *M. tuberculosis*, but the reliability of these criteria has not been demonstrated for guiding the treatment of disseminated MAC infections. Heifets and Iseman (71) have proposed alternate criteria based on the C_{max} of the drug and the corresponding interpretive criteria for *M. tuberculosis*. However, these criteria have not been correlated with therapeutic efficacy in either an animal model or in clinical trials in humans.

As more effective antimicrobial agents are identified for treating MAC infections, in vitro susceptibility tests may be more meaningful. At pres-

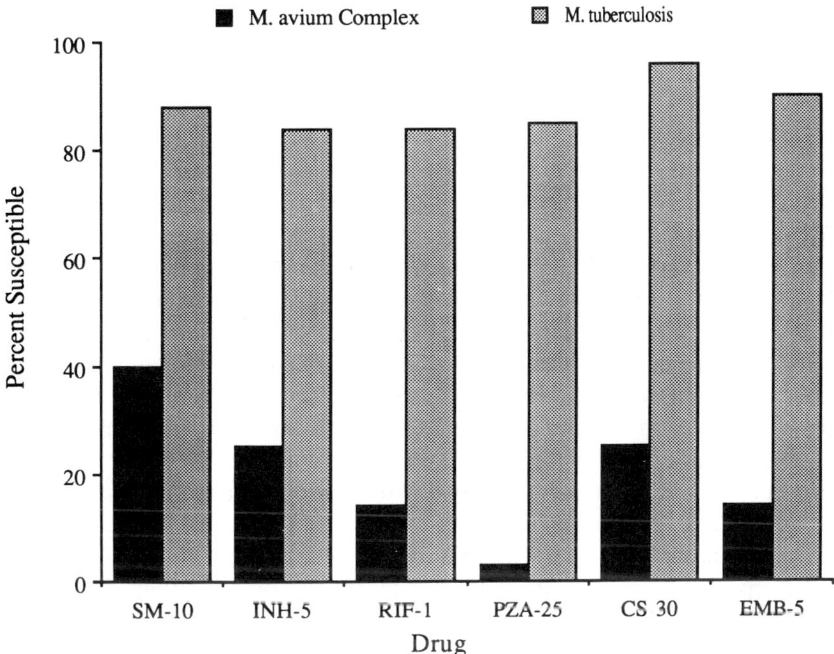

Figure 1 SM-10, streptomycin at 10 μg/ml; INH-5, isoniazid at 5 μg/ml; RIF-1, rifampin at 1 μg/ml; PZA-25, pyrazinamide at 25 μg/ml; CS-30, cycloserine at 30 μg/ml; and EMB-5, ethambutol at 5 μg/ml. (Data taken from Good, RC, Silcox, VA, Kilburn, JO, Plikaytis BD. Clin Microbiol Newsletter, 1985; 7:133-6.)

ent the following conventional agents may be tested: rifampin, ethambutol, amikacin, and clofazimine. Other agents to consider are rifabutin, ethionamide, and the new macrolides, clarithromycin and azithromycin. Criteria for interpretation of the macrolides might be better based on tissue levels than serum levels. It may also be useful to test ciprofloxacin or other fluoroquinolones. Although ciprofloxacin is not active in an animal model of disseminated MAC (90), in vitro, it is active against approximately 30% of MAC isolates.

Although the proportion method of susceptibility testing is most commonly used to test MAC isolates in clinical laboratories, broth dilution test methods that yield a discrete MIC may provide more useful information (89). We recommend using a broth dilution method such as the Bactec™ method or possibly a broth microdilution method (89) and reporting the results as MICs (μg/ml). If the MIC results are interpreted in terms of "susceptible" or "resistant," the interpretive data should be provided with the report to the clinician.

IV. PATHOGENESIS

A. Clinical Epidemiology

For the period 1981 to 1987, the incidence of disseminated nontuberculous mycobacterial infections in AIDS patients as reported by the Centers for Disease Control (CDC) was 5.5% (85). This data was primarily limited to cases of disseminated MAC that were AIDS-defining, and, therefore, this data underestimates the overall prevalence of disseminated disease. Data gathered from autopsy series indicate that the prevalence of disseminated disease varies anywhere from 47%, in one longitudinal study, to as great as 88% (18,164). CDC data indicate that the geographic distribution of MAC in patients is fairly uniform throughout the United States (85). Limited epidemiological data suggest that prior BCG vaccination may provide some protective immunity to infection with MAC (97). There is no apparent sex discrimination. Caucasian, non-Hispanic, HIV-infected patients are more frequently infected with MAC compared with Hispanic, Haitian, and African-American HIV-infected individuals. However, the incidence of tuberculosis is slightly higher in these latter groups (85,119,135). Parenthetically, the incidence of disease due to MAC in non-AIDS patients also is increasing (6,29,129,182), but less than 50% of these cases are caused by the *M. avium* species; i.e., there are significantly more *M. intracellulare* strains isolated from these patients (Fig. 2). This fact may account for the reports of differences in the in vitro susceptibility of MAC isolates from AIDS patients versus non-AIDS patients (23).

Immune deficiency due to HIV infection appears to be the single most significant risk factor for disseminated MAC disease. Less than 20% of MAC infections represent the AIDS-defining illness, while the remainder of cases usually occur late in the course of AIDS. The absolute number of CD4+ cells appears to inversely correlate with the incidence of disseminated infection (80). Several studies suggest that patients with CD4+ counts greater than 100/mm^3 are at less immediate risk for MAC bacteremia than patients with lower CD4 counts (26,81,86,100). There are undoubtedly other complex host factors that have not been elucidated that influence the course of infection either independent of the nature of the infecting strain of MAC or in combination.

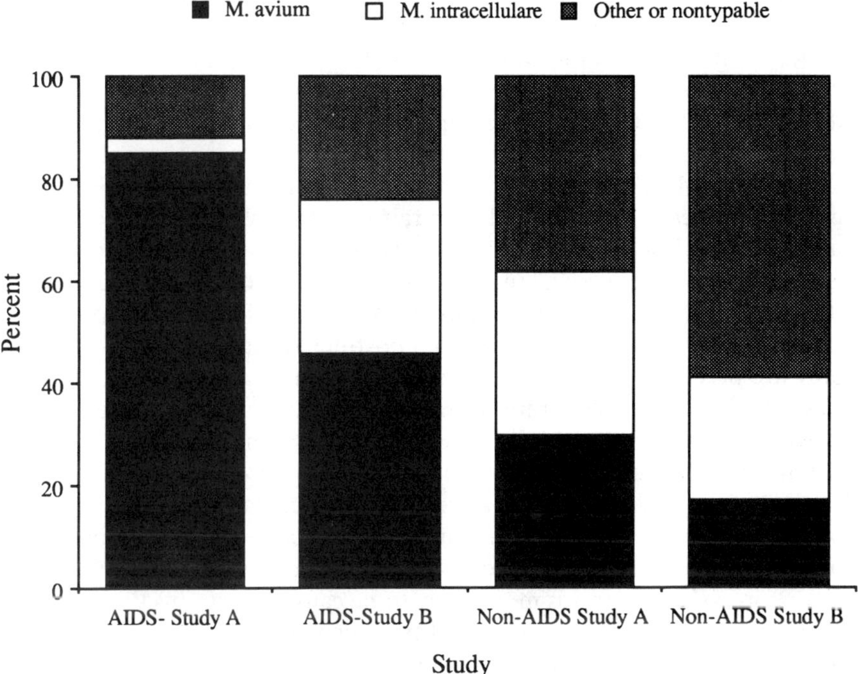

Figure 2 Distribution of *M. avium* and *M. intracellulare* in AIDS and non-AIDS patients based on serovar including all body sites. (Data taken from Yakrus MA and Good RC. J Clin Microbiol 1990; 28:926-9, and Horsburgh et al., Antimicrob Agents Chemother 1986; 30:955-7.)

MAC infection also may be more common in patients from developed countries, like the United States and Europe, than from Third World countries (85). For example, disseminated MAC is uncommon in AIDS patients in Africa (130). An epidemiologically important factor may be the incidence of tuberculosis in Third World populations. Tuberculosis occurs relatively early during the course of HIV infection in comparison with nontuberculous mycobacterial disease, reflecting the greater severity of immune dysfunction necessary to allow nontuberculous disease. In geographical areas with a high incidence of tuberculosis and a high tuberculosis-associated mortality rate, patients may not survive long enough to develop disseminated MAC.

Geographic and species-related differences may also account for different prevalence rates in various populations. MAC strains isolated from patients with AIDS in the United States (103,178,182) and Australia (36) were shown to be predominantly serovars 1, 4, and 8. In contrast, although disseminated MAC disease is comparatively uncommon in Sweden, the predominant serovar isolated from AIDS patients in that country is 6 (77).

Although MAC can be readily isolated from the stools of healthy humans, it is unclear whether all these strains are capable of causing disseminated disease. For example, *M. intracellulare* made up 13% of respiratory isolates in one large survey, but only 1.3% of blood isolates and none of the stool isolates (178). Based on a restriction fragment length polymorphism (RFLP) analysis, Hampson et al. (65) postulated that AIDS patients not only are predominantly infected with *M. avium*, but are infected with a single highly conserved strain of *M. avium*. This intriguing observation suggests that certain strains of MAC possess virulence factors that more readily lead to infection and dissemination. This observation led these investigators to postulate that MAC isolates, which cause disease in AIDS patients, are not simply "opportunistic" gut microflora that gratuitously penetrate the intestine (65). It seems plausible that disseminated MAC infection in AIDS patients is more likely to be caused by strains that possess virulence factors that confer an ability to penetrate and multiply within tissue and contribute to an immune suppression that assures survival within macrophages and other host cells (11,17,31,32,79,126,156,161). Implicit in this postulate is the assumption that there are host immune defects related directly or indirectly to the underlying HIV infection, perhaps in concert with other underlying host factors, that predispose AIDS patients to disseminated infection.

B. Acquisition of Infection

While the initial routes of infection and pathogenesis of dissemination have not yet been fully defined, some authors believe that MAC disease represents a primary infection rather than reactivation (as is typical of tuberculosis); however, the data are often conflicting. For example, Farber et al. found that AIDS patients with disseminated disease lacked antibody to MAC (46); yet others have shown that up to 44% of HIV-positive and 33% of HIV-negative homosexual males have elevated levels of antibodies to type-specific glycopeptidolipid MAC antigens, suggesting frequent exposure to this organism in these individuals (108). In the latter study only 2% of controls had antibodies to the MAC antigens; however, the control group was dissimilar to the experimental groups in several important features. While these data may suggest that homosexual men are more frequently exposed to or colonized with this organism, it is possible that patients who lack antibody are at greater risk of developing disseminated disease.

Both the respiratory and gastrointestinal tracts are suspected portals of entry of infection. Although disseminated disease may be preceded by colonization (68,84), this has not been a uniform observation (157). Some authors have suggested that the gastrointestinal tract is the more likely portal of entry given the high frequency of positive stool cultures in some series, the high frequency of gastrointestinal involvement in autopsy series, the frequent marked degree of mycobacterial gastrointestinal infiltration on histopathological specimens, and a suggested resemblance to Whipple's disease (34,105,141,164,182). Much of these data were collected, however, in patients with disseminated disease.

Although there is little direct evidence that MAC may disseminate from the lung, a smaller series demonstrated that sputum cultures were twice as likely to be positive than stool cultures (66% vs. 33%) (84). Progression to dissemination occurred with equal frequency (33%) in patients with positive respiratory or stool isolates during a mean observation period of 5 months. In another series, 23 of 30 patients with positive respiratory or urine specimens either had or subsequently demonstrated disseminated disease (84). A single nonrandomized trial suggested that early treatment of respiratory isolates prevented dissemination (1). Three of three untreated patients subsequently developed positive blood cultures in contrast to none of three patients treated with a four-drug regimen.

C. Immunological Mechanisms

Impaired cell mediated immunity, impaired oxidative killing, and cytokine disturbances are each important in the pathogenesis of MAC infection in patients with AIDS. However, the specific mechanisms remain undefined. Lymphocyte proliferation and cytokine production are impaired in the presence of mycobacterial antigens (123). Both cytotoxic T cells and normal NK cells kill mycobacterial-laden monocytes (13,99). However, activation of NK cells is impaired in patients with AIDS, in part due to diminished production of IL-2 (112,173). In the presence of MAC, activation of monocyte-macrophages is inadequate and monocyte-macrophage intracellular killing is impaired (9). One author suggested that serum from patients with AIDS may lack a factor that effectively suppresses intracellular mycobacterial growth in normal host macrophages (31). TNF-α and granulocyte-macrophage colony stimulating factor (GM-CSF) stimulate superoxide anion production and modestly increase intracellular killing of MAC, but IL-2 alone does not (10,15,136). Defects in vitamin D metabolism may mediate macrophage production of TNF-α and GM-CSF (14). Anti-GM-CSF antibody markedly impaired 1,25(OH$_2$)-D$_3$-dependent macrophage activation, but there was only modest inhibition by anti-TNF antibody.

Data on INF-γ is conflicting. Increased phagocytosis and decreased intracellular growth occurred in response to IFN-γ (15,37,150), particularly in the presence of indomethacin and vitamin D$_3$, but an initial period of enhanced replication was observed in one study (15). IL-1, IL-3, and M-CSF also appear to enhance replication (37). A recently identified heat-shock protein from MAC selectively interferes with superoxide anion production, diminishes macrophage responses to IFN-γ, and interferes with host cell transcriptional activity (7,8). The clinical significance of these observations remains to be determined, but may provide exciting avenues for future immunotherapy.

V. CLINICAL MANIFESTATIONS IN PATIENTS WITH AIDS

A. Focal Disease

MAC is not uncommonly isolated from respiratory and stool culture specimens obtained from patients with severe HIV disease, and such isolation should prompt a more thorough search for evidence of focal or disseminated disease (68,180). Distinction between primary infection without disease (colonization), primary infection with disease, and secondary infection as a manifestation of dissemination is, at times, difficult. As these organisms are ubiquitous in nature, especially in water, culture contamination is possible (64). Patients may have transient respiratory colonization with a single positive culture or episodic excretion of MAC without disease. There is, at present, no controlled data that indicates whether therapy is of benefit in these patients.

Signs and symptoms of MAC pulmonary disease, including cough, dyspnea, and fever, are nonspecific, but the presentation is generally milder than that of tuberculosis (119,167). Recommended diagnostic criteria for patients with noncavitary pulmonary disease caused by nontuberculous mycobacteria include 1) the presence of two or more sputum specimens that are AFB smear-positive or that produce heavy growth on culture, and 2) failure to clear cultures with good pulmonary toilet or 2 weeks of antimycobacterial therapy (167). These guidelines may not, however, apply to severely immunocompromised patients. In the absence of adequate clinical data, HIV-positive patients with sputum repeatedly culture-positive for MAC and persistent respiratory symptoms or evidence of radiographic disease, not attributable to another pathogen, should be considered candidates for antimycobacterial therapy.

B. Disseminated Disease

Signs and symptoms of disseminated MAC in persons with AIDS are nonspecific, but patients characteristically present with recurrent daily episodes of fever, frequently with very high temperatures, chills, profuse night sweats, weakness, malaise, anorexia, and inexorably progressive weight loss (100,119,164). Between episodes of fever, the patient may look and feel relatively well. Diarrhea occurs in almost one-half of the patients and nausea and vomiting in less than one-fourth. Intractable, crampy abdominal pain occurs in some patients, possibly due to gastrointestinal, hepatosplenic, or retroperitoneal nodal involvement. Severe anemia may be a predictor of disseminated MAC disease, and patients may require frequent transfusions (26,80). On examination, hepatosplenomegaly is not uncommon, but significant peripheral lymphadenopathy (< 1.0 cm) is unusual ($< 10\%$ of cases). Unusual sites of infection include skin (127), bone and joints (19), eyes (68), large airways (131), and brain. Isolation of MAC from cerebrospinal fluid is unusual, but may occur in disseminated disease (93).

C. Delayed Identification of AFB Smears or Cultures

More problematic is the delayed identification of AFB visualized by smear from respiratory secretions, tissue specimens or stool smears. Several clues may facilitate the evaluation of the patient with infection with an unidentified mycobacterium (Table 1). Although there is no apparent age or sex discrimination, Caucasian, non-Hispanic patients are more likely to be infected with MAC, whereas Hispanic, Haitian, and African-American individuals are more likely to be infected with *M. tuberculosis* (85,119, 135). Tuberculosis may be slightly more common in inner city intravenous drug users as well as women (49) than in otherwise similar risk groups.

Chest roentgenograms are abnormal in more than 80% of patients with tuberculosis, whereas pneumonitis, with evidence of patchy or nodular infiltrates, occurs in only 4-9% of patients with MAC (119,142). Media-

Table 1 Pertinent Clinical, Radiographic, and Laboratory Features Relevant to the Differentiation of Disease in an HIV-Infected Patient with an Unidentified Mycobacterium

M. avium complex	*M. tuberculosis*
Caucasian, non-Hispanic individuals are more likely to have MAC	African-Americans, Hispanics, Haitians, and intravenous drug users are more likely to have tuberculosis
>90% have preexisting AIDS	The majority do not have AIDS (70%)
CD4 counts are rarely >100/mm^3	Occurs at any level of immunity
Pneumonitis is unusual (4-10%)	Pulmonary involvement occurs in 70%
Abnormal chest roentgenograms are uncommon (25%)	Chest roentgenograms are frequently abnormal (83%)
Cavitary disease, hilar lymphadenopathy, and effusions are unusual	Hilar lymphadenopathy is common (25%), and cavitary disease and pleural effusions may occur
Sputum smears may be positive (16%)	Sputum smears are frequently positive (60%)
Sputum cultures may be positive (25%)	Sputum cultures are frequently positive (70%)
Extrapulmonary disease is common	Extrapulmonary disease is common
Stool smears and cultures are positive in 40-50%	Stool smears and cultures are positive in 40-50%
Bacteremia occurs in >85% of patients with disseminated disease	Bacteremia occurs in 2-12%
Blood cultures may be positive within 6-14 days	Blood cultures may take 4-8 weeks

Source: Refs. 85,119,167.

stinal and hilar lymphadenopathy is unusual and cavitary disease and pleural effusions are rare in patients with MAC. Cavities caused by MAC tend to be thin walled and with less surrounding infiltrate than those caused by *M. tuberculosis*. The presence of pneumonitis in a patient with positive sputum or lavage cultures for MAC more likely signals concurrent infection with a second pathogen (113). In patients with positive respiratory cultures, sputum smears are more likely to be positive in patients with tuberculosis than MAC (83% vs. 25%). Blood cultures are frequently positive in disseminated MAC, commonly within 6-14 days (reflecting the unusually high grade of bacteremia), in contrast to patients with tuberculosis. However, MAC and *M. tuberculosis* are visualized in smears and isolated with fairly equal frequency from lymph nodes, bone marrow, and stool specimens.

Furthermore, the onset of mycobacterial disease relative to the onset of AIDS may be helpful in distinguishing between tuberculosis and MAC disease. Tuberculosis characteristically precedes the diagnosis of AIDS

40-67% of the time, and occurs as the AIDS-defining illness or concurrent with AIDS 26% of the time (119,151). In contrast, only 3-13% of MAC infections represent the AIDS-defining illness, frequently concurrent with another opportunistic infection, and the remainder of cases usually occur late in the course of AIDS. Several studies suggest that patients with CD4+ counts greater than 100/mm³ are at less immediate risk for MAC bacteremia than patients with lower CD4+ counts (26,81,86,100). A recent study demonstrated that three consecutive blood cultures yielded MAC at least once in 14 of 39 (36%) symptomatic HIV-infected patients with CD4 counts less than 100/mm³ versus none of the 41 symptomatic patients with CD4+ counts greater than 100/mm³ (66).

VI. TREATMENT OF INFECTION

A. Therapeutic Agents

To date, the agents most commonly used in clinical trials include orally administered ciprofloxacin, clofazimine, ethambutol, isoniazid, rifampin, and parenterally administered amikacin (Table 2). Clofazimine is an analine dye with a remarkably long elimination half-life (56). It is orally administered in a 100- to 200-mg daily dose (300-mg daily doses have been used in the treatment of other diseases), and it is very well-tolerated with few dose limiting adverse effects. It is a mainstay of leprosy therapy, is highly concentrated within tissues, and has considerable in vitro activity against most MAC isolates. In the beige mouse model, it remains one of the most effective mycobacterial agents at serum concentrations achievable in humans, particularly in combination with amikacin (55,111). In vitro susceptibility data suggest that *M. avium* and *M. intracellulare* are similar in their susceptibility to clofazimine (159). The MIC 90% (MIC which inhibits 90% of strains tested) values for clofazimine against *M. avium* are 1.6 and 3.13 μg/ml for environmental source and human isolates, respectively; against *M. intracellulare* the MIC 90% is 1.6 μg/ml.

Ethambutol is a dextro-2,2′-(ethylenediimino)-di-1-butanol-dihydrochloride with a high degree of antituberculous activity. It is well tolerated in the treatment of MAC disease and is commonly administered in a dosage of 15 mg/kg weight per day, usually as a single orally administered dose. Higher doses (25 mg/kg weight) have been used, but may be associated with ocular complications such as retrobulbar neuritis. These side effects are uncommon, typically associated with long-term use (longer than one month), and, in most cases, are reversible. A recent analysis

Table 2 Antimycobacterial Agents Commonly Used in the Treatment of *M. avium* Complex Infection in Patients with AIDS

Agent	Adult dose	Pediatric dose	Adverse effects
Amikacin	7.5 mg/kg QD-BID IV	7.5 mg/kg QD-BID IV	Ototoxicity, nephrotoxicity
Ciprofloxacin	750 mg BID	Not approved for under 18 yr	Anorexia, nausea, vomiting, abdominal pain, diarrhea, rash, rarely mental status changes, seizure
Clofazimine	100-300 mg/day	No recommendation	Skin discoloration, ichthyosis, anorexia, nausea, vomiting, abdominal pain, rarely ocular changes
Ethambutol	15 mg/kg/day (25 mg/kg max)	10-15 mg/kg/day	Anorexia, nausea, vomiting, diarrhea, rash, optic neuritis, mental status changes
Rifampin	10 mg/kg/day (600 mg/day max)	10 mg/kg/day (600 mg/day max)	Anorexia, nausea, vomiting, diarrhea, rash rarely hepatitis
Alternative agents			
Ethionamide	30 mg/kg/day (250 mg BID initially, 1.0 g/day max)	15-20 mg/kg/day	Anorexia, nausea, vomiting, diarrhea, rash, hepatitis, mental status changes, seizures, neuropathy
Cycloserine	500-1000 mg/day (250 mg BID initially, 1 g/day max)	10-20 mg/kg/day (1 g/day max)	Somnolence, headache, vertigo, tremor, mental status changes, visual changes, seizures
New agents			
Rifabutin	300-600 mg/day	No recommendation	Nausea, dyspepsia, diarrhea, abdominal pain, fever, flulike symptoms, headache, rash, leukopenia
Azithromycin	300-600 mg/day	10 mg/kg/day (max 600 mg/day)	Nausea, diarrhea, abdominal pain, vomiting
Clarithromycin	500-1000 mg BID	No recommendation	Nausea, diarrhea, abdominal pain, vomiting

demonstrated that only 7% of MAC isolates were sensitive to 5 μg/ml of ethambutol, but 76% of isolates were sensitive to 10 μg/ml (114). Additional in vitro studies showed MIC 90% values for ethambutol against *M. avium* were 25 and 50 μg/ml for environmental source and human isolates, respectively. Against *M. intracellulare* these values were 12.5 and 25 μg/ml, respectively (159). Although these results suggest that ethambutol is not active against many strains as a single agent, ethambutol may potentiate the activity of other agents (177) because of the influence of this agent on cell wall permeability (78,98).

Rifampin is a 3-4(4-methylpiperazinyl-iminomethylidene)-rifamycin SV and is in the rifamycin group of antimicrobials. The recommended dose for the treatment of MAC disease is 600 mg as a single daily dose for patients weighing 50 kg or more (typically 10 mg/kg weight). It is well absorbed when taken without food, and a peak serum concentration of approximately 10 μg/ml occurs within 2 hours of administration. It is fairly well tolerated in patients with AIDS, but approximately 10-15% of patients will demonstrate dose-limiting intolerance (100,151). The concentrations in tissues are significantly higher than serum concentrations; rifampin concentration is five times the extracellular concentration in human monocytes and four times that in mouse macrophages (145). Differences in serovars and in human versus environmental strains greatly impact susceptibility data (159), but many isolates demonstrate high levels of resistance with MIC values greater than 100 μg/ml (114).

Ciprofloxacin and other fluoroquinolones (e.g., sparfloxacin, temafloxacin, and WIN 57273) have shown variable in vitro activity against MAC (73,90,109,181). In the treatment of MAC, ciprofloxacin is commonly administered in a dosage of 750 mg twice daily, and it is fairly well tolerated, although dose-limiting side effects occur in up to 15% of patients. In vitro susceptibility data suggest that *M. avium* may be slightly more susceptible to the fluoroquinolones than *M. intracellulare*. The MIC 90% values of ciprofloxacin against *M. avium*, as determined by broth dilution susceptibility tests, are 6.25 and 12.5 μg/ml for environmental and human isolates, respectively; against *M. intracellulare*, 12.5 μg/ml (159).

Amikacin, one of the first agents shown to be active against the MAC, remains one of the most bactericidal agents in vitro and in the animal model (53,55,90). Amikacin is a semisynthetic aminoglycoside antibiotic derived from kanamycin. Amikacin is not orally absorbed from the gastrointestinal tract and is administered by either the intravenous or intramuscular route in a dosage of 7.5-15 mg/kg body weight/day. The most significant adverse effects are otoxicity and nephrotoxicity, which develop in approximately 13% of aptients with AIDS (100). Ototoxicity consists of primarily cochlear dysfunction and occasional vestibular dysfunction, both of which are usually irreversible. These toxicities are commonly associated with prolonged administration, elevated peak serum concentrations greater than 30 μg/ml, and persistently elevated trough serum concentrations greater than 10 μg/ml. Analysis of in vitro susceptibilities with clinical isolates indicate that only 9% of MAC isolates are susceptible to 12 μg/ml of amikacin, but 75% of MAC isolates are susceptible to 30 μg/ml (114).

Rifabutin, another rifamycin, has slightly better in vitro activity against MAC compared with rifampin. It has been used in a few modestly successful combination regimens, but the individual contribution of this agent is unknown (1,86). It is well absorbed from the gastrointestinal tract, and serum concentrations are approximately one-tenth that of rifampin. Although plasma levels are low, tissue concentrations are several times higher—15 times the extracellular concentration within human monocytes (145).

Although isoniazid has been used as a component of combination therapies, the drug is inactive in vitro against a majority of MAC isolates (89) and the inclusion of this agent in a specifically anti-MAC treatment regimen must be questioned. Similarly, pyrazinamide, *p*-aminosalicylic acid, and capreomycin should not be considered for treatment of MAC infections.

B. Therapeutic Recommendations

Although several previous clinical trials have demonstrated some degree of clinical and microbiological efficacy, there is no generally accepted therapy for disseminated MAC infection in patients with AIDS (Table 3) (1,3,28,86,100,114,166). Combination regimens of at least two to six antimycobacterial agents have been recommended based on data in non-AIDS patients with MAC pulmonary disease, which suggests a relationship between the number of agents administered and efficacy (44). Some authors have recommended an "induction" regimen of 4-6 agents for 1-2 months, followed by a less toxic "maintenance" regimen of two to three agents (182). However, such intensive regimens may not result in any greater microbiological efficacy and are frequently administered at the expense of ease and tolerance. Thus, while the ultimate goal of therapy is eradication of systemic disease, until the development of better regimens, a more reasonable goal of therapy may be suppression of clinical symptoms using as few agents as possible. In this regard, the selection of therapy is frequently individualized with the aggressiveness of therapy modulated by individual patient considerations.

In the past, without controlled data suggesting clinical benefit, prolonged survival, or enhanced quality of life, some physicians elected to forgo therapy (25,106). Recent data contradict this practice. Case-control studies have identified disseminated MAC as an independent risk factor for early mortality (26) and indicated that treatment may enhance survival (81). Several studies confirm a decrease in survival of AIDS patients with disseminated MAC compared with noninfected controls (80,94). Furthermore, a reduction in the degree of MAC bacteremia with therapy may be associated with amelioration of clinical symptoms (28,100). In two limited surveys, quantitative colony counts were variably reduced by combinations of isoniazid, ethambutol, ethionamide, rifampin, ansamycin, clofazimine, and amikacin (68,100). Two recent studies indicate that significant reductions in colony counts can be achieved as early as the second week of therapy (28,100). The first of these trials, utilizing a combination of rifampin, ethambutol, ciprofloxacin, and amikacin, demonstrated reduction in colony counts of 1.5 log cfu/ml by the fourth week of therapy (28). In a subsequent trial, a comparable reduction was seen when orally administered clofazimine was substituted for amikacin (100).

Based on the favorable clinical and microbiological results of this and another recent trial, combination therapy with ciprofloxacin, clofazimine, ethambutol, and rifampin has been recommended for patients with disseminated MAC disease (80,100). In one multicenter trial, approximately 75% of the patients demonstrated a significant clinical response (despite evidence of persistent low-grade bacteremia in some), and 42% became blood culture negative (100). However, clinical response did not usually occur until the third to fourth week of therapy. Opportunistic infection, other than MAC, was documented in 70% of patients with continued or recurrent fever after 4 weeks of therapy. Thus, the occurrence of fever beyond 4 weeks should prompt a search for etiologies other than MAC.

Even with this entirely oral regimen, adverse effects of therapy were common, and almost one-half of the patients were forced to discontinue at least one agent because of intolerance (100). The condition of several patients was adversely impacted by the institution of therapy and, despite the beneficial effect observed, most patients continued to have progressive weight loss. For these reasons, we recommend starting with two well-tolerated agents, with gradual sequential addition of one or more agents (as tolerated) during the first 1-2 weeks. Parenterally administered amikacin or other second-line therapies should probably be reserved for those patients who remain symptomatic after 4 weeks of oral therapy. Although there is little evidence that in vitro susceptibility data correlates to any

Table 3 Clinical and Microbiological Results of Patients with *Mycobacterium avium* Complex Bacteremia Treated with Various Combination Antimycobacterial Regimens

Method of evaluation	No. of patients	Daily therapeutic regimen	Duration of therapy	Clinical results	Microbiological results	Ref.
Review	26	Ansamycin 150-300 mg, clofazimine 300 mg, ethionamide 750 mg or ethambutal 15 mg/kg, (± rifampin, isoniazid, etc.)	Variable, 4-30 weeks, (mean 6 wks)	—	2/26 blood culture negative (but with disease at autopsy), 3 others with decreased counts	68
Prospective	13	Ansamycin 150-300 mg; clofazimine 100 mg (± amikacin 15 mg/kg)	Variable	1/13 with clinical improvement	6/13 blood culture negative (2 with later recurrence)	114
Review	25	Ansamycin 300-600 mg, clofazimine 100 mg, ethambutol 15 mg/kg, isoniazid 300 mg	Indefinite, 6-74 weeks (median 38 weeks)	21/25 with clinical improvement	22/25 blood culture negative (6 with later recurrence)	86

Prospective trial	7	Ansamycin 150 mg, clofazimine 100 mg, ethambutol 15 mg/kg, isoniazid 300 mg	Indefinite	6/7 with clinical improvement	6/7 blood culture negative (1 with later recurrence)	1
Prospective trial	17	Amikacin 7.5 mg/kg (d0-28) ciprofloxacin 750 mg BID, ethambutol 1000 mg rifampin 600 mg	12 weeks	7/17 with clinical improvement	Colony counts decreased $-1.5 \log_{10}$ at wk 4 and $-2.1 \log_{10}$ at wk 12; 3/17 culture negative	28
Prospective trial	16	Ciprofloxacin 750 mg BID, clofazimine 100 mg, ethambutol 400 mg BID, rifampin 300 BID	Variable, 4-24 weeks	12/16 with clinical improvement	—	82
Prospective trial	31	Ciprofloxacin 750 mg BID, clofazimine 100-200 mg, ethambutol 15 mg/kg, rifampin 600 mg, (amikacin 7.5 mg/kg, d29-56 in a subset of patients)	12 weeks (mean 8 weeks)	27/31 with clinical improvement	Colony counts decreased $-1.5 \log_{10}$ at wk 4 and $-2.1 \log_{10}$ at wk 12; 13/31 blood culture negative	100

significant degree with in vivo efficacy, it may provide a guide for further modification of therapy in certain cases (72,82). Quantitative mycobacterial cultures may provide a marker of microbiological efficacy. Both pieces of information, however, lag behind the real-time need for clinical decision making.

Many clinicians, when faced with a febrile patient at risk for disseminated MAC infection, offer empiric antimycobacterial therapy. This may be reasonable in certain cases provided other causes of fever have been eliminated, adequate cultures obtained, and the need for continued therapy reevaluated on an ongoing basis.

The optimal duration of treatment in patients with disseminated MAC has yet to be determined. Limited evidence suggests that there is a rapid resurgence of bacteremia upon discontinuation of therapy (100). Therefore, therapy should probably be continued indefinitely or, at a minimum, for several months after sterilization of blood cultures. Concurrent anti-retroviral therapy should be continued as tolerated and may act to further enhance the microbiological response (5).

Children with disseminated MAC infection present with signs and symptoms that are similar to those of adults and are usually comparably severely immunodeficient (22,87); however, there is little data on the optimal management of these individuals.

C. Newer Therapeutic Avenues

Several clinical centers and laboratories are currently evaluating the contribution of individual agents to combination therapy as well as the predictive value of in vitro susceptibility testing. Agents currently under investigation include clofazimine, ethambutol, rifampin, ansamycin, sparfloxacin, trospectomycin, liposomal-encapsulated gentamicin, azithromycin, and clarithromycin. Improved formulations of combination therapy await these results.

Clarithromycin, a macrolide similar in structure to erythromycin, inhibited 90% of strains tested in vitro at MIC values that are therapeutically achievable (50,125). When tested in a murine model of disseminated MAC disease, clarithromycin treatment resulted in a significant decrease in the number of mycobacteria in tissue and blood (50). In a recent clinical trial, 6 of 8 patients who received 6 weeks of clarithromycin therapy alone had negative blood cultures, but 5 of 6 patients had low-level bacteremia ($\leqslant 27$ cfu/ml) at baseline (35). In another trial, a combination of clarithromycin and clofazimine resulted in clearance of bacteremia in all 11 patients after 1 week of therapy (144).

Azithromycin, another new generation macrolide (azalide), is a very promising agent with a remarkable ability to penetrate tissues and concentrate within macrophages (12,58,59). The in vitro activity of azithromycin in broth appears modest with MICs 16- to 32-fold above the serum concentration of the drug; however, the tissue concentrations of azithromycin may reach 2000 μg/g (or higher) without toxicity. A recent uncontrolled clinical trial showed that when patients received 20-30 days of azithromycin (500 mg/day) there was a significant decrease in the mycobacteremia and amelioration of fever, night sweats, and splenomegaly (183). The results of additional and expanded clinical trials with both clarithromycin and azithromycin are eagerly awaited. Liposomal encapsulated agents, including amikacin, gentamicin, and clofazimine analogs, also are currently under investigation. Finally, there is growing interest in the role of immunomodulator therapy as an adjunct to antimicrobial therapy, especially the use of GM-CSF.

ACKNOWLEDGMENTS

This work was supported in part by a contract from the National Institute of Allergy and Infectious Diseases, AI-73637, and the California University-wide AIDS Research Program, R91-CC86SD.

REFERENCES

1. Agins BD, Berman DS, Spicehandler D, El-Sadr W, Simberkoff MS, Rahal JJ. Effect of combined therapy with ansamycin, clofazimine, ethambutol, and isoniazid for *Mycobacterium avium* infection in patients with AIDS. J Infect Dis 1989; 159:784–7.

2. Allwright S, Chapman P, Antico V, Gruenewald S. Cutaneous gallium uptake in patients with AIDS with *Mycobacterium avium-intracellulare* septicemia. Clin Nucl Med 1988; 13:506-8.

3. Bach MC. Treating disseminated *Mycobacterium avium-intracellulare* infection. Ann Intern Med 1989; 110:169-70.

4. Baess I. Deoxyribonucleic acid relationships between different serovars of *Mycobacteriuim avium, Mycobacterium intracellulare,* and *Mycobacterium scrofulaceum.* Acta Pathol Microbiol Immunol Scand 1983; 91:201-3.

5. Bautista G, Alcid D, Gocke D. Quantitative blood culture (QBC) for mycobacteria in patients with acquired immunodeficiency syndrome (AIDS). In: Program and abstracts of the 31st Interscience Conference on Antimicrobial Agents and Chemotherapy, Chicago, 1991:139.

6. Bennett C, Vardiman J, Golomb H. Disseminated atypical mycobacterial infection in patients with hairy cell leukemia. Am J Med 1986; 80:891–6.

7. Bermudez L, Claesgens J, Young LS, Wu M. 33KDa protein from *Mycobacterium avium* complex (MAC) binds to macrophage DNA and interferes with cytokine-mediated stimulation. In: Abstracts of the 91st General Meeting of the American Society of Microbiology, Dallas, 1991:U-48.

8. Bermudez LE, Petrofsky M, Young LS, Martinelli J. Stress conditions upregulate the expression of virulence *Mycobacterium avium* complex (MAC) proteins. In: Abstracts of the 91st General Meeting of the American Society of Microbiology, Dallas, 1991; U-51.

9. Bermudez LE, Young LS. Phagocytosis and intracellular killing of *Mycobacterium avium* complex by human and murine macrophages. Braz J Med Biol Res 1987; 20:191–201.

10. Bermudez LE, Young LS. Recombinant granulocyte-macrophage colony-stimulating factor activates human macrophages to inhibit growth or kill *Mycobacterium avium* complex. J Leuk Biol 1990; 48:67–73.

11. Bermudez LEM, Wu M, Young LS. Intracellular killing of *Mycobacterium avium* complex by rifapentine and liposome-encapsulated amikacin. J Infect Dis 1987; 156:510–3.

12. Bermudez LEM, Young LS. Activities of amikacin, roxithromycin, and azithromycin alone or in combination with tumor necrosis factor against *Mycobacterium avium* complex. Antimicrob Agents Chemother 1988; 32:1149–53.

13. Bermudez LEM, Young LS. Natural killer cell-dependent mycobacteriostatic and mycobactericidal activity in human macrophages. J Immunol 1991; 146:265–70.

14. Bermudez LEM, Young LS, Gupta S. 1,25 Dihydroxyvitamin D_3-dependent inhibition of growth or killing of *Mycobacterium avium* complex in human macrophages is mediated by TNF and GM-CSF. Cell Immunol 1990; 127:432–41.

15. Bermudez LM, Young LS. Tumor necrosis factor, alone or in combination with IL-2, but not IFN-g, is associated with macrophage killing of *Mycobacterium avium* complex. J Immunol 1988; 140:3006–13.

16. Bertram MA, Inderlied CB, Yadegar S, Kolanski P, Yamada JK, Young LS. Confirmation of the beige mouse model for study of disseminated infection with *Mycobacterium avium* complex. J Infect Dis 1986; 154:194.

17. Black CM, Bermudez LE, Young LS, Remington JS. Co-infection of macrophages modulates interferon gamma and tumor necrosis factor-induced activation against intracellular pathogens. J Exp Med 1990; 172:977–80.

18. Blaser MJ, Cohn DL. Opportunistic infections in patients with AIDS: clues to the epidemiology of AIDS and the relative virulence of pathogens. Rev Infect Dis 1986; 8:21-30.

19. Blumenthal DR, Zucker JR, Hawkins CA. *Mycobacterium avium* complex-induced septic arthritis and osteomyelitis in a patient with the acquired immunodeficiency syndrome. Arthritis Rheum 1990; 33:757–8.

20. Brennan PJ. Structures of the typing antigens of atypical mycobacteria: a brief review of present knowledge. Rev Infect Dis 1981; 3:905–13.

21. Brennan PJ. Structure of mycobacteria: recent developments in defining cell wall carbohydrates and proteins. Rev Infect Dis 1989; 11:S420–30.

22. Butler KM, Husson RN, Mueller BU, Fowler CL, Pizzo PA. Defining the population of HIV-infected children at risk for *Mycobacterium avium intracellulare* (MAI). In: Program and Abstracts of the 31st Interscience Conference on Antimicrobial Agents and Chemotherapy, Chicago, 1991:139.

23. Byrne SKG, Geddes GL, Isaac-Renton JL, Black WA. Comparison of in vitro antimicrobial susceptibilities of *Mycobacterium avium-M. intracellulare* strains from patients with acquired immunodeficiency syndrome (AIDS), patients without AIDS, and animal sources. Antimicrob Agents Chemother 1990; 34:1390–2.

24. Carson LA, Petersen NJ, Favero MS, Aguero SM. Growth characteristics of atypical mycobacteria in water and their comparative resistance to disinfectants. Appl Environ Microbiol 1978; 36:839–46.

25. Chaisson RE, Hopewell PC. Mycobacteria and AIDS mortality. Am Rev Respir Dis 1989; 139:1–3.

26. Chaisson RE, Keruly J, Richman DD, Creagh-Kirk T, Moore RD. Incidence and natural history of *Mycobacterium avium* complex infection in advanced HIV disease treated with zidovudine. Am Rev Respir Dis 1991; 143:A278.

27. Chapman JS. The ecology of the atypical mycobacteria. Arch Environ Health 1976; 22:41–6.

28. Chiu J, Nussbaum J, Bozette S, Tilles JG, Young LS, Leedom J, Heseltine PNR, McCutchan JA. Treatment of disseminated *Mycobacterium avium* complex infection in AIDS with amikacin, ethambutol, rifampin, and ciprofloxacin. Ann Intern Med 1990; 113:358–61.

29. Contreras MA, Chenung OT, Sanders DE, Goldstein RS. Pulmonary infection with nontuberculous mycobacteria. Am Rev Respir Dis 1988; 137:149–52.

30. Crawford JT, Bates JH. Analysis of plasmids in *Mycobacterium avium-intracellulare* isolates from persons with acquired immunodeficiency syndrome. Am Rev Respir Dis 1986; 134:659–61.

31. Crowle AJ, Cohn DL, and Poche P. Defects in sera from acquired immunodeficiency syndrome (AIDS) patients and from non-AIDS patients from *Mycobacterium avium* complex infection which decrease macrophage resistance to *M. avium*. Infect Immunol 1989; 57:1445–51.

32. Crowle AJ, Dahl R, Ross E, May MH. Evidence that vesicles containing living, virulent *Mycobacterium tuberculosis* or *Mycobacterium avium* in cultured human macrophages are not acidic. Infect Immunity 1991; 59:1823–31.

33. D'Amato RF, Isenberg HD, Hochstein L, Mastellone AJ, Alperstein P. Evaluation of the Roche Septi-Chek AFB system for recovery of mycobacteria. J Clin Microbiol 1991; 29:2906–8.

34. Damsker B, Bottone EJ. *Mycobacterium avium-Mycobacterium intracellulare* from the intestinal tracts of patients with acquired immunodeficiency syndrome: concepts regarding acquisition and pathogenesis. J Infect Dis 1985; 151:179–81.

35. Dautzenberg B, Truffot C, Legris S, Meyohas M-C, Berlie HC, Mercat A, Grosset J. Activity of clarithromycin against *Mycobacterium avium* infection in patients with the acquired immune deficiency syndrome. Am Rev Respir Dis 1991; 144:564–9.

36. Dawson DJ. Infection with *Mycobacterium avium* complex in Australian patients with AIDS. Med J Aust 1990; 153:466–8.

37. Denis M, Gregg EO. Recombinant tumor necrosis factor-alpha decreases whereas recombinant interleukin-6 increases growth of a virulent strains of *Mycobacterium avium* in human macrophages. Immunol 1990; 71:139–41.

38. Drake TA, Herron RM, Hindler JA, Berlin OGW, Bruckner DA. DNA probe reactivity of *Mycobacterium avium* complex isolates from patients without AIDS. Diagn Microbiol Infect Dis 1988; 11:125–8.

39. Dryden MS, Shanson DC. The microbial causes of diarrhoea in patients infected with the human immunodeficiency virus. J Infect 1988; 17:107–14.

40. DuMoulin GC, Stottmeier KD. Waterborne mycobacteria: an increasing threat to health. ASM News 1986; 52:525–9.

41. DuMoulin GC, Stottmeier KD, Pelletier PA, Tsang AY, W JH. Concentration of *Mycobacterium avium* by hospital hot water systems. J Am Med Assoc 1988; 260:1599–1602.

42. Ellner PD, Kiehn TE, Cammarata R, Hosmer M. Rapid detection and identification of pathogenic mycobacteria by combining radiometric and nucleic acid probe methods. J Clin Microbiol 1988; 26:1349–52.

43. Eng RHK, Bishburg E, Smith SM, Mangia A. Diagnosis of *Mycobacterium* bacteremia in patients with acquired immunodeficiency syndrome by direct examination of blood films. J Clin Microbiol 1989; 27:768–9.

44. Etzkorn ET, Sigfredo A, McAllister CK, Matthels J, Ognebene AJ. Medical therapy of *Mycobacterium avium-intracellulare* pulmonary disease. Am Rev Respir Dis 1986; 134:442–5.

45. Falkinham JO, Parker BC, Groft H. Epidemiology of infection by nontuberculous mycobacteria. 1. Geographic distribution in the Eastern United States. Am Rev Respir Dis 1980; 121:931–7.

46. Farber C-M, Yernault J-C, Legros F, Debruyn J, Van Hooren J-P. Detection of anti-p32 mycobacterial IgG antibodies in patients with AIDS. J Infect Dis 1990; 162:279–80.

47. Farhi DC, Mason UG 3d, Horsburgh CR Jr. The bone marrow in disseminated *Mycobacterium avium-intracellulare* infection. Am J Clin Pathol 1985; 83:463–8.

48. Farhi DC, Mason UG 3d, Horsburgh CR Jr. Pathologic findings in disseminated *Mycobacterium avium-intracellulare* infection. A report of 11 cases. Am J Clin Pathol 1986; 85:67–72.

49. Farizo KM, Buehler JW. Pulmonary mycobacterial infections in persons with HIV infection. In: Program and Abstracts of the 31st Interscience Conference on Antimicrobial Agents and Chemotherapy, Chicago, 1991:139.

50. Fernandes PB, Hardy DJ, McDaniel D, Hanson CW, Swanson RN. In vitro and in vivo activities of clarithromycin against *Mycobacterium avium*. Antimicrob Agents Chemother 1989; 33:1531–4.

51. Flepp M, Vurma-Rapp U, Rhyner K, Luthy R. Sensitivity (S) of acid-fast smears (AFS) of sputum, lymph node tissues and stools in AIDS patients with disseminated *Mycobacterium avium* complex (MAC) infection or extra-pulmonary tuberculosis caused by *M. tuberculosis* (TBC). In Program and Abstracts of the IV International Conference on AIDS, Stockholm, vol. 2, abstract 7550, 1988.

52. Fry KL, Meissner PS, Falkinham JO 3d. Epidemiology of infection by nontuberculous mycobacteria. VI. Identification and use of epidemiologic markers for studies of *Mycobacterium avium, M. intracellulare,* and *M. scrofulaceum.* Am Rev Respir Dis 1986; 134:39–43.

53. Gangadharam PR, Kesavalu L, Rao PNR, Perumal VK, Iseman MD. Activity of amikacin against *Mycobacterium avium* complex under simulated in vivo conditions. Antimicrob Agents Chemother 1988; 32:886–9.

54. Gangadharam PR, Perumal VK, Crawford JT, Bates JH. Association of plasmids and virulence of *Mycobacterium avium* complex. Am Rev Respir Dis 1988; 137:212–4.

55. Gangadharam PRJ, Perumal VK, Rao PNR, Kesavalu L, Iseman MD. In vivo activity of amikacin alone or in combination with clofazimine or rifabutin or both against acute experimental *Mycobacterium avium* complex infections in beige mice. Antimicrob Agents Chemother 1988; 32:1400–3.

56. Garrelts JC. Clofazimine: a review of its use in leprosy and *Mycobacterium avium* complex infection. Ann Pharmacol 1991; 25:525–31.

57. Gill VJ, Park CH, Stock F, Gosey LL, Witebsky FG, Masur H. Use of lysis-centrifugation (Isolator) and radiometric (BACTEC) blood culture systems for the detection of mycobacteria. J Clin Microbiol 1985; 22:543–6.

58. Girard AE, Girard D, English AR, Gootz TD, Cimochowski CR, Faiella JA, Haskell SL, Retsema JA. Pharmokinetic and in vivo studies with azithro-

mycin (CP-62,993), a new macrolide with an extended half-life and excellent tissue distribution. Antimicrob Agents Chemother 1987; 31:1948-54.

59. Gladue RP, Isaacson RE, Newborg MF. In vitro and in vivo uptake of azithromycin (CP-62,993) by phagocytic cells: possible mechanism of delivery and release at sites of infection. Antimicrob Agents Chemother 1989; 33: 277-82.

60. Godwin JC, Stopeck A, Chang VT, Godwin TA. Mycobacteremia in acquired immune deficiency syndrome: rapid diagnosis based on inclusions in the peripheral blood smear. Am J Clin Pathol 1991; 95:369-75.

61. Gonzalez R, and Hanna BA. Evaluation of Gen-Probe DNA hybridization systems for the identification of *Mycobacterium tuberculosis* and *Mycobacterium avium-intracellulare*. Diagn Microbiol Infect Dis 1987; 8:69-77.

62. Good RC. Opportunistic pathogens in the genus *Mycobacterium*. Ann Rev Microbiol 1985; 39:347-69.

63. Goslee S, and Wolinsky E. Water as a source of potentially pathogenic mycobacteria. Am Rev Respir Dis 1976; 113:287-92.

64. Graham L Jr, Warren NG, Tsang AY, Dalton HP. *Mycobacterium avium* complex pseudobacteriuria from a hospital water supply. J Clin Microbiol 1988; 26:1034-6.

65. Hampson SJ, Thompson J, Moss MT, Portaels F, Green EP, Herman-Taylor, J, McFadden JJ. DNA probes demonstrate a single highly conserved strain of *Mycobacterium avium* infecting AIDS patients. Lancet 1989; 1:65-8.

66. Havlik JA, Horsburgh CR, Metchock B, Williams P, Thompson SE. Clinical risk factors for disseminated *Mycobacterium avium* complex infection (DMAC) in persons with HIV infection. In: Program and Abstracts of the VI International Conference on AIDS, San Francisco, Vol. 1, abstract Th. B. 515, 1990.

67. Havlir DV, Keyes L, Davis C. Measurement of *Mycobacterium avium* bacteremia; quantitative Isolator lysis centrifugation versus BACTEC 13A blood culture systems. In: Program and Abstracts of the 31st Interscience Conference on Antimicrobial Agents and Chemotherapy, Chicago, 1991:209.

68. Hawkins CC, Gold JWM, Whimby E, Kiehn TE, Brannon P, Cammarata BA, Brown AE, Armstrong D. *Mycobacterium avium* complex infections in patients with the acquired immunodeficiency syndrome. Ann Intern Med 1986; 105:184-8.

69. Heifets L. MIC as a quantitative measurement of the susceptibility of *Mycobacterium avium* strains to seven antituberculosis drugs. Antimicrob Agents Chemother 1988; 32:1131-6.

70. Heifets L. Quantitative and quantitative drug-susceptibility tests in mycobacteriology. Am Rev Respir Dis 1988; 137:1217-22.

71. Heifets LB, Iseman MD. Choice of antimicrobial agents for *M. avium* disease based on quantitative tests of drug susceptibility. N Engl J Med 1990; 323: 419–20.

72. Heifets LB, Iseman MD. Individual therapy versus standard regimens in the treatment of *Mycobacterium avium* infections. Am Rev Respir Dis 1991; 144:1–2.

73. Heifets LB, Lindholm LP. MICs and MBCs of Win 57273 against *Mycobacterium avium* and *M. tuberculosis*. Antimicrob Agents Chemother 1990; 34:770–4.

74. Heifets LB, Lindholm-Levy PJ, Iseman MD. Rifabutine: minimal inhibitory and bactericidal concentrations for *Mycobacterium tuberculosis*. Am Rev Respir Dis 1988; 137:719–21.

75. Hellyer TJ, Brown IN, Dale JW, Easmon CS. Plasmid analysis of *Mycobacterium avium-intracellulare* (MAI) isolated in the United Kingdom from patients with and without AIDS. J Med Microbiol 1991; 34:225-31.

76. Hoffner SE. Improved detection of *Mycobacterium avium* complex with the Bactec radiometric system. Diagn Microbiol Infect Dis 1988; 10:1–6.

77. Hoffner SE, Kallenius G, Petrini B, Brennan PJ, Tsang AY. Serovars of *Mycobacterium avium* complex isolated from patients in Sweden. J Clin Microbiol 1990; 28:1105–7.

78. Hoffner SE, Kratz M, Olsson-Liljequist B, Svenson SB, Kallenius G. In-vitro synergistic activity between ethambutol and fluorinated quinolones against *Mycobacterium avium* complex. J Antimicrob Chemother 1989; 24: 317–24.

79. Hooper LC, Barrow WW. Decreased mitogenic response of murine spleen cells following intraperitoneal injection of serovar-specific glycopeptidolipid antigens from the *Mycobacterium avium* complex. Adv Exp Med Biol 1988; 239:309–25.

80. Horsburgh CR Jr. *Mycobacterium avium* complex infection in the acquired immunodeficiency syndrome. N Engl J Med 1991; 324:1332–8.

81. Horsburgh CR Jr, Havlik JA, Ellis DA, Kennedy E, Fann SA, DuBois RE, Thompson SE. Survival of patients with acquired immune deficiency syndrome and disseminated *Mycobacterium avium* complex infection with and without antimycobacterial chemotherapy. Am Rev Respir Dis 1991; 144:557–9.

82. Horsburgh CR, Havlik JA, Heifets L, Flory M, Metchock B, Thompson SE. Response to therapy of *Mycobacterium avium* complex (MAC) infection in AIDS correlates with in vitro susceptibility testing. Program and Abstracts of the 31st Interscience Conference on Antimicrobial Agents and Chemotherapy, Chicago, 1991:211.

83. Horsburgh CR Jr, Mason UG 3d, Heifets LB, Southwick K, Labrecque J, Iseman MD. Response to therapy of pulmonary *Mycobacterium avium-in-*

tracellulare infection correlates with results of in vitro susceptibility testing. Am Rev Respir Dis 1987; 135:418–21.

84. Horsburgh CR, Metchock BG, McGowan JE, Thompson SE. Progression to disseminated infection in HIV-infected persons colonized with mycobacteria other than tuberculosis (MOTT). Am Rev Respir Dis 1991; 143:A279.

85. Horsburgh CR Jr, Selik RM. The epidemiology of disseminated nontuberculous mycobacterial infection in the acquired immunodeficiency syndrome (AIDS). Am Rev Respir Dis 1989; 139:4–7.

86. Hoy J, Mijch A, Sandland M, Grayson L, Lucas R, Dwyer B. Quadruple-drug therapy for *Mycobacterium avium-intracellulare* bacteremia in AIDS patients. J Infect Dis 1990; 161:801–5.

87. Husson RN. Mycobacterial infections. In: PA Pizzo and CM Wilfert, eds. Pediatric AIDS. The challenge of HIV infection in infants, children, and adolescents, Baltimore: Williams & Wilkins, Inc., 1991:209–24.

88. Ichiyama S, Shimokata K, Tsukamura M. The isolation of *Mycobacterium avium* complex from soil, water, and dusts. Microbiol Immunol 1988; 32:733–9.

89. Inderlied CB. Antimycobacterial agents: in vitro susceptibility testing, spectrums of activity, mechanisms of action and resistance, and assays for activity in biological fluids. In: V Lorian, ed. Antibiotics in laboratory medicine. Baltimore: Williams & Wilkins, Inc., 1991; 134–97.

90. Inderlied CB, Kolonoski PT, Wu M, Young LS. Amikacin, ciprofloxacin, and imipenem treatment for disseminated *Mycobacterium avium* complex infection of beige mice. Antimicrob Agents Chemother 1989; 33:176-80.

91. Inderlied CB, Young LS, Yamada JK. Determination of in vitro susceptibility of *Mycobacterium avium* complex isolates to antimicrobial agents by various methods. Antimicrob Agents Chemother 1987; 31:1697–702.

92. Isenberg HD, D'Amato RF, Heifets L, Murray PR, Scardamaglia M, Jacobs MC, Alperstein P, Niles A. Collaborative feasibility study of biphasic system (Roche Septi-Chek AFB) for the rapid detection and isolation of mycobacteria. J Clin Microbiol 1991; 29:1719–22.

93. Jacobs C, Henein S, Heurich A, Kamholz S. Nontuberculous mycobacterial meningitis in patients with AIDS. Am Rev Respir Dis 1991; 143:A279.

94. Jacobson MA, Hopewell PC, Yajko DM, Hadley WK, Lazarus E, Mohanty PK, Modin GW, Feigal DW, Cusick PS, Sande MA. Natural history of disseminated *Mycobacterium avium* complex infection in AIDS. J Infect Dis 1991; 164:994-8.

95. Jensen AG, Bebbedsen J, Rosdahl VT. Plasmid profiles of *Mycobacterium-avium-intracellulare* isolated from patients with AIDS or cervical lymphadenitis and from environmental samples. Scand J Infect Dis 1989; 21:645-9.

96. Jucker MT, Falkinham JOI. Epidemiology of infection by nontuberculous mycobacteria IX. Evidence for two DNA homology groups among small plasmids in *Mycobacterium avium, Mycobacterium intracellulare,* and *Mycobacterium scrofulaceum.* Am Rev Respir Dis 1990; 142:858–62.

97. Kallenius G, Hoffner SE, Svenson SB. Does vaccination with Bacille Calmette-Guerin protect against AIDS? Rev Infect Dis 1989; 11:349–51.

98. Kallenius G, Svenson SG, Hoffner SE. Ethambutol: a key for mycobacterium avium complex chemotherapy. Am Rev Respir Dis 1989; 140:264.

99. Katz P, Yeager H Jr, Whalen G, Evans M, Swartz RP, Roecklein J. Natural killer cell-mediated lysis of *Mycobacterium avium* complex infected monocytes. J Clin Immunol 1990; 10:71-7.

100. Kemper CA, Meng TC, Nussbaum J, Chiu J, Fiegal DF, Bartok AE, Leedom JM, Tilles JG, Deresinski SC, McCutchan JA. Treatment of *Mycobacterium avium* complex bacteremia in AIDS with a four-drug oral regimen: rifampin, ethambutol, clofazimine and ciprofloxacin. Ann Int Med 1992; (in press).

101. Kiehn TE, Cammarata R. Laboratory diagnosis of mycobacterial infections in patients with acquired immunodeficiency syndrome. J Clin Microbiol 1986; 24:708–11.

102. Kiehn TE, and Cammarata R. Comparative recoveries of *Mycobacterium avium-M. intracellulare* from Isolator lysis-centrifugation and BACTEC 13A blood culture systems. J Clin Microbiol 1988; 26:760–1.

103. Kiehn TE, Edwards FF, Brannon P, Tsang AY, Maio M, Gold JW, Whimbey E, Wong B, McClatchy JK, Armstrong D. Infections caused by *Mycobacterium avium* complex in immunocompromised patients: diagnosis by blood culture and fecal examination, antimicrobial susceptibility tests, and morphological and seroagglutination characteristics. J Clin Microbiol 1985; 21:168–73.

104. Kirihara JM, Hillier SL, Coyle MB. Improved detection times for *Mycobacterium avium* complex and *Mycobacterium tuberculosis* with the BACTEC radiometric system. J Clin Microbiol 1985; 22:841–5.

105. Klatt EC, Jensen DF, Meyer PR. Pathology of *Mycobacterium avium-intracellulare* infection in acquired immunodeficiency syndrome. Hum Pathol 1987; 18:709–14.

106. Kuitert LM, Thomas MG, Ellis-Pegler RB. Outcome of untreated *Mycobacterium avium-intracellulare* complex infection in AIDS. J AIDS 1991; 5:1036–8.

107. Kunze ZM, Wall S, Appelberg R, Silva MT, Portaels F, McFadden JJ. IS901, a new member of a widespread class of atypical insertion sequences, is associated with pathogenicity in *Mycobacterium avium.* Mol Microbiol 1991; 5:2265–72.

108. Lee B-Y, Chatterjee D, Bozic CM, Brennan PJ, Cohn DL, Bales JD, Harrison SM, Andron LA, Orme IM. Prevalence of serum antibody to the type-specific glycopeptidolipid antigens of *Mycobacterium avium* in human immunodeficiency virus-positive and -negative individuals. J Clin Microbiol 1991; 29:1026–9.

109. Leysen DC, Haemers A, Pattyn SR. Mycobacteria and the new quinolones. Antimicrob Agents Chemother 1989; 33:1–5.

110. Lim SD, Todd J, Lopez J, Ford E, Janda JM. Genotypic identification of pathogenic *Mycobacterium* species by using a nonradioactive oligonucleotide probe. J Clin Microbiol 1991; 29:1276–8.

111. Lindholm-Levy PJ, Heifets LB. Clofazimine and other rimino-compounds: Minimal inhibitory and minimal bactericidal concentrations at different pH's for *Mycobacterium avium* complex. Tubercle 1988; 69:179–86.

112. Maggi E, Macchia D, Parronchi P, Mazzetti M, Ravina A, Milo D, Romagnani S. Reduced production of interleukin-2 and interferon-g and enhanced helper activity for IgG synthesis by cloned CD4 + T cells from patients with AIDS. Eur J Immunol 1987; 17:1685–90.

113. Marinelli DL, Albelda SM, Williams TM, Kern JA, Iozza RV, Miller WT. Nontuberculous mycobacterial infection in AIDS: Clinical, pathologic, and radiologic features. Thoracic Rad 1986; 160:77–86.

114. Masur H, Tuazon C, Gill V, Grimes G, Baird B, Fauci AS, Lane HC. Effect of combined clofazimine and ansamycin therapy on *Mycobacterium avium-Mycobacterium intracellulare* bacteremia in patients with AIDS. J Infect Dis 1987; 155:127–9.

115. Meissner G, Anz W. Sources of *Mycobacterium avium* complex infection resulting in human disease. Am Rev Resp Dis 1977; 166:1057–64.

116. Meissner PS, Falkinham JO 3d. Plasmid DNA profiles as epidemiological markers for clinical and environmental isolates of *Mycobacterium avium, Mycobacterium intracellulare,* and *Mycobacterium scrofulaceum.* J Infect Dis 1986; 153:325–31.

117. Mizuguchi Y, Fukunaga M, Taniguchi H. Plasmid deoxyribonucleic acid and translucent-to-opaque variation in *Mycobacterium intracellulare* 103. J Bacteriol 1981; 146:656–9.

118. Mizuguchi Y, Udou T, Yamada T. Mechanism of antibiotic resistance in *Mycobacterium intracellulare.* Microbiol Immunol 1983; 27:425–31.

119. Modilevsky T, Sattler FR, Barnes PF. Mycobacterial disease in patients with human immunodeficiency virus infection. Arch Intern Med 1989; 149:2201–5.

120. Monsour HP Jr, Quigley EM, Markin RS, Dalke DD, Goldsmith JC, Harty RF. Endoscopy in the diagnosis of gastrointestinal *Mycobacterium avium-intracellulare* infection. J Clin Gastroenterol 1991; 13:20.

121. Morris SL, Rouse DA, Malik A, Chaparas SD, Witebsky FG. Characterization of plasmids extracted from AIDS-associated *Mycobacterium avium* isolates. Tubercle 1990; 71:181-5.

122. Motyl MR, Saltzman B, Levi MH, McKitrick JC, Friedland GH, Klein RS. The recovery of *Mycobacterium avium* complex and *Mycobacterium tuberculosis* from blood specimens of AIDS patients using the nonradiometric Bactec NR 660 medium. Am J Clin Pathol 1990; 94:84-6.

123. Murray HW, Scavuzzo DA, Chapras SD, Roberts RB. T lymphocyte responses to mycobacterial antigen in AIDS patients with disseminated *Mycobacterium avium-Mycobacterium intracellulare* infection. Chest 1988; 93:922-5.

124. Musail CE, Tice LS, Stockman L, Roberts GD. Identification of mycobacteria from culture by using the Gen-Probe Rapid Diagnostic system for *Mycobacterium avium* complex and *Mycobacterium tuberculosis* complex. J Clin Microbiol 1988(Oct):2120-3.

125. Naik S, Ruck R. In vitro activities of several new macrolide antibiotics against *Mycobacterium avium* complex. Antimicrob Agents Chemother 1989; 33:1614-6.

126. Nakamura RM, Goto Y, Kitamura K, Tokunaga T. Two types of suppressor T cells that inhibit delayed-type hypersensitivity to *Mycobacterium intracellulare* in mice. Infect Immun 1989; 57:779-84.

127. Noel SB, Ray MC, Greer DL. Cutaneous infection with *Mycobacterium avium-intracellulare scrofulaceum* intermediate: a new pathogenic entity. J Am Acad Dermatol 1988; 19:492-5.

127a. Northelt DW, Mayer A, Kaplan LD, Abrams DI, Hadley WK, Yajko DM, Heindler BG. The usefulness of diagnostic bone marrow examination in patients with human immunodeficiency virus (HIV) infection. J AIDS 1991; 4:659-66.

128. Nussbaum JM, Dealist C, Lewis W, Heseltine PNR. Rapid diagnosis by buffy coat smear of disseminated *Mycobacterium avium* complex infection in patients with acquired immunodeficiency syndrome. J Clin Microbiol 1990; 28:631-2.

129. O'Brien RJ, Geiter LJ, Snider DE Jr. The epidemiology of nontuberculous mycobacterial diseases in the United States. Results from a national survey. Am Rev Respir Dis 1987; 135:1007-14.

130. Okello DO, Sewankambo N, Goodgame R, Aisu TO, Kwezi M, Morrissey A, Ellner J. Absence of bacteremia with *Mycobacterium avium-intracellulare* in Ugandan patients with AIDS. J Infect Dis 1990; 162:208-10.

131. Packer SJ, Cesario T, Williams JH Jr. *Mycobacterium avium* complex infection presenting as endobronchial lesions in immunosuppressed patients. Ann Intern Med 1988; 109:389-93.

132. Parker BC, Ford MA, Grutt H, Falkinham JO. Epidemiology of infection by non-tuberculous mycobacteria IV. Preferential aerosolization of *M. intracellulare* from natural waters. Am Rev Resp Dis 1983; 128:652–6.

133. Peterson EM, Lu R, Floyd C, Nakasone A, Friedly G, de la Maza L. Direct identification of *Mycobacterium tuberculosis, Mycobacterium avium,* and *Mycobacterium intracellulare* from amplified primary cultures in BACTEC media using DNA probes. J Clin Microbiol 1989; 27:1543–7.

134. Picken RN, Plotch SJ, Wang Z, Lin BC, Donegan JJ, Yang HL. DNA probes for Mycobacteria. I. Isolation of DNA probes for the identification of *Mycobacterium tuberculosis* complex and for mycobacteria other than tuberculosis (MOTT). Mol Cell Probes 1988; 2:111–24.

135. Pitchenik AE, Cole C, Russell BW, Fischl MA, Spira TJ, Snider DE Jr. Tuberculosis, atypical mycobacteriosis, and the acquired immunodeficiency syndrome among Haitian and non-Haitian patients in south Florida. Ann Intern Med 1984; 101:641–5.

136. Pluda JM, Yarchoan R, Smith PD, McAtee N, Shay LE, Oette D, Maha M, Wahl SM, Myers CE, Broder S. Subcutaneous recombinant granulocyte-macrophage colony-stimulating factor used as a single agent and in an alternating regimen with azithymidine in leukopenic patients with severe human immunodeficiency virus infection. Blood 1990; 76:463–72.

137. Poropatich CO, Labriola AM, Tuazon CU. Acid-fast smear and culture of respiratory secretions, bone marrow, and stools as predictors of disseminated *Mycobacterium avium* complex infection. J Clin Microbiol 1987; 25:929–30.

138. Radin DR. Intraabdominal *Mycobacterium tuberulosis* vs. *Mycobacterium avium-intracellulare* infections in patients with AIDS: distinction based on CT findings. Am J Roentgenol 1991; 156:487–91.

139. Rastogi N, Frehel C, Ryter A, Ohayon H, Lesourd M, David HL. Multiple drug resistance in *Mycobacterium avium*: is the wall architecture responsible for the exclusion of antimicrobial agents? Antimicrob Agents Chemother 1981; 20:666–77.

140. Roberts MC, McMillan C, Coyle MB. Whole chromosomal DNA probes for rapid identification of *Mycobacterium tuberculosis* and *Mycobacterium avium* complex. J Clin Microbiol 1987; 25:1239–43.

141. Roth RI, Owen RL, Keren DF, Volberding PA. Intestinal infection with *Mycobacterium avium* in acquired immune deficiency syndrome (AIDS): pathological and clinical comparison with Whipple's disease. Dig Dis Sci 1985; 30:497–504.

142. Ruf B, Schuermann D, Brehmer W, Pohle HD II. Pulmonary manifestations due to *Mycobacterium avium-Mycobacterium intracellulare* (MAI) in AIDS patients. Am Rev Respir Dis 1991; 141:A611.

143. Runyon EH. Ten mycobacterial pathogens. Tubercle 1974; 55:235–40.

144. Saint-Marc T, Touraine JL. Clinical experience with a combination of clarithromycin and clofazimine in the treatment of disseminated *M. avium* infections in AIDS. In: Program and abstracts of the 31st Interscience Conference on Antimicrobial Agents and Chemotherapy, Chicago, 1991:138.

144a. Saito H, Tomioka H, Sato K, Tasaka H, Dawson DJ. Identification of various serovar strains of *Mycobacterium avium* complex by using DNA probes specific for Mycobacterium avium and *Mycobacterium intracellulare*. J Clin Microbiol 1990; 28:1694-7.

145. Saito H, Sato K, Tomioka H. Comparative in vitro and in vivo activity of rifampin and rifampicin against *Mycobacterium avium* complex. Tubercle 1988; 69:187–92.

146. Saito H, Tomioka H. Susceptibilities of transparent, opaque, and rough colonial variants of *Mycobacterium avium* complex to various fatty acids. Antimicrob Agents Chemother 1988; 32:400–2.

147. Salfinger M, Stoll EW, Piot D, Heifets L. Comparison of three methods for recovery of *Mycobacterium avium* complex from blood specimens. J Clin Microbiol 1988; 26:1225–6.

148. Schaefer WB, Davis CL, Cohn ML. Pathogenicity of transparent, opaque, and rough variants of *Mycobacterium avium* in chickens and mice. Am Rev Respir Dis 1970; 102:499–506.

149. Sherman I, Harrington N, Rothrock A, George H. Use of a cutoff range in identifying mycobacteria by the Gen-Probe Rapid Diagnostic system. J Clin Microbiol 1989; 27:241–4.

150. Shiratsuchi H, Johnson JL, Toba H, Ellner JJ. Strain- and donor-related differences in the interaction of *Mycobacterium avium* with human monocytes and its modulation by interferon-γ. J Infect Dis 1990; 162:932-8.

151. Small PM, Schector GF, Goodman PC, Sande MA, Chaisson RE, Hopewell PC. Treatment of tuberculosis in patients with advanced human immunodeficiency virus infection. N Engl J Med 1991; 324:289–94.

152. Songer JG. Environmental sources of *Mycobacterium avium* for infection in animals and man. Proc Ann Meeting US Anim Health Assoc 1980; 84:528-35.

153. Stanley MW, Horwitz CA, Burton LG, Weisser JA. Negative images of bacilli and mycobacterial infection: a study of fine needle aspiration smears from lymph nodes in patients with AIDS. Diagn Cytopathol 1990; 6:118–21.

154. Stormer RS, Falkinham JO III. Differences in antimicrobial susceptibility of pigmented and unpigmented colonial variants of *Mycobacterium avium*. J Clin Microbiol 1989; 27:2459–65.

155. Strand CL, Epstein C, Verzosa S, Effatt E, Hormozi P, Siddiqi SH. Eval-

uation of a new blood culture medium for mycobacteria. Am J Clin Pathol 1989; 91:316–8.

156. Takashima T, Collins FM. T-cell-medicated immunity in persistent *Mycobacterium intracellulare* infections in mice. Infect Immun 1988; 56:2782–7.

157. Tenholder MF, COL, Moser RJ III, MAJ, Tellis CJ COL. Mycobacteria other than tuberculosis: pulmonary involvement in patients with acquired immunodeficiency syndrome. Arch Intern Med 1988; 148:953–5.

158. Timple A, Runyon EH. The relationship of "atypical" acid-fast bacteria to human disease. J Lab Clin Med 1954; 44:202–9.

159. Tomioka H, Sato K, Saito H, Yamada Y. Susceptibility of *Mycobacterium avium* and *Mycobacterium intracellulare* to various antibacterial agents. Microbiol Immunol 1989; 33:509–14.

160. Tsang AY, Drupa I, Goldberg M, McClatchy JK, Brennan PJ. Use of serology and thin layer chromatography for the assembly of an authenticated collection of serovars within the *Mycobacterium avium-Mycobacterium intracellulare-Mycobacterium scrofulaceum* complex. Int J Sys Bact 1983; 33:285–92.

161. Tsuyuguchi I, Shiratsuchi H, Okuda Y, Yamamoto Y. An analysis of in vitro T cell responsiveness in nontuberculous mycobacterial infection. Chest 1988; 94:822–9.

162. Uribe-Botero G, Prichard JG, Kaplowitz HJ. A comparison of fluorescent staining and cultures in the detection of mycobacteria. Am J Clin Path 1989; 91:313–5.

163. von Reyn CF, Hennigan S, Niemczyk S, Jacobs NJ. Effect of delays in processing on the survival of *Mycobacterium avium-M. intracellulare* in the Isolator blood culture system. J Clin Microbiol 1991; 29:1211–4.

164. Wallace JM, Hannah JB. *Mycobacterium avium* complex infection in patients with the acquired immunodeficiency syndrome: a clinicopathologic study. Chest 1988; 93:926–32.

165. Wallace RJ Jr. Nontuberculous mycobacteria and water: a love affair with increasing clinical importance. Infect Dis Clin North Am 1987; 1:677-86.

166. Wallace RJ, Glassroth J, O'Brien R. A plea for clinical trials to resolve the issue of optimal therapy in the treatment of *Mycobacterium avium* infection. Am Rev Respir Dis 1991; 144:3–4.

167. Wallace RJ Jr, Obrein R, Glassroth J, Raleigh J, Dutt A. Diagnosis and treatment of disease caused by nontuberculous mycobacteria. Am Rev Respir Dis 1990; 142:940–53.

168. Wasem CF, McCarthy CM, Murray LW. Multilocus enzyme electrophoresis analysis of the *Mycobacterium avium* complex and other mycobacteria. J Clin Microbiol 1991; 29:264–71.

169. Wayne LG. The "atypical" mycobacteria: recognition and disease association. CRC Crit Rev Microbiol 1985; 12:185–222.

170. Wayne LG, Anderson B, Chetty K, Light RW. Antibodies to mycobacterial peptidoglycolipid and to crude protein antigens in sera from different categories of human subjects. J Clin Microbiol 1988; 26:2300–6.

171. Wayne LG, Young LS, Bertram M. Absence of mycobacterial antibody to AIDS patients. Eur J Clin Microbiol 1986; 5:363–5.

172. Wendt SL, George KL, Parker BC, Groft H, Falkinham JO. Epidemiology of infection by nontuberculous mycobacteria. III Isolation of potentially pathogenic mycobacteria from aerosols. Am Rev Resp Dis 1980; 122:259–63.

173. Winkelstein A, Kingsley LA, Klein RS, Lyter DW, Evans TL, Rinaldo CR Jr, Weaver LD, Machen LL, Schadle RC. Defective T-cell colony formation and IL-2 receptor expression at all stages of HIV infection. Clin Exp Immunol 1988; 71:417–22.

174. Winter SM, Bernard EM, Gold JW, Armstrong D. Humoral response to disseminated infection by *Mycobacterium avium-Mycobacterium intracellulare* in acquired immunodeficiency syndrome and hairy cell leukemia. J Infect Dis 1985; 151:523–7.

175. Wong B, Edwards FF, Kiehn TE, Whimby E, Donnelly H, Bernard EM, Gold JWM, Armstrong D. Continuous high-grade *Mycobacterium avium-intracellulare* bacteremia in patients with the acquired immune deficiency syndrome. Am J Med 1985; 78:35–40.

176. Yagupsky P, Menegus MA. Cumulative positivity rates of multiple blood cultures for *Mycobacterium avium-intracellulare* and *Cryptococcus neoformans* in patients with the acquired immunodeficiency syndrome. Arch Pathol Lab Med 1990; 114:923–5.

177. Yajko DM, Kirihara J, Sanders C, Nassos P, Hadley WK. Antimicrobial synergism against *Mycobacterium avium* complex strains isolated from patients with acquired immune deficiency syndrome. Antimicrob Agents Chemother 1988; 32:1392–5.

178. Yakrus MA, Good RC. Geographic distribution, frequency, and specimen source of *Mycobacterium avium* complex serotypes isolated from patients with acquired immunodeficiency syndrome. J Clin Microbiol 1990; 28: 926–9.

179. Yoshimura HH, Graham DY. Nucleic acid hybridization studies of mycobactin-dependent mycobacteria. J Clin Microbiol 1988; 26:1309–12.

180. Young LS. *Mycobacterium avium* complex infection. J Infect Dis 1988; 157:863–7.

181. Young LS, Berlin OG, Inderlied CB. Activity of ciprofloxacin and other flourinated quinolones against mycobacteria. Am J Med 1987; 82:23–6.

182. Young LS, Inderlied CB, Berlin OG, Gottlieb MS. Mycobacterial infections in AIDS patients, with an emphasis on the *Mycobacterium avium* complex. Rev Infect Dis 1986; 8:1024–33.

183. Young LS, Wiviott L, Wu M, Kolonoski P, Bolan R, Inderlied CB. Azithromycin for treatment of *Mycobacterium avium-intracellulare* complex infection in patients with AIDS. Lancet 1991; 338:1107–9.

7

Foscarnet Therapy for AIDS-Related Opportunistic Herpesvirus Infections

Mark A. Jacobson

*University of California—San Francisco,
and San Francisco General Hospital,
San Francisco, California*

Parts of this chapter were originally published in Jacobson MA, O'Donnell JJ. Approaches to the treatment of cytomegalovirus retinitis: ganciclovir and foscarnet. J AIDS 1991; 4: S11-S15.

I. INTRODUCTION

On September 27, 1991, foscarnet became the second antiviral agent to be approved by the U.S. Food and Drug Administration (FDA) for the therapy of AIDS-related cytomegalovirus (CMV) retinitis (ganciclovir was licensed by the FDA in 1989). The availability of foscarnet as an alternate therapy for CMV retinitis represents a major therapeutic advance for patients who are clinically and virologically resistant to ganciclovir's CMV-suppressive activity or who are intolerant of ganciclovir's myelo-suppressive effects. Although data available to date from clinical trials suggest that the efficacy of foscarnet appears to be identical to that of ganciclovir in halting progression of CMV retinitis, this new agent has a very different toxicity profile from ganciclovir. Possibly due to foscarnet's antiretroviral activity, survival was observed to be longer for foscarnet-treated retinitis patients with normal renal function than for ganciclovir-treated patients in a recent multicenter, randomized trial. However, survival was worse with foscarnet among the subgroup in this trial who had an estimated creatinine clearance < 1.2 ml/min/kg. Thus, for specific retinitis patients without a history of ganciclovir resistance or intolerance, the key to rational decision making in choosing which of these two drugs will be optimal therapy lies in understanding the differences in their adverse effects.

In addition to treatment for CMV retinitis, foscarnet is the only antiviral agent to have established efficacy in the therapy of AIDS-associated acyclovir-resistant mucocutaneous herpes simplex virus disease. Also, preliminary uncontrolled data suggest a potential beneficial role for foscarnet in the therapy of AIDS-associated CMV colitis and esophagitis, as well as for acyclovir-resistant varicella-zoster virus disease. In addition, data from human trials have demonstrated that foscarnet has in vivo antiviral effects in controlling HIV-1 infection and HIV-associated Epstein-Barr virus infection; however, the clinical implications of these latter two observations are still not clear.

II. MECHANISM AND ANTIVIRAL SPECTRUM

Foscarnet (trisodium phosphonophormate, Foscavir) is an antiviral agent that selectively inhibits the DNA polymerase of all human herpesviruses at concentrations less than one hundredth of that required to inhibit eukaryotic DNA polymerase (1). As a pyrophosphate analog that inhibits viral DNA polymerase by binding directly to the polymerase pyrophosphate binding site, foscarnet, unlike other antiherpes agents such as ganciclovir and acyclovir, does not require preliminary intracellular metabolism (i.e., phosphorylation) for its antiviral activity. This difference in mechanism results in foscarnet retaining its antiviral activity against clinical herpesvirus isolates that have developed decreased susceptibility to acyclovir or ganciclovir.

Foscarnet inhibits replication of all human herpesviruses at concentrations that are easily achievable in plasma with intravenous administration. This antiviral spectrum is similar to that of ganciclovir but is in marked contrast to that of acyclovir, which similarly inhibits herpes simplex 1 and 2, varicella-zoster virus, and Epstein-Barr virus but has little activity against CMV at plasma achievable levels. Table 1 summarizes the concentrations of acyclovir, ganciclovir, and foscarnet that inhibited in vitro CMV plaque formation by 50% when clinical CMV isolates were added to cell cultures (2–5). In addition, nearly all clinical strains of acyclovir-resistant herpes simplex virus and varicella-zoster virus isolated from patients with chronic mucocutaneous lesions unresponsive to acyclovir therapy as well as of ganciclovir-resistant CMV isolated from patients with

Table 1 In vitro Inhibition of Clinical Cytomegalovirus Isolates by Acyclovir, Ganciclovir, and Foscarnet and Peak Plasma Concentrations Achievable with Intravenous Therapy

	ACV	GCV	PFA
ED_{50} for CMV (μg/ml)			
Range	23-46	0.2-3.0	15-242
Most clinical isolates	>23	<1.5	<61
C_{max} (μg/ml)	10-25	10	125-250

ACV = acyclovir; GCV = ganciclovir; PFA = foscarnet; C_{max} = peak plasma concentration; ED_{50} = concentration that inhibits in vitro plaque formation by 50%.

CMV retinitis unresponsive to ganciclovir therapy have been susceptible to foscarnet in vitro (6–8).

Foscarnet also has been reported to inhibit in vitro HIV replication completely at plasma achievable levels, while ganciclovir has little activity against HIV (9). Using HIV p24 antigen as an in vivo marker for antiretroviral activity, foscarnet has demonstrated anti-HIV activity as well in several small, uncontrolled clinical trials. Seven p24 antigenemic patients who received foscarnet induction therapy for CMV retinitis all had decreases in serum p24 antigen concentration with a mean decrease of 55% ($p = 0.01$) between initiation and completion of a 2-week course of foscarnet 60 mg/kg every 8 hours (10). When foscarnet was added to zidovudine therapy in six patients with persistent p24 antigenemia after 9–27 weeks of high-dose zidovudine therapy, serum p24 antigen concentrations decreased in all six by a mean 55% ($p = 0.005$) between initiation and completion of a 2-week course of foscarnet 30 mg/kg every 8 hours (11). No such in vivo antiretroviral effects have been reported with ganciclovir therapy. However, the clinical implications of foscarnet's antiretroviral activity, as discussed below, remain to be elucidated.

III. PHARMACOLOGY

The half-life of foscarnet in plasma is in the range of 3–4 hours, the drug is cleared only by renal excretion without any hepatic metabolism, and it achieves cerebrospinal fluid levels approximately 40% of simultaneous plasma concentrations (12,13). This pharmacokinetic profile is virtually identical to that of ganciclovir. For both drugs, intracellular half-lives are probably more pertinent to drug efficacy than plasma half-lives. For ganciclovir, the intracellular half-life of the active metabolite ganciclovir-triphosphate is known to be in the range of >18 hours, suggesting that once-daily dosing might have clinical efficacy (14). The intracellular half-life of foscarnet is unknown, but likely exceeds plasma half-life. Both drugs are poorly bioavailable by the oral route. In the case of foscarnet, oral administration is also limited by dose-related diarrhea (13). Even with ranitidine-induced decreased gastric acidity, absorption of oral foscarnet is inadequate to achieve effective plasma concentrations (15). Foscarnet can be co-administered with zidovudine without important changes in the pharmacokinetic disposition of either agent (16).

Foscarnet has several additional unique chemical and pharmacokinetic characteristics that impact on clinical therapeutics. Because the drug is only 5% soluble in water and has low pKa values (7.27, 3.41, and 0.49), which limit cellular penetration of drug, large volumes and large doses of drug must be administered in order to achieve an in vivo antiviral effect (1). Also, 10-28% of initial foscarnet doses are deposited in bone where the drug has a long terminal half-life, possibly on the order of months (1).

IV. FOSCARNET EFFICACY IN CMV RETINITIS

The efficacy of antiviral therapy for CMV retinitis has been most objectively evaluated in clinical trials by prospective serial funduscopic examinations of the retina. When such serial exams have been performed during therapy, a particularly useful measure of the therapeutic efficacy has been the time to retinitis progression, usually defined as the interval between a baseline funduscopic examination and the first follow-up examination in which a new retinal lesion or significant increase in size of an old lesion is noted. The median time to retinitis progression for groups of retinitis patients has been determined by calculating survival curves with the product-limit method.

Since most previously untreated individuals with AIDS-associated CMV retinitis respond to the initial 2- to 3-week induction course of ganciclovir or foscarnet therapy (17,18), the efficacy measure of greatest clinical relevance has been time to retinitis progression after initiating maintenance antiviral therapy. For patients first initiating maintenance therapy with ganciclovir, time to retinitis progression has been reported to be 32–58 days with treatment regimens of 5 mg/kg, 5 days/week (25 mg/kg/week), and 75 days with a regimen of 5 mg/kg/day (35 mg/kg/week) in uncontrolled studies (19–21). For patients first initiating maintenance therapy with foscarnet, time to retinitis progression has been reported to be 39–123 days with doses of 60–120 mg/kg/day (420–840 mg/kg/week) in uncontrolled studies (22–24). Based on these trials, time to retinitis progression appeared to be similar for ganciclovir and foscarnet maintenance treatment regimens. Preliminary analysis of a recently completed, multicenter, collaborative National Eye Institute and National Institute of Allergy and Infectious Diseases–sponsored trial of 240 AIDS patients with newly diagnosed CMV retinitis randomly assigned to initiate therapy with either ganciclovir or foscarnet has confirmed the equivalent efficacy of these two drugs in controlling retinitis (25).

Surprisingly, this NEI/NIAID collaborative trial showed that among patients with a baseline estimated creatinine clearance of ≥ 1.2 ml/min/kg, those initially assigned to foscarnet primary therapy for their CMV retinitis had a significant survival advantage; conversely, a survival advantage was observed for ganciclovir among those patients who entered the trial with an estimated creatinine clearance < 1.2 ml/min/kg. The survival advantage with ganciclovir among patients with abnormal renal function could plausibly be related to foscarnet's known nephrotoxic potential (see below). However, the reason for a survival advantage with foscarnet among patients with normal renal function is not entirely clear. Whereas ganciclovir has no direct antiretroviral activity, foscarnet is known to have significantly lower anti-HIV p24 antigen concentrations in vivo (10). In addition, foscarnet has as additive or synergistic antiretroviral activity when combined in vitro or in vivo with zidovudine (11). Thus, foscarnet's antiretroviral activity could be the primary mechanism accounting for the improved survival observed in this study. On the other hand, ganciclovir was less frequently co-administered with antiretroviral agents than was foscarnet in this trial, largely because of ganciclovir's known myelosuppressive toxicity and the lack of other licensed and easily available non-myelosuppressive agents or myeloid-stimulating factors. Thus, an alternative explanation of the survival results is that suboptimal antiretroviral therapy was received by the ganciclovir-assigned group. Since this study was not designed to address the impact of antiretroviral therapy on survival (ganciclovir and foscarnet were the only therapeutic interventions randomly assigned), subgroup analysis of concomitant antiretroviral therapies cannot satisfactorily determine the extent to which either of these two equally plausible hypotheses is correct.

Although the precise role of foscarnet in primary therapy for CMV retinitis remains to be fully elucidated, the drug is clearly indicated for patients who are intolerant of ganciclovir myelosuppressive toxicity or who have had retinitis progression occur despite ganciclovir therapy in association with excretion of ganciclovir-resistant CMV. The latter situation may be more common among patients receiving chronic ganciclovir therapy than was initially appreciated. In a prospective study by Drew et al. (26) 72 AIDS patients treated with ganciclovir for CMV disease were evaluated for excretion of drug-resistant virus. No ganciclovir-resistant strains were isolated prior to or during the first 3 months of ganciclovir therapy. Of these 72 patients receiving ganciclovir for >3 months, 18% were excreting CMV, and overall 7.6% were excreting ganciclovir-resistant CMV. We recently reported two cases in which rapid retinitis progression despite optimal ganciclovir dosing was associated with excretion of ganciclovir-resistant, foscarnet-sensitive CMV (6). In both cases, institution of foscarnet therapy resulted in a 6- to 12-fold increase in the time to subsequent retinitis progression. Thus it may be reasonable to assume that patients whose retinitis progresses rapidly during ganciclovir therapy in association with CMV excretion have ganciclovir-resistant CMV and are likely to benefit from foscarnet therapy. Preliminary data from a multicenter, Phase II trial of foscarnet therapy confirms that such a clinical definition does describe patients whose retinitis is better controlled with foscarnet than ganciclovir (27).

In both primary and salvage therapy for CMV retinitis, foscarnet has generally been administered in two phases: an initial intensive induction therapy for 14-21 days with intravenous drug infusions administered every 8–12 hours with the goal of completely halting viral replication and permitting retinal inflammation to decrease, followed by chronic, generally life-long, daily intravenous infusions (maintenance therapy) with the chemosuppressive goal of preventing further retinal necrosis. The typical induction and maintenance regimens currently utilized with each drug are summarized in Table 2. However, no prospective trials have compared initiating therapy with an intensive induction regimen versus initiating therapy with the once-daily maintenance infusion regimen. Thus, the current practice of induction followed by maintenance, though theoretically appealing, has not been objectively established as more effective than a single daily dosing regimen. European investigators have recently reported preliminary data suggesting a >90% response rate with acceptable toxicity rates in patients induced with a 100 mg/kg infusion every 12 hours (28). It may be that for some individuals initiating foscarnet therapy with an every-12-hour dosing regimen may be as effective as an every-8-hour regimen.

Foscarnet therapy was approved by the FDA for chronic maintenance therapy of CMV retinitis at a dose of 90 mg/kg/day to be administered

Table 2 Foscarnet Therapeutic Regimen for CMV Retinitis

Induction: 60 mg/kg IV q 8 hr × 14 days. Administer as a 1-hour infusion by infusion pump only.

CrCl[a]	Dose	CrCl[a]	Dose
>1.6	60	1.5	56.5
1.4	53	1.3	49.4
1.2	45.9	1.1	42.4
1.0	38.9	0.9	35.3
0.8	31.8	0.7	28.3
0.6	24.8	0.5	21.2
0.4	17.7		

Maintenance: 60-120 mg/kg IV qd. Administer as a 2-hour infusion by infusion pump only; co-administration of 1 liter normal saline may decrease risk of nephrotoxicity.

CrCl[a] (ml/min/kg)	Dose (mg/kg) q 24 h		
>1.4	60	90	120
1.2-1.4	52	78	104
1.0-1.2	50	75	100
0.8-1.0	47	71	94
0.6-0.8	42	63	84
0.4-0.6	38	57	76

$^{a}CrCl = \dfrac{(140 - age)}{72} \times$ serum creatinine ($\times$ 0.85 for females)

as a 2-hour intravenous infusion (with dosage reduction for creatinine clearance < 1.4 ml/min/kg) (Table 2). In individuals who progress at this maintenance dose, it is recommended that a 2-week reinduction course be instituted (60 mg/kg every 8 hours) followed by maintenance therapy at an increased dose of 120 mg/kg/day. For some individuals who tolerate foscarnet well during primary induction therapy, a primary maintenance dose of 120 mg/kg/day may be optimal.

V. FOSCARNET TOXICITY

The most common serious adverse effect of foscarnet is nephrotoxicity, occurring as a dose-limiting toxicity in 10–23% of patients treated (29). Although the mechanism of foscarnet-induced nephrotoxicity is not well characterized, increases in serum creatinine are common, and cases of acute renal failure have been reported (18,30,31). In order to limit foscarnet-induced nephrotoxicity, clinicians are advised to keep patients receiving this drug well hydrated. Intravenous sodium loading with co-administered normal saline has been reported to reduce risk of nephrotoxicity in an uncontrolled trial (32). Since foscarnet is exclusively excreted by the kidneys, excessively high plasma levels of foscarnet can be avoided by careful monitoring of renal function and frequent adjustment of foscarnet dose per a nomogram based on estimated creatinine clearance (see Table 2).

Hypocalcemia is the second most common serious toxicity of foscarnet therapy. Severe and even fatal hypocalcemia has been reported in individuals receiving foscarnet co-administered with parenteral pentamidine (33). Foscarnet appears to complex with free, unbound serum calcium, resulting in transient ionized hypocalcemia (34). In one study, plasma ionized calcium concentrations decreased acutely in all of 17 individuals evaluated before and immediately after receiving foscarnet infusions of 90–120 mg/kg over 2 hours (34). This decrease was dose-related (mean 0.17 mmol/liter in patients receiving the 90 mg/kg dose vs. 0.28 mmol/liter in those receiving the 120 mg/kg dose, $p = 0.0016$). This phenomenon might explain occasional arrhythmias and seizures reported in conjunction with foscarnet therapy as well as mental status changes and other forms of neurotoxicity reported in association with foscarnet therapy.

Benign, self-limiting hyperphosphatemia has been described with foscarnet therapy (30), and mild worsening of anemia is common. Hypokalemia, hypomagnesemia, and nephrogenic diabetes insipidus have also been reported (35). In addition, acute penile ulcerations have been associated with foscarnet therapy and are thought to be due to either a fixed drug eruption or drug-induced contact dermatitis (36).

VI. ADMINISTERING AND MANAGING FOSCARNET THERAPY

Foscarnet is formulated as a 24 mg/ml solution in a 250- or 500-ml vial at pH = 7. At this concentration, foscarnet may be directly infused via a central venous catheter. However, for administration via a peripheral vein, dilution in dextrose or saline fluid to a concentration of 8–12 mg/ml is required. Because of the severe toxicity of acute overdoses or too rapid infusions leading to acute ionized hypocalcemia, which can result in seizure or arrhythmia, foscarnet therapy must be administered intravenously via an infusion pump. Serum creatinine, calcium, magnesium, potassium, phosphorus, and hemoglobin should be monitored two or three times per week during induction foscarnet therapy and weekly during maintenance. The foscarnet dose should be recalculated two or three times a week during induction and weekly during maintenance based on estimated creatinine clearance and weight (37). As mentioned above, co-administered intravenous saline infusions appear to decrease the risk of nephrotoxicity (32). Known nephrotoxic drugs, particularly aminoglycosides, amphotericin, and parenteral pentamidine, must be avoided during foscarnet therapy.

VII. FOSCARNET THERAPY FOR CMV GASTROINTESTINAL DISEASE

Preliminary reports from several uncontrolled series of patients prospectively treated with foscarnet for CMV gastrointestinal disease suggest another potential role for this drug. In England, Nelson et al. (38) reported complete control of esophagitis symptoms in 15 of 18 episodes of histologically confirmed CMV eosphagitis and partial control of diarrhea in 11 of 18 episodes of confirmed CMV colitis following 3 weeks of foscarnet therapy. In the United States, Dieterich et al. (39) reported that foscarnet therapy resulted in improvement in symptoms in 11 (79%) of 14 AIDS patients and elimination of CMV cytopathic changes from repeat biopsies in 9 (64%) of AIDS patients with CMV gastrointestinal disease who had clinically failed prior ganciclovir therapy.

VIII. FOSCARNET THERAPY FOR ACYCLOVIR-RESISTANT HERPES SIMPLEX OR VARICELLA-ZOSTER VIRUS DISEASE

AIDS patients with chronic ulcerative mucocutaneous lesions that failed to heal with acyclovir therapy and from which acyclovir-resistant herpes simplex virus (HSV) type 2 was recovered were first described in 1989 (7). Virtually all of these and subsequent similar patients have been infected with HSV strains that were resistant to acyclovir due to a lack of viral thymidine kinase activity yet retained susceptibility in vitro to vidaribine and foscarnet, which of course does not require phosphorylation. Since these cases were first described, those individuals reported to receive treatment with foscarnet (40–60 mg/kg every 8 hours) have invariably had dramatic cutaneous ulcer healing (40,41), generally within 2 weeks. In a recently published, randomized prospective trial comparing vidarabine to foscarnet therapy for acyclovir-resistant HSV lesions in AIDS patients, the study was terminated after only 14 subjects had been enrolled because of the highly significant, superior efficacy and less frequent serious toxicity observed with foscarnet (41). Unfortunately, most of these patients eventually have recurrences of acyclovir-resistant HSV lesions, which do require foscarnet retreatment (41).

AIDS patients with unusual nonhealing hyperkeratotic lesions occurring at cutaneous sites of previous zoster outbreaks, failing to heal with acyclovir therapy, and from which acyclovir-resistant varicella-zoster virus was recovered were first described in 1990 (8). Virtually all of these and subsequent similar patients have been infected with varicella-zoster virus strains that were also resistant to acyclovir due to a lack of viral thymidine kinase activity, yet retained susceptibility in vitro to vidaribine and foscarnet. Since these cases were first described, several individuals have been reported to receive treatment with foscarnet (40 mg/kg every 8 hours) with beneficial clinical outcomes (though less dramatic than that reported for acyclovir-resistant HSV cases) (42). The optimal dose of foscarnet for this uncommon condition may be greater than 40 mg/kg every 8 hours.

IX. FOSCARNET EFFECT ON HIV-ASSOCIATED EPSTEIN-BARR VIRUS INFECTION

Serological evidence of Epstein-Barr virus (EBV) infection is present in most HIV-infected individuals, and EBV has been implicated as a cofactor in AIDS-related lymphoma and in HIV disease progression. In a small, randomized study of HIV-infected patients, undergoing serial cultures of throat washings for EBV transformation of fetal cord blood cells, foscarnet demonstrated more in vivo anti-EBV activity than acyclovir, zidovudine, or didanosine (43). The clinical implications of foscarnet's anti-EBV activity remain to be elucidated.

X. COMBINED FOSCARNET AND GANCICLOVIR THERAPY

Two recently published reports document that a combination of ganciclovir and foscarnet can increase in vitro eficacy against human strains of CMV (44,45). Interactions between two antiviral drugs, such as ganciclovir and foscarnet, used simultaneously can be evaluated by the fractional inhibitory concentration (FIC) method in which the FIC for each combination of two specific drug concentrations is calculated by the formula FIC = (IC of drug X in combination/IC of drug X alone) + (IC of drug Y in combination/IC of drug Y alone) (44). Using this method, Manischewitz et al. (44) reported a mean FIC = 0.72 and Freitas et al. (45) reported a mean FIC = 0.64 when ganciclovir and foscarnet were combined to inhibit CMV replication in cell culture. These in vitro data suggest that ganciclovir and foscarnet in combination result in an additive or synergistic inhibition of CMV replication.

Since the major reported adverse effects of ganciclovir and foscarnet are mutually exclusive (i.e., myelosuppression for ganciclovir versus nephrotoxicity and hypocalcemia for foscarnet), reduced-dose combination therapy might provide a means to treat CMV retinitis patients with as much or more efficacy while reducing drug toxicity. Clinical trials of such combined regimen are currently being implemented.

XI. CONCLUSION

Foscarnet is a major therapeutic advance in the management of antiviral drug-resistant opportunistic herpesvirus infections. In addition, recent survival data from a large, randomized multicenter trial suggest that foscarnet may be the best initial treatment for AIDS patients with CMV retinitis who have normal renal function.

REFERENCES

1. Oberg B. Antiviral effects of phosphonoformate. Pharmac Ther 1983; 19:387–415.

2. Matthews T, Boehme R. Antiviral activity and mechanism of action of ganciclovir. Rev Infect Dis 1988; 10:S490-4.

3. Verheyden JPH. Evolution of therapy for cytomegalovirus infections. Rev Infect Dis 1988; 10:S477–89.

4. Plotkin SA, Drew WL, Felsenstein D, Hirsch MS. Sensitivity of clinical isolates of human cytomegalovirus to 9-(1,3-dihydroxy-2-propoxymethyl)guanine. J. Infect Dis 1985; 152:833–4.

5. Akesson-Johansson A, Lernestedt JO, Ringden O, Lonnqvist B, Wahren B. sensitivity of cytomegalovirus to intravenous foscarnet treatment. Bone Marrow Transplant 1986; 1:215–20.

6. Jacobson MA, Drew WL, Feinberg J, O'Donnell JJ, Whitmore PV, Miner RD, Parenti D. Foscarnet therapy for ganciclovir-resistant cytomegalovirus retinitis. J Infect Dis 1991; 163:1348–50.

7. Erlich KS, Mills J, Chatis P, et al. Acyclovir-resistant herpes simplex virus infections in patients with the acquired immunodeficiency syndrome. N Engl J Med 1989; 320(5):293–6.

8. Jacobson MA, Berger TG, Fikrig S, et al. Acyclovir-resistant varicella zoster virus infection after chronic oral acyclovir therapy in patients with the acquired immunodeficiency syndrome. Ann Intern Med 1990; 112:187–91.

9. Sandstrom EG, Byington RE, Kaplan JE, Hirsch MS. Inhibition of human T cell lymphotropic virus type III in vitro by phosphonoformate. Lancet 1985; 1:1480–2.

10. Jacobson MA, Crowe S, Levy J, et al. Effect of foscarnet therapy in infection with human immunodeficiency virus in patients with AIDS. J Infect Dis 1988; 158:862–5.

11. Jacobson MA, van det Horst C, Causey DM, et al. In vivo additive antiretroviral effect of combined zidovudine and foscarnet therapy for human immunodeficiency virus infection (ACTG Protocol 053). J Infect Dis 1991; 163: 1219–22.

12. Sommadossi JP, Bevan R, Long T, et al. Clinical pharmacokinetics of ganciclovir in patients with normal and impaired renal function. Rev Infect Dis 1988; 10:S507–14.

13. Sjovall J, Karlsson A, Ogenstad S, Sandstrom E, Saarimaki M. Pharmacokinetics and absorption of foscarnet after intravenous and oral administration to patients with human immunodeficiency virus. Clin Pharmacol Ther 1988; 44:65–73.

14. Smee DR, Boehme R, Chernow M, et al. Intracellular metabolism and enzymatic phosphorylation of 9-(1,3-dihydroxy-2-propoxymethyl)guanine and acyclovir in herpes simplex virus-infected and uninfected cells. Biochem Pharmacol 1985; 34:1049–56.

15. Barditch-Crovo P, Petty BG, Gambertoglio J, et al. The effect of increasing gastric PH upon the bioavailability of orally-administered phosphonoformic acid (foscarnet) [abstract]. VII International Conference on AIDS, 1991, Florence, Italy, Abstr. W.B.2115.

16. Aweeka FT, Gambertoglio J, van der Horst C, Jacobson MA. Pharmacokinetics (PK) of concomitantly administered foscarnet (F) and zidovudine (Z) in the treatment of patients with AIDS. (submitted for publication).

17. Collaborative DHPG Treatment Study Group. Treatment of serious cytomegalovirus infections with 9-(1,3-dihydroxy-2-propoxymethyl)guanine in patients with AIDS and other immunodeficiencies. N Engl J Med 1986; 314: 801–5.

18. Walmsley SL, Chew E, Fanning MM, et al. Treatment of cytomegalovirus retinitis with trisodium phosphonoformate hexahydrate (foscarnet). J Infect Dis 1988; 157:569–72.

19. Jacobson MA, O'Donnell JJ, Brodie HR, Wofsy C, Mills J. Randomized prospective trial of ganciclovir maintenance therapy for cytomegalovirus retinitis. J Med Virol 1988; 25:339–49.

20. Rozenbaum W, Gharakhanian S, Zazoun L, et al. Efficacy and toxicity of ganciclovir maintenance treatment in AIDS-related CMV retinitis. V International Conference on AIDS, 1989, Montreal, Canada. Abstr. M.B.P.132.

21. Feinberg J, Katz D, Mastre B, DeArmond B. Ganciclovir in AIDS patients with immediately sight-threatening CMV retinitis: initial summary of "Treatment IND" data. VI International Conference on AIDS, 1990, San Francisco, CA. Abstr. Th.B.432.

22. Katlama C, Dohin E, Massin-Cochereau I, et al. Prophylaxis of CMV retinitis relapse: evaluation of foscarnet in maintenance therapy [abstract]. V International Conference on AIDS, 1989, Montreal, Canada. Abstr. M.B.P.117.

23. Jacobson MA, Causey D, Polsky B, et al. Dose-ranging study of daily intravenous maintenance foscarnet therapy for cytomegalovirus retinitis in AIDS patients. VI International Conference on AIDS, 1990, San Francisco, CA. Abstr. F.B.96.

24. Palestine AG, Polis M, de Smet M, et al. A randomized controlled trial of foscarnet in the treatment of cytomegalovirus retinitis [abstract]. In Proceedings of The Association for Research in Vision and Opthalmology, 1990, Sarasota, FL, Abstr. 1802.

25. Study of Ocular Complications of AIDS Research Group. Foscarnet-ganciclovir cytomegalovirus retinitis trial: 2. Mortality (submitted for publication).

26. Drew WL, Miner RC, Busch DF, et al. Prevalence of resistance in patients receiving ganciclovir for serious cytomegalovirus infection. J Infect Dis 1990; 163:716–9.

27. Jacobson MA, Wulfson M, Feinberg J, Davis R, Power M, Crumpacker CS. Phase 2 dose-ranging study of foscarnet salvage therapy for cytomegalovirus retinitis in patients intolerant of or resistant to ganciclovir therapy (ACTG Protocol 093) [abstract]. 31st Interscience Conference on Antimicrobial Agents and Chemotherapy, 1991, Chicago, IL, Abstr. 296.

28. Gentilini M, Dohin E, Cochereau I, et al. Foscarnet in acute therapy of CMV retinitis: experience with a twice daily intermittent regimen [abstract]. VII International Conference on AIDS, 1991, Florence, Italy, Abstr. W.B.2257.

29. Jacobson MA, unpublished data.

30. Jacobson MA, O'Donnell JJ, Mills J. Foscarnet treatment of cytomegalovirus retinitis in patients with acquired immunodeficiency syndrome. Antimicrob Agents Chemother 1989; 33:736–41.

31. Cacoub P, Deray G, Baumelou A, et al. Acute renal failure induced by foscarnet: 4 cases. Clin Nephrol 1988; 29:315–8.

32. Deray G, Martinez F, Katlama C, et al. Foscarnet nephrotoxicity: mechanism, incidence and prevention. Am J Nephrol 1989; 9:316–21.

33. Youle MS, Clarbour J, Gazzard B, Chanas A. Severe hypocalcemia in AIDS patients treated with foscarnet and pentamidine [letter]. Lancet 1988; 1:1455–6.

34. Jacobson MA, Gambertoglio JG, Aweeka FT, Causey DM, Portale AA. Foscarnet-induced hypocalcemia and effects on calcium metabolism. J Clin Endocrinol Metab 1991; 72:1130–5.

35. Farese RV, Schambelan M, Hollander H, Stringari S, Jacobson MA. Nephrogenic diabetes insipidus associated with foscarnet treatment of cytomegalovirus retinitis in a patient with acquired immunodeficiency syndrome. Ann Intern Med 1990; 11:955–6.

36. Fegueux S, Salmon D, Picard C, et al. Penile ulcerations with foscarnet. Lancet 1990; 1:547–8.

37. Aweeka F, Gambertoglio J, Mills J, Jacobson MA. Pharmacokinetics of intermittently administered intravenous foscarnet in the treatment of acquired immunodeficiency syndrome patients with serious cytomegalovirus retinitis. Antimicrob Agents Chemother 1989; 33:742–5.

38. Nelson M, Connolly G, Hawkins D, et al. Foscarnet in the treatment of cytomegalovirus infection of the oesophagus and colon [abstract]. VII International Conference on AIDS, 1991, Florence, Italy, Abstr. W.B.2262.

39. Dieterich D, Dicker M, Tepper R. Foscarnet treatment of cytomegalovirus gastrointestinal infections in AIDS patients who have failed ganciclovir [abstract]. VII International Conference on AIDS, 1991, Florence, Italy, Abstr. W.B.2293.

40. Erlich KS, Jacobson MA, Koehler JE, et al. Foscarnet therapy for severe acyclovir-resistant herpes simplex virus type-2 infections in patients with the acquired immunodeficiency syndrome (AIDS). Ann Intern Med 1989; 110(9): 710–3.

41. Safrin S, Crumpacker C, Chatis P, et al. A controlled trial comparing foscarnet with vidarabine for acyclovir-resistant mucocutaneous herpes simplex in the acquired immunodeficiency syndrome. N Engl J Med 1991; 325(8): 551–5.

42. Safrin S, Berger TG, Gilson I, et al. Foscarnet therapy in five patients with AIDS and acyclovir-resistant varicella-zoster virus infection. Ann Intern Med 1991; 115(1):19–21.

43. Van der Horst C, Fiscus S, Jacobson MA, et al. Epstein-Barr virus in HIV patients: antiviral therapy [abstract]. 30th Interscience Conference on Antimicrobial Agents and Chemotherapy, 1990, Chicago, IL, Abstr. 548.

44. Manischewitz JF, Quinnan GV, Lane HC, Wittek AE. Synergistic effect of ganciclovir and foscarnet on cytomegalovirus replication in vitro. Antimicrob Agents Chemother 1990; 34:373–5.

45. Freitas VR, Fraser-Smith EB, Matthews TR. Increased efficacy of ganciclovir in combination with foscarnet against cytomegalovirus and herpes simplex virus type 2 in vitro and in vivo. Antiviral Res 1989; 12:205–12.

8

Pathophysiology of the AIDS Wasting Syndrome

Carl Grunfeld
University of California—San Francisco, and Department of Veterans Affairs Medical Center, San Francisco, California

Donald P. Kotler
College of Physicians and Surgeons, Columbia University, and St. Luke's–Roosevelt Hospital Center, New York, New York

I. INTRODUCTION

Progressive weight loss and debilitation are common consequences of
human immunodeficiency virus (HIV) infection, and malnutrition has
long been recognized as a major cause of morbidity in this disease (1–3).
AIDS in Africa was first known as ''slim disease'' because of a syndrome
of severe wasting that preceded death (4). Weight loss of greater than 10%
of body weight associated with fever or diarrhea of more than 30 days
duration and the presence of antibody against HIV are sufficient criteria
to make the diagnosis of AIDS in the absence of specific AIDS-defining
complications (5). Despite the use of antiretroviral agents, improvements
in therapy and prophylaxis against many of the major disease complications, the prevalence of the wasting syndrome is increasing.

Many characteristic features of the wasting syndrome in AIDS are similar to those seen in other chronic infections and malignancies. Studies
over the past several years have defined the general features of wasting
associated with HIV infection, the underlying pathophysiological mechanisms and the general responses to nutritional support programs. A role

for interventions specifically directed at the wasting syndrome itself is increasingly being explored. The aims of this chapter are to describe the effects of malnutrition upon body composition in HIV-infected individuals, to present the biochemical and physiological mechanisms underlying wasting, and to discuss the status of nutritional support.

II. THE CLINICAL SYNDROME OF WASTING

A. Studies of Body Composition

Many studies have documented significant weight loss in AIDS patients. While readily available and easily measured, body weight may not be a precise measure of nutritional status in clinically ill patients due to confounding effects of vomiting, diarrhea, decreased fluid intake, or hydration therapy, which may change weight substantially without affecting the underlying nutritional status. A more relevant measure of the amount of functional protoplasm is the body cell mass, which is the nonadipose cellular mass (1). The major components of the body cell mass are the muscles and viscera.

Patients with AIDS have been shown to be depleted of body cell mass using a variety of methods, such as determining total body potassium content, intracellular water volume, and total body nitrogen content, the latter implying protein depletion (1,6). Body cell mass depletion occurs out of proportion to loss of body weight (1). The difference is due to an increase in extracellular water volume. Similar results have been seen in other models of protein-calorie malnutrition and are due, at least in part, to the effects of hypoalbuminemia. However, some AIDS patients have normal body cell mass measurements, indicating that AIDS is not caused by malnutrition and that malnutrition is not a universal phenomenon (1). Thus, the development of malnutrition must represent the effect of a complication of AIDS rather than AIDS itself.

Body fat content in HIV infection also has been measured, and the results differ from the effects on body cell mass (1,6). While many patients are fat depleted, other malnourished patients may have normal or even increased body fat contents. Excess body fat, like excess extracellular water, may mask significant body cell mass depletion. Depletion of body cell mass without fat depletion is the opposite response of what would be expected in uncomplicated semistarvation, in which nitrogen sparing and predominant utilization of fat for energy occurs (1,7–9). Thus, wasting in AIDS is different from starvation.

While the use of body weight for assessment of nutritional status is possible in many clinical illnesses, the process may be insensitive in detecting malnutrition in AIDS due to a relative excess in extracellular water volume or body fat. It is important to remember the predilection of patients with AIDS to become malnourished and to maintain a high index of suspicion. Despite a lack of sensitivity, however, progressive changes in weight, especially in the setting of prior stability, indicate the likely presence of an active disease complication and mandates an evaluation for the cause.

B. Relationship Between the Magnitude of Wasting and Survival

The relationship between the degree of wasting and death was analyzed retrospectively in patients dying with a wasting syndrome in the absence of formal nutritional support (1). Body cell mass depletion, analyzed as a function of time before death, had a linear relationship to survival. The extrapolated body cell mass at death was 54% of normal, which corresponded to a body weight at death of 66% of ideal. Historical studies of death by starvation also found that the risk of dying rose as body weight fell to about one third below ideal (1). On the other hand, body weight as percent of ideal, extrapolated to 100 days before death, was within the normal range (91% of ideal), though body cell mass depletion was found (71% of normal). Body fat content bore no identifiable relationship to time of death (1). Another study also found a relationship between survival and wasting (3). Similar relationships have been found in other diseases such as cancer (10). The implication of these studies is that death from wasting may be due to the degree of wasting rather than the specific cause of the wasting process itself. If so, then maintenance of a nutritional status above this critical point should lead to prolonged survival. This latter point has not been tested.

III. PATHOGENETIC MECHANISMS UNDERLYING WASTING

A. Multifactorial Nature

Caloric balance is most simply viewed as the interactions between calorie intake and absorption versus intermediary metabolism. If the former factors are greater, excess energy is available to be stored as body cell mass or fat. On the other hand, if the needs of intermediary metabolism are greater than the amount of energy consumed or absorbed, an energy deficit occurs, which must be balanced by converting body cell mass or fat to energy. The normal homeostatic controls of these processes are important in maintaining health.

The mechanisms that underlie wasting can be divided into three categories: those that impair nutrient intake, those that interfere with nutrient absorption, and those that produce metabolic derangements (Table 1). An important feature of HIV infection is the multifactorial nature of malnutrition. Since AIDS is a disease of weakened resistance to infection and malignancy, several complications may occur simultaneously and promote the development of malnutrition by different mechanisms. A single disease also can affect nutritional status by more than one mechanism. The situation is complicated further, since the disease complications may change during the clinical course of AIDS, and the mechanisms underlying malnutrition may also change.

B. Metabolic Abnormalities

Several aspects of intermediary metabolism have been studied in HIV-infected individuals in relationship to the wasting process, and it is generally felt that metabolic alterations may play an important role in malnutrition at many stages of the disease. Many studies have shown that cytokines, hormones that mediate immune and inflammatory responses, can mediate the metabolic disturbances and wasting in infections and

Table 1 Theoretical Mechanisms of Wasting

Decreases in nutrient intake
Anorexia
Dementia
Mechanical obstruction
Decreased nutrient absorption
Malabsorption
Metabolic disturbances
Wasting of protein
Hypermetabolism
Inappropriate use of substrates
Futile cycling
The fat cell and the cachectin hypothesis

cancers (11,12). Progress in this area of inquiry has proceeded relatively slowly due to its great complexity, incomplete knowledge of the systems studied, and poor understanding of the mechanisms of wasting in any disease model.

The following sections will discuss the emerging field of cytokine regulation of metabolism in detail. This will be followed by a review of the results of metabolic studies in HIV-infected individuals, including studies of cytokines.

C. The Cachectin Hypothesis

Wasting is a characteristic feature of chronic infections. The lack of correlation between infective burden and the degree of wasting (13) and the reproduction of the metabolic effects of infection by administering nonviable extracts of infectious origin (14,15) suggested that the metabolic response to infection may be mediated by endogenous host processes. Cytokine infusions in humans and experimental animals (12) reproduce the constitutional symptoms associated with infections (Table 2). These include some that are prominent in AIDS. Cytokines also mediate shock (12).

Certain infections are characterized by both weight loss and severe hypertriglyceridemia (16). The alterations in lipid metabolism are associated with increased hepatic fatty acid synthesis and VLDL production and decreased clearance rates for triglycerides (11–13). The latter abnormality

Table 2 Symptoms of AIDS
Reproduced by Cytokine Therapy

Fever
Myalgia
Fatique
Lethargy
Nausea
Anorexia
Diarrhea
Anemia
Leukopenia
Headache
Confusion
Tachycardia

is associated with decreased activity of lipoprotein lipase (LPL), the enzyme responsible for clearing circulating triglycerides. Because a decrease in the clearance of triglycerides could theoretically lead to decreased storage of fat in adipose tissue, a factor (named cachectin) was sought that might produce both wasting and hypertriglyceridemia by inducing adipose tissue catabolism (16). The media from endotoxin-simulated macrophages contained a factor that could induce weight loss in animals and decrease LPL activity. The culture supernatant also decreased the de novo synthesis of lipids in cultured fat cells and promoted lipolysis (16). Postulating that a single factor was responsible for both the wasting and hypertriglyceridemia, the material was purified based on its ability to inhibit LPL in cultured fat cells; upon sequencing, cachectin was found to be the cytokine tumor necrosis factor (TNF). Further studies demonstrated the ability of TNF to mediate many of the effects of cachectin. Purified recombinant TNF decreased the synthesis of LPL and the de novo synthesis of fatty acids in cultured fat cells, while promoting lipolysis (11,17). The actions of TNF occur at both transcriptional and posttranscriptional levels. The initial studies (17) led to the advancement of the cachectin hypothesis, in which TNF was considered to be the cause of wasting in infections and tumors. However, many further studies have indicated a far more complex system of metabolic regulation.

The catabolic effects of cytokines on cultured fat cells are not limited to TNF but are also found with interleukin-1 (IL-1) and interferons-alpha, -beta, and -gamma (11,17–19). These cytokines decrease LPL, inhibit de novo lipogenesis, and increase lipolysis in culture. Thus, multiple cytokines share the ability to reproduce the effect of cachectin on fat cell metabolism in vitro.

However, effects of TNF can be separated from the effects of cachectin. For example, rodents progressively lose weight when injected with the same daily dose of crude cachectin (20). In contrast, when daily or even twice daily injections of purified recombinant TNF are given to rats, the weight loss is transient (11,21–29). Decreased food intake, decreased water intake, and increased urine output account for the acute loss in weight (28), then the animals become tachyphylactic to the anorectic and diuretic effects of TNF. Thus, the syndrome of cachexia cannot be reproduced with injection of pure TNF. However, chronic TNF treatment produces persistent hypertriglyceridemia irrespective of the weight changes (28). Thus, the metabolic disturbances that lead to hypertriglyceridemia are not inevitably linked to wasting.

D. Cytokine-Induced Changes in Lipid Metabolism In Vivo

Serum triglycerides increase rapidly after TNF administration to rats in vivo, associated with an increase in very low-density lipoprotein (VLDL) of normal composition (30). This finding cannot be explained by the known effects of TNF on cultured fat cells in vitro. The effect of TNF upon LPL activity in the epididymal fat pad does not occur until several hours after serum triglycerides have risen (31–33), and no decrease is seen in muscle LPL (31,32). In fact, total postheparin lipolytic activity is increased by TNF treatment (31). As a consequence, there is no effect of TNF on the clearance of chylomicrons or VLDL despite TNF-induced hypertriglyceridemia (33–36). Therefore, the effect of TNF on fat cells cannot be the cause of TNF-induced hypertriglyceridemia. Likewise, it is also not possible to demonstrate an effect of IL-1 on triglyceride clearance in vivo (37).

Recent studies have shown that TNF and IL-1 increase plasma triglycerides by increasing hepatic lipogenesis and VLDL production (30,33,37,38). The time course for TNF stimulation of de novo fatty acid synthesis in liver parallels the increase in serum triglycerides (30). In addition to TNF, IL-1, IL-6, and interferon-alpha also increase hepatic fatty acid synthesis (37–40). TNF and IL-1 stimulate hepatic fatty acid synthesis at concentrations that are similar to those that induce fever (endogenous pyrogen activity), implying that the effect of cytokines upon fatty acid synthesis occurs during the normal response to infection (39).

E. Futile Cycling

Some of the metabolic disturbances that occur during infection lead directly to energy losses and could potentially contribute to wasting. For example, in septic dogs, hypertriglyceridemia is not due to decreases in LPL and triglyceride clearance (41) but to enhanced VLDL production. Fatty acids, mobilized from the periphery, are reesterified into triglyceride and secreted as VLDL (41) and not oxidized, as occurs during exercise or fasting.

In rodents, TNF acutely increases serum free fatty acids (36,42). Phenylisopropyladenosine, which is known to block fat cell lipolysis, prevents both the TNF-induced rise in fatty acids and the increase in serum triglycerides (36), implying that the fatty acids mobilized by TNF are substrates for hepatic VLDL synthesis.

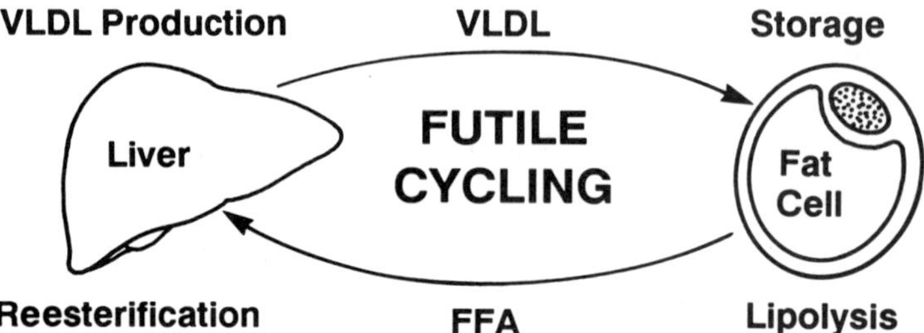

Figure 1 A fatty acid/triglyceride futile cycle that wastes energy during infection. Lipolysis mobilizes fatty acids from peripheral fat cells, returning them to the liver. The fatty acid, rather than being oxidized to produced energy in the hepatocyte, is reesterified into triglyceride and resecreted in VLDL. The VLDL returns to adipose tissue where its triglyceride is hydrolyzed by lipoprotein lipase and the fatty acids are stored again as triglyceride within the fat cells. Each extra synthesis of triglyceride (either intrahepatic and intraadipose) wastes energy. [Reproduced with permission from C. Grunfeld, Mechanisms of wasting in infection and cancer: An approach to cachexia in AIDS. In: *Gastrointestinal and Nutritional Manifestations of the Acquired Immunodeficiency Syndrome*, D.P. Kotler (ed.), Raven Press, Ltd., New York, 1991, p. 220.]

The two studies described above illustrate the process of substrate or futile cycling (Fig. 1). Fatty acids released from adipose tissue stores are resynthesized into VLDL, requiring ATP. When the resultant VLDL is broken down by LPL in the periphery and fatty acids are taken back up into fat and muscle, ATP is again required to synthesize triglyceride. The energy expended in shuttling the fatty acid between liver and periphery is not compensated for by fatty acid oxidation, and the result is energy loss rather than energy gain. Other potential futile cycles exist in carbohydrate and protein metabolism.

F. Inappropriate Use of Substrates

Efficient use of energy sources is necessary for homeostasis. When excess nutrients are available, the body stores energy in the most efficient form possible on a weight basis, as triglycerides. However, some energy is utilized transforming glucose into fatty acid for storage. When needs are increased, fatty acid decreases and fat is oxidized for energy. Thus, the increase in de novo hepatic fatty acid (and subsequent VLDL synthesis) induced by TNF, IL-1, IL-6, and interferon-alpha are inappropriate when caloric needs are increased or exceed intake.

Another possible inefficient use of substrate deals with storage and metabolism of glucose. Glucose can be taken up into liver by a direct or an indirect pathway, which requires more energy.

G. Protein Wasting

Loss of muscle mass or protein is a more problematic aspects of cachexia than loss of fat mass. These changes distinguish cachectin patients from those with pure starvation, such as anorexia nervosa (1). In response to decreased caloric intake, the body normally can differentially regulate the catabolism of muscle and fat. As illustrated in Figure 2, an acute fast of 24 hours in a 70-kg man results in the oxidation of about of 60 g of protein and 150 g of fat (7–9). With prolonged fasting (Fig. 2), the body is able to reduce protein loss by about two thirds (8,9). The compensation probably accounts for some of the decrease seen in the resting energy expenditure (REE) seen during chronic caloric restriction (7–9). Sepsis dramatically increases protein losses (Fig. 3), which may reach levels as high as 125 g/day (9). The protein-conservation mechanism is not effec tive in the presence of sepsis after caloric restriction, and protein losses of up to 90 g/day are found (9).

The factors responsible for the increase in muscle protein degradation during sepsis have not yet been clearly defined. Endotoxin-stimulated macrophages produce a substance(s) that can induce the acute degradation of muscle protein in vitro (25). However, no single cytokine or combination has been shown to reproduce this acute proteolysis in muscle cells.

H. The Hypermetabolic State

Acute sepsis is accompanied by increases in REE or basal metabolic rate (9,43,44). While futile cycling and inappropriate use of substrate contribute to the increase in REE, much of the increase comes from unknown pathways (41). Multiple cytokines including TNF, IL-1, and the interferons induce fever (11,12); hyperthermia per se is a known cause of increased REE. The ability of cytokines such as TNF and IL-1 to increase REE is still being debated. In contrast to what is seen during infection, cancer patients are not always hypermetabolic (45,46).

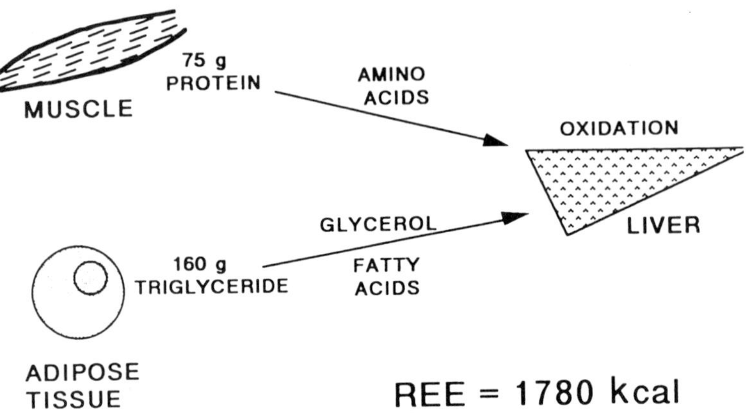

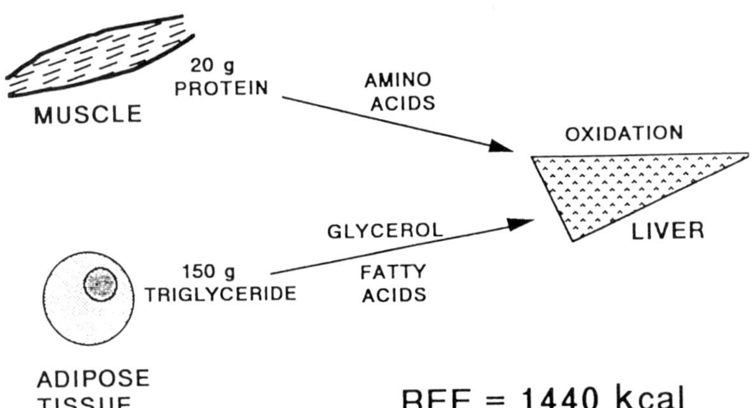

Figure 2 Fuel homeostasis during fasting. Over the course of a 24-hr fast, a 70-kg subject utilizes 75 g muscle protein and 160 g triglyceride to provide energy needs. After chronic fasting, protein is conserved, as over the course of 24 hr only 20 g of protein but 150 g of triglyceride are used. Initial REE is 1780 kcal, but with chronic fasting REE falls to 1440 kcal. (Reproduced with permission from C. Grunfeld and D. P. Kotler, *Wasting in the Acquired Immunodeficiency Syndrome. Seminars in Liver Disease.* Thieme, Inc., New York, 1992.)

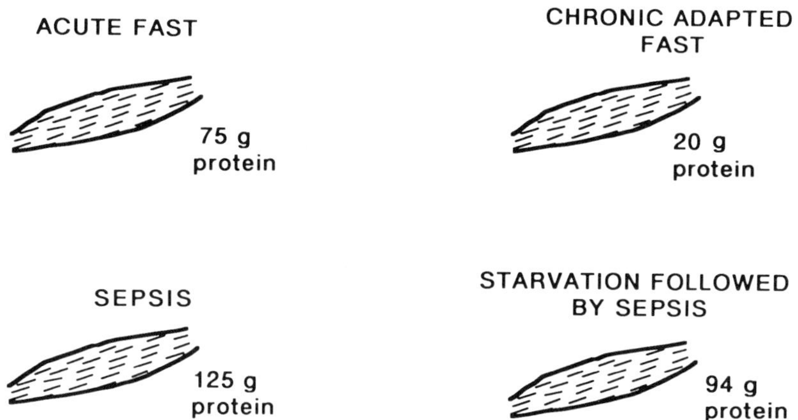

Figure 3 Protein metabolism during fasting and sepsis. As shown in Figure 2, over a 24-hr acute fast, 75 g of protein are consumed but with chronic fasting, mechanisms conserve protein and 24-hr utilization decreases. During acute sepsis, protein catabolism increases compared to an acute fast. When chronic caloric deprivation precedes sepsis, protein catabolism is blunted compared to sepsis in a nutritionally replete patient, but still exceeds that during an acute fast and far exceeds the level of conservation seen during chronic fasting without sepsis. (Reproduced with permission from C. Grunfeld and D. P. Kotler, *Wasting in the Acquired Immunodeficiency Syndrome. Seminars In Liver Disease.* Thieme, Inc., New York, 1992.)

I. Anorexia, Cytokines, and Wasting

Cytokines also have profound effects upon food intake. Experimental and clinical therapy with cytokines produces anorexia. In experimental animals, TNF decreases gastric motility, leading to retention of food in the stomach and small intestine (21,47). However, animals became refractory to the anorectic effects of TNF (21–29). In contrast, IL-1 can induce continuous anorexia with failure to maintain normal weight in rodents (48,49). The use of IFN-alpha and -gamma in cancer chemotherapy may also be accompanied by anorexia (50–52).

As discussed above, it is unlikely that TNF or any other cytokine is the sole cause of cachexia during infection and that the metabolic effects of cytokines (i.e., disturbances in lipid metabolism hypertriglyceridemia) do not inevitably cause wasting. On the other hand, anorexia may be a major contributor to weight loss. When TNF doses are sequentially escalated reaching levels that would be lethal in previously unexposed animals, the TNF-treated rats lose weight; however, pair-fed rats show the same rate of weight loss (22). Continuous infusion of TNF through chronic indwelling catheters also produces anorexia and sustained weight loss, but again the changes are similar in pair-fed rats (53). Finally, a tumor genetically engineered to secrete TNF induces both anorexia and cachexia (54). Serum TNF levels are readily detectable before the onset of weight loss, when intake is normal; with large tumor burdens, high levels of TNF, anorexia and weight loss occur (55).

Additionally, interferon-gamma has been proposed to mediate anorexia and weight loss in other animal tumor models (56). In contrast, circulating TNF is not found in humans with cancer cachexia (57,58).

Tisdale has recently studied multiple colon cancers, which induce similar metabolic effects to those seen during infection, including excess hepatic fatty acid synthesis (59), but do not necessarily induce cachexia. The tumor-bearing animals that maintained adequate weight increased their caloric intake to compensate for the tumor-induced disturbances in metabolism. In contrast, those animals that lost weight did not increase their intake. The inappropriate increase in hepatic fatty acid synthesis continued in the face of anorexia (59). Thus, it appears that a combination of anorexia and metabolic disturbances drives cachexia in this animal model.

J. Other Potential Effects of Cytokines

The mechanism behind other metabolic defects and the cytokines involved are not yet understood. Cytokines have a wide variety of metabolic effects on glucose and amino acid metabolism (see Ref. 11). In addition, cytokines are known to induce levels of key catabolic hormones including glucagon, ACTH, glucocorticoids, and catecholamines (11). Administration of some cytokines reduces plasma thyroxine and triiodothyronine levels (11).

IV. METABOLIC ABNORMALITIES IN HIV-INFECTED PATIENTS

A. Energy Expenditure

Several groups have reported that REE is elevated in AIDS and HIV infection (60–64). One group found an increase in REE in HIV-seropositive individuals with normal T-helper lymphocyte counts (62). Another study found increased REE early in HIV infection, with a further increase in REE seen later in AIDS (63). Finally, AIDS patients with secondary infection, particularly those with *Mycobacterium avium-intracellulare*, may be severely hypermetabolic (64). While some of the increase in REE seen in AIDS may be due to undetected opportunistic infections (63), the increase in REE in asymptomatic HIV-infected individuals without AIDS, who have no opportunistic infections (62,63), suggests that some of the increase in REE alteration may be related to the underlying HIV infection itself. However, no correlations have been found between increased REE and short-term weight loss (60,63) or other measures of wasting.

Hypermetabolism is not a universal phenomenon in AIDS. One group of AIDS patients selected to be clinically stable and studied prospectively was found to maintain body cell mass over a 6-week period (65). Caloric intake was normal, while mild-moderate malabsorption was found in the AIDS group, as compared to controls. REE was significantly lower in the AIDS group than in the control group, indicating an appropriate compensatory response (65). Caloric restriction is known to decrease REE in the absence of infection (7–9) (see Fig. 2). This group of AIDS patients maintained their weight in the presence of malabsorption by decreasing REE.

B. Serum Cytokine Concentrations in AIDS

Soon after sensitive assays for TNF were developed, a report of increased circulating TNF levels in AIDS patients was published (66). It was proposed that TNF was responsible for wasting in AIDS (66–68). However, no relationship between the degree of weight loss and the levels of circulating TNF was shown (66). Several of the patients with elevated TNF concentrations had active ongoing infections, such as pneumocystis (66). Subsequent studies were unable to demonstrate elevated TNF levels in AIDS (60,69–73). Reddy et al. (69) did find an increase in TNF levels in AIDS patients with a history of intravenous drug abuse, due to a small number of patients with strikingly elevated levels. However, when studying more clinically relevant controls (HIV-seronegative patients on methadone maintenance), the differences disappeared; HIV-negative intravenous drug addicts had the same high levels of TNF as HIV-positive addicts; HIV-negative homosexual controls had levels similar to homosexual AIDS patients (69).

Serum TNF levels are more likely to be elevated in overwhelming infections, acute sepsis, and acute parasitic infections than in chronic infections

(57,74–76). Increased serum TNF levels were not found during the chronic phases of other infections that lead to wasting (57,76). Likewise, patients with cancer cachexia do not have detectable TNF in the circulation (57,58).

C. Lipid Metabolism in AIDS

Early clinical observations noted turbidity of the serum in HIV-infected patients, which led to the discovery of fasting hypertriglyceridemia. Serum triglycerides and body composition were measured in patients with AIDS, HIV-infected non-AIDS patients, and controls (77). Serum triglyceride levels were higher in the AIDS group than in controls, while levels in HIV-infected patients were intermediate. Serum cholesterol concentrations were not elevated and did not correlate with triglyceride levels. Fifty percent of the AIDs group had abnormally elevated triglyceride concentrations, as did 50% of the HIV-infected group. Hypertriglyceridemia was chronically elevated in patients whose sera were followed longitudinally.

No correlations were found between the presence or level of hypertriglyceridemia or the presence of body cell mass depletion, as measured by total body potassium counting or altered fat content. In addition, patients often maintained their body cell mass over time despite persistent hypertriglyceridemia (77). Thus, just as seen with chronic TNF treatment (28), disturbances in triglyceride metabolism do not inevitably lead to wasting.

There also was no correlation between wasting and cholesterol levels (77). Recent data indicate that decreases in plasma cholesterol levels occur early in HIV infection and persist through the development of AIDS (71). Decreases are found in both LDL and HDL. The lack of correlation between hypertriglyceridemia and wasting is important, and suggests that the body is capable of compensating for the deleterious effects of some metabolic alterations.

In follow-up studies, the correlations between serum triglyceride concentrations and plasma concentrations of selected cytokines were determined (70,71). A significant correlation was found between serum interferon-alpha concentration and triglyceride concentration. Some of the variance can be accounted for by genetic factors. AIDS subjects with the apolipoprotein E3/2 phenotype are more susceptible to hypertriglyceridemia (78). No correlations were found with circulating TNF concentrations. Interleukin-1 beta was not detected in serum (70).

At least two mechanisms contribute to hypertriglyceridemia in AIDS. First, there is a decrease in the triglyceride clearance rate in HIV-infected individuals, which likely is due to inhibition of lipoprotein lipase activity (71). Second, these patients show an increase in fasting and postprandial hepatic lipogenesis (73). The presence and concentration of interferon-alpha in serum correlated even more strongly with the slowing of triglyceride clearance and with the increase in fasting de novo hepatic lipogenesis (71, 73). It is not clear whether circulating interferon-alpha in AIDS directly induces hypertriglyceridemia or whether interferon-alpha is merely a marker of immunological activity; another cytokine or cytokines participating in the immune response may mediate the hypertriglyceridemia.

The increase in de novo hepatic fatty acid synthesis seen in AIDS and HIV infection is inappropriate usage of energy, although it is also quantitatively small (73). In the single study to date, there was no increase in glucose stored by the less efficient indirect pathway in AIDS (79). The role of futile cycling has not yet been defined in AIDS. In addition, the role of futile cycling in any form of wasting is not clear. Futile cycling per se should not cause wasting. Theoretically, an increase in caloric intake could compensate for the energy lost in futile cycling. However, the effect of extra alimentation on futile cycling has not been studied. In addition, the known amount of futile cycling in sepsis or burns does not represent a major energy loss, accounting for only 15% of the increase in resting energy expenditure (40).

D. Protein Metabolism

The data on protein metabolism in AIDS are limited. Protein losses are not dramatically accelerated in many patients with AIDS (79). Both protein synthesis and protein degradation are nearly equally depressed, with perhaps a slightly greater decrease in the synthetic rate. This pattern is more like starvation than the increased turnover of sepsis and may make it difficult to maintain or regain lean muscle mass. In addition, anorexia with decreased caloric intake does not induce conservation of protein metabolism as efficiently in AIDS patients as in controls, especially in the presence of secondary infection (80). Just as conservation of REE may occur in a subset of patients with AIDS (65), it is possible that varying degrees of protein loss and protein conservation are seen in AIDS depending upon the clinical situation.

E. Malabsorption

Intestinal nutrient malabsorption in AIDS patients was an early observation and remains a serious problem in many cases. When present, small intestinal injury may be severe and associated with significant functional impairment (81,82). Nutrient malabsorption occurs secondary to decreased intestinal surface area, functional defects in pathogen-damaged cells, and functional immaturity of villus epithelial cells associated with rapid cell turnover (83,84).

A cross-sectional study demonstrated partial vilus atrophy and crypt hyperplasia in a subgroup of AIDS patients. Villus and crypt abnormalities correlated with the presence of protozoal infections (81). In contrast, most patients without small intestinal pathogens had normal villus and crypt measurements and normal D-xylose absorption, the latter a reflection of intestinal surface area (82). Small intestinal injury has been found by other groups, but the relationship to parasitic infection was not analyzed specifically (85–87). Villus atrophy with hypoplastic crypts was reported in one study (86).

Several enteric pathogens have been shown to cause small bowel injury and malabsorption in AIDS as a result of epithelial cell damage. Villus atrophy and decreased mucosal surface area occurs despite compensatory crypt hyperplasia. As a result of the crypt hyperplasia, however, cell migration and turnover on the villus is accelerated, which results in functional immaturity, with further adverse effects upon the absorption of lactose and fats (88,89).

Cryptosporidiosis is the most common identifiable cause of small bowel injury and malabsorption, occuring in up to 10% of cases (90). Cryptosporidiosis causes a self-limited diarrheal illness in immunocompetent people, while patients with AIDS usually develop a protracted enteropathy (91). No effective antiparasitic treatment is known. Small intestinal injury and malabsorption also is a consequence of isosporiasis in AIDS (91,92). Isosporiasis can be treated with trimethoprin-sulfamethoxazole, although chronic suppressive therapy is needed. Microsporidia also are an important cause of small intestinal injury and malabsorption. Initially reported to occur in 1985, the infection has been increasingly recognized worldwide and may be responsible for up to 10% of cases of severe malabsorption AIDS (90–94). Definitive diagnosis of microsporidia requires electron microscopy due to their small size. There is no known effective treatment for microsporidiosis.

Myocobacterium avium complex (MAC) infection of the intestine in AIDS patients also is associated with malabsorption. The mechanism appears to involve infiltration of the lamina propria and lymphatics with infected macrophages, producing a physical block to solute absorption plus exudative enteropathy (95). Intestinal MAC usually is associated with systemic involvement, including liver, spleen, bone marrow, and retroperitoneal lymph nodes. Multidrug antimycobacterial regimens have been capable of suppressing the clinical manifestations of the disease (96).

The term "AIDS enteropathy" has been used to describe idiopathic diarrhea and small intestinal injury (with or without malabsorption) for which no etiological agent is found on evaluation. Evidence of HIV in intestinal mucosa by molecular hybridization or immunohistological techniques has been reported by several laboratories (87,97–100). Retroviral infection has produced a severe enteropathy in a feline model (101). A direct role for HIV in producing small intestinal injury has not been demonstrated.

Mild-to-moderate degrees of malabsorption are commonly found in AIDS patients and may not be associated with identifiable enteric pathogens. Abnormal lactose breath tests, elevated fecal fat content, and D-xylose malabsorption have been reported in the absence of diarrhea and weight loss (102,103). Vitamin B_{12} malabsorption may be a common occurence and related to subnormal serum concentrations. Vitamin B_{12} malabsorption may precede the development of AIDS and may occur in the absence of identifiable pathogens (103–105). Excess bile salt deconjugation, implying ileal dysfunction, also was found in a group of AIDS patients with or without intestinal disease (106,107). The absorption of other micronutrients has not been reported but would be expected to be affected by severe mucosal injury. Other reported alterations in intestinal function that might affect absorption include hypochlorhydria and increased intestinal permeability. Protein-energy malnutrition by itself may impair absorption by promoting gut hypoplasia (108). In contrast, pancreatic function appears normal in the absence of specific pancreatic pathology (109).

F. Anorexia

Several studies of food intake have been performed in clinically stable HIV-infected individuals that documented normal macronutrient and micronutrient intake (60,63). However, subjects with weight loss have significant anorexia; many of these patients also have active secondary opportunistic or bacterial infections (63). In contrast, caloric intake of AIDS patients who are gaining weight is above normal. A strong correlation was found between caloric intake and short-term weight change (63).

Decreased food intake may occur by several mechanisms, including local pathology in the oral cavity, hypopharynx, or esophagus. Food intake also may be adversely affected in patients with malabsorptive disorders, profound diarrhea, systemic infections, medications, organic mental syndrome, or psychosocial factors that limit access to food. The specific problems affecting intake have been reviewed elsewhere (110).

G. Other Metabolic Changes in AIDS

Current data indicate that catecholamines, glucocorticoids, and glucagon are not elevated in AIDS patients (60). In addition, it appears that conversion of thyroxine of triiodothyronine is decreased in patients with AIDS and anorexia and weight loss (80), similar to that seen in the euthyroid sick syndrome (111). This decrease in triiodothyronine should theoretically help conserve protein and decrease energy expenditure (111). However, the patients with decreased triodothyronine levels did not show a compensatory decrease in protein turnover (80), suggesting that the euthyroid sick conservation mechanism does not work adequately during infection in AIDS.

H. Potential Role of Synergy Between Cytokines in Cachexia of AIDS

While the pathogenesis of cachexia in AIDS is uncertain, the results of animal experiments and studies in AIDS suggest a possible mechanism. It appears that neither TNF nor any other cytokine is the single cause of cachexia during infection. However, synergistic effects of multiple cytokines acting in concert might produce wasting. Synergistic effects entail multiplicative rather than additive interactions. The potential mechanisms for type of synergy are being explored. Although TNF, IL-1, IL-6, and interferon-alpha induce similar metabolic disturbances, such as the increase in de novo hepatic fatty acid synthesis, interferon-alpha acts by a different mechanism from TNF and the interleukins (112). As a consequence, interferon-alpha shows striking synergy with either TNF or IL-1 in stimulating hepatic fatty acid synthesis (112). Thus, while the body could potentially adapt to the effects of a single cytokine, multiple cytokines working by different mechanisms may produce more drastic changes in metabolism that could induce wasting. Likewise, synergy between TNF and IL-1 produces septic shock at low doses of both cytokines (113).

In two of the three models of TNF-induced anorexia/cachexia discussed above (53,54), weight loss potentially was due to synergy between cytokines. For example, rats that are chronically catheterized develop inflammation around catheter site and often fail to grow normally. Cytokines

or other inflammatory products that are generated at the catheter insertion site could act synergistically with the continuous infusion of TNF
to induce anorexia/cachexia. Earlier experiments using TNF secretion
from surgically implanted ALZET minipumps, where inflammation at the
insertion site subsides more rapidly, did not produce cachexia (J. Patton,
personal communication). Likewise, a tumor that secretes TNF may secrete other unidentified tumor products that could interact synergistically
with TNF. It has previously been shown that tumor-bearing animals are
more sensitive to the toxic effects of TNF (114). Also, the local production of TNF could interact with products of tumor macrophages. Similar
tumors engineered to secrete IL-6 also produce weight loss (115). In other
tumors, interferon-gamma (but not TNF) is associated with weight loss
(56).

Rapid wasting with anorexia occurs in AIDS during secondary infection (63). Bacterial and fungal infections can induce monokines such as
TNF and IL-1, although the ability to detect these monokines in the circulation may only be transient. It is possible that the induction of monokines during these secondary infections allows for synergy with the interferon-alpha that is found in the circulation of subjects with AIDS. Thus,
while AIDS patients can compensate for the metabolic effects of interferon-alpha (including the associated disturbances in lipid metabolism) and
do not undergo wasting, they may be unable to compensate for the effects
produced by the combination of the monokines with interferon-alpha.

V. STRATEGIES TO REVERSE WASTING IN AIDS

A. Treatment of Infection Improves Nutritional Status

Since wasting may result from specific disease complications such as infection (63), it is logical that effective treatment of infection should promote repletion of body mass. This hypothesis has been tested in a study
of patients receiving ganciclovir for cytomegalovirus colitis. Ganciclovir
treatment prolongs survival in CMV-infected patients (116). Successfully
treated patients showed an increase in body weight, body cell mass as measured by total body potassium, body fat, and serum albumin, whereas untreated historic controls with CMV infection showed decreases in these
parameters (117). The treated group showed a difference of more than 600
kcal/day in energy balance greater than the untreated patients based upon calculations made from average daily changes in body cell mass and
body fat content.

A key early study demonstrating the effectiveness of zidovudine (AZT) in preventing disease progression to AIDS documented a 3-kg weight gain during therapy (118). Thus, treatment of HIV infection itself may improve energy balance.

Since it appears that secondary infection is a major cause of rapid wasting in AIDS and that successful treatment of infections in patients with AIDS can reverse or at least blunt the wasting process, a careful search for treatable infections and/or malignancies is warranted in patients with AIDS and the wasting syndrome.

B. Nutritional Support

The ability of nutritional support programs to prevent or reverse wasting in chronic infections and malignancies and AIDS is uncertain as it has not been determined whether nutritional support will overcome metabolic aberrations such as futile cycling or inappropriate use of substrates. Several previous studies in oncological models suggested that alimentation may not lead to nutritional repletion and, under certain circumstances, may cause morbidity.

Hyperalimentation has been studied most during cancer chemotherapy. Intake falls during chemotherapy, and malnutrition is associated with poor prognosis in cancer. Several groups studied the ability of hyperalimentation during chemotherapy to prolong survival in cancer patients. A meta-analysis of these studies suggest that parenteral nutritional support during chemotherapy may decrease long-term survival in cancer; the odds ratio for survival was 0.81 ($p = 0.05$) suggestive of decreased survival (119). These authors also found a fourfold increased risk of infection in patients receiving hyperalimentation. Infection is also increased when central venous catheters are used in AIDS patients (120, 121).

However, data on parenteral nutrition in the absence of chemotherapy are more relevant to AIDS. Hyperalimentation of patients with lymphoma and weight loss who do not have anorexia leads to significant weight gain, but the weight gain is primarily fat, with no significant increase in muscle mass (122). In contrast, nutritional support in malignancies accompanied by decreased food intake (such as gastric or esophageal carcinoma) may decrease the rate of protein breakdown towards normal (123). Thus, when decreased food intake is the primary driving force in cancer cachexia, alimentation may lead to maintenance of or improvement in muscle mass.

C. Effect of Alimentation upon Nutritional Status in AIDS

Few studies have carefully examined the effect of alimentation in AIDS, but those that have been published suggest that the situation may be similar to that described for cancer in the preceding section. Severely malnourished AIDS patients who had documented decreased food intake were given formula diets at a rate of 500 kcal/day more than predicted requirements through a percutaneous gastrostomy (124). This enteric alimentation induced significant increases in body cell mass, fat, total lymphocytes, and serum albumin in these patients (124).

However, body cell mass repletion does not occur in all patients. In another study, total parenteral nutrition was given for a median of 14 weeks to 12 patients with AIDS and the wasting syndrome (125). In AIDS patients with wasting due to decreased food intake or severe malabsorption, hyperalimentation produced increases in body cell mass as well as body fat (125). In contrast, AIDS patients with severe and ineffectively treated systemic infections (including cytomegalovirus and MAC) showed only gains in body fat with no increases in body cell mass (125). Preliminary data from other groups also suggest that fat rather than muscle is formed during enteral alimentation in unselected subjects (126).

Experimental appetite stimulation with megesterol acetate has been proposed (127). Preliminary data from large studies indicate that most patients gain weight with a dose-dependent relationship to drug (128,129), but it remains to be determined whether this is lean body mass or fat.

D. Role of Lethargy and Fatigue in Wasting

As detailed above, AIDS usually is not characterized by unremittent wasting and severe protein catabolism (60,63,65,77,79). Most subjects with AIDS have periods of relative stability interspersed with bouts of rapid wasting, such as during secondary infection. As the disease progresses, recovery from these episodes of rapid wasting is less complete with chronic loss of body cell mass.

The constitutional symptoms of lethargy and fatigue may play an important role in this process. When weight is stable, total energy expenditure must equal caloric intake (TEE = CI). Total energy expenditure equals resting energy expenditure plus dietary thermogenesis plus energy expended in activity (TEE = REE + DT + EEA). In subjects with HIV disease and AIDS who have stable weight, REE may be increased, yet caloric intake is normal, i.e., caloric intake is not increased to compensate for the increase in REE (63). In these subjects, de novo hepatic lipogenesis increases with feeding, which should increase dietary thermogenesis (73). Therefore, to maintain total energy expenditure equal to caloric intake, these subjects must have a decrease in their energy expended in activity. Thus the lethargy and fatigue of infection serves to maintain weight in the face of increased REE.

However, decreased activity, while maintaining weight, is detrimental in the long term. Activity is required for maintenance of muscle mass, the most important component of body cell mass. Inactivity may lead to the inability to maintain muscle mass. Decreased muscle mass increases the frequency of fatigue, hence the activity of food preparation and even eating becomes more difficult. Finally, aggressive alimentation in the face of inactivity will produce fat storage disproportionate to muscle mass, as has been found in several studies (122,125,126).

VI. CONCLUSIONS AND FUTURE DIRECTIONS

Wasting in AIDS is a complex, multifactorial process. Metabolic disturbances are common but do not inevitably cause rapid wasting. Short-term weight loss is usually accompanied by decreased caloric intake and is often associated with secondary infections. It is likely that cytokines, the hormones that mediate the immune and inflammatory responses, are responsible for the metabolic disturbances and anorexia. However, no single cytokine can been linked to wasting in AIDS.

The relative role of malabsorption needs to be explored in well-characterized patient groups. Likewise, larger, randomized trials of appetite stimulation and enteric or parenteral feeding are necessary. Anabolic agents may be able to block infection-induced disturbances in metabolism and promote positive nitrogen balance. Other therapeutic approaches may decrease resting energy expenditure or dietary thermogenesis. Finally, specific therapies for the lethargy and fatigue of infection may lead to increases in muscle mass as well as improvement in the quality of life.

When weight loss is due to decreased nutrient intake (decreased food intake or malabsorption) in the absence of severe systemic infection, therapeutic intervention to increase nutrient intake may replete body cell mass. However, subjects with untreated systemic infection appear resistant to nutritional therapy. Therefore, any patient with rapid weight loss should be rigorously examined for treatable infections or malignancies.

ACKNOWLEDGMENTS

Supported in part by grants from the NIH (DK40990 and AI21414), the UCSF AIDS Clinical Research Center (University Wide Task Force on AIDS #91RCC86-SF), and Department of Veterans Affairs.

REFERENCES

1. Kotler DP, Wang J, Pierson R. Studies of body composition in patients with the acquired immunodeficiency syndrome. Am J Clin Nutr 1985; 42:1255–65.

2. Kotler DP, Tierney AR, Francisco A, Wang J, Pierson Jr RN. The magnitude of body cell mass depletion determines the timing of death from wasting in AIDS. Am J Clin Nutr 1989; 50:444-7.

3. Chlebowski RT, Grosvenor MB, Bernhard NH, Morales LS, Bulcavage LM. Nutritional status, gastrointestinal dysfunction, and survival in patients with AIDS. Am J Gastroenterol 1989; 84:1288-93.

4. Serwadda D, Sewankambo NK, Carswell JW, Bayley AC, Tedder RS, Weiss RA, Mugerwa RD, Lwegaba A, Kirya GB, Downing RG, Clayden SA and Dalgleish AG. Slim disease: a new disease in Uganda and its association with HTLV-III infection. Lancet 1985; ii:850-2.

5. Centers for Disease Control. Revision of the CDC case surveilance definition for acquired immunodeficiency syndrome. MMWR 1987; 36(Suppl 1S):3S-14S.

6. Kotler DP, Tierney AR, Dilmanian FA, et al. Correlation between total body potassium and total body nitrogen in patients with acquired immunodeficiency syndrome. Clin Res 1991; 39:649A.

7. Keys A, Brozek J, Henschel A, Mickelson O, Taylor HL. The biology of human starvation. Minneapolis: University of Minnesota Press, 1950.

8. Cahill GF. Starvation in man. N Engl J Med 1970; 282:668-75.

9. Brennan MF. Uncomplicated starvation versus cancer cachexia. Cancer Res 1977; 37:2359-64.

10. Heymsfield SB, McManus C, Smith J, Stevens V, Nixon DW. Anthropometric measurement of muscle mass: revised equations for calculating bone-free arm muscle area. Am J Clin Nutr 1982; 36:680-90.

11. Grunfeld C, Feingold KR. The metabolic effects of tumor necrosis factor and other cytokines. Biotherapy 1991; 3:143-58.

12. Grunfeld C, Palladino MA. Tumor necrosis factor: immunologic, antitumor, metabolic and cardiovascular activities. Adv Int Med 1990; 35:45-72.

13. Beisel WR. Metabolic response to infection. Ann Rev Med 1975; 26:9-20.

14. Kaufmann RL, Matson CG, Beisel WR. Hypertriglyceridemia produced by endotoxin: role of impaired triglyceride disposal mechanisms. J Infect Dis 1976; 133:548-55.

15. Lang CH, Bagby GJ, Spitzer JJ. Glucose kinetics and body temperature after lethal and nonlethal doses of endotoxin. Am J Physiol 1985; 248:R471-8.

16. Beutler B, Cerami A. Cachectin and tumor necrosis factor as two sides of the same biological coin. Nature 1986; 320:584-8.

17. Patton JS, Shepard HM, Wilking H, Lewis G, Aggarwal BB, Eessalu TE, Gavin LA, Grunfeld C. Interferons and tumor necrosis factors have similar catabolic effects on 3T3-L1 cells. Proc Natl Acad Sci USA 1986; 83:8313-7.

18. Beutler BA, Cerami A. Recombinant interleukin-1 suppresses lipoprotein lipase activity in 3T3-L1 cells. J Immunol 1986; 135:3969-71.

19. Feingold KR, Doerrler W, Dinarello CA, Fiers W, Grunfeld C. Stimulation of lipolysis in cultured fat cells by TNF, IL-1 and the interferons is blocked by inhibition of prostaglandin synthesis. Endocrinology 1992; 130:10–6.

20. Cerami A, Ikeda Y, Latrang N, Hotez PGA, Beutler B. Weight loss associated with an endotoxin induced mediator from peritoneal macrophages: the role of cachectin (tumor necrosis factor). Immunol Lett 1985; 11:173–7.

21. Patton JS, Peters PM, McCabe J, Crase D, Hansen S, Chen AB. Development of partial tolerance to the gastrointestinal effects of high doses of recombinant tumor necrosis factor alpha in rodents. J Clin Invest 1987; 80: 1587–96.

22. Tracey KJ, Wei H, Manogue KR. Cachectin/tumor necrosis factor induces cachexia, anemia and inflammation. J Exp Med 1988; 167:1211–27.

23. Socher SH, Friedman A, Martinez D. Recombinant human-tumor necrosis factor induces acute reductions in food-intake and body-weight in mice. J Exp Med 1988; 167:1957–62.

24. Stovroff MC, Fraker DL, Swedenborg JA, Norton JA. Cachectin/tumor necrosis factor, a possible mediator of cancer anorexia in the rat. Cancer Res 1988; 48:920–5.

25. Kettelhut IC, Goldberg AL. Tumor necrosis factor can induce fever in rats without activating protein breakdown in muscle or lipolysis in adipose tissue. J Clin Invest 1988; 81:1384–9.

26. Kramer SM, Aggarwal BB, Eessalu TE, McCabe SE, Ferraiolo BL, Figari IS, Palladino Jr MA. Characterization of the *in vitro* and *in vivo* species preference of human and murine tumor necrosis factor alpha. Cancer Res 1988; 48:920–5.

27. Mahony SM, Tisdale MJ. Induction of weight loss and metabolic alterations by human recombinant tumor necrosis factor. Br J Cancer 1988; 58:345–9.

28. Grunfeld C, Wilking H, Neese R, Gulli R, Gavin LA, Moser AH, Serio MK, Feingold KR. Persistence of the hypertriglyceridemic effect of tumor necrosis factor despite development of tachyphylaxis to its anorectic/cachectic effects in rats. Cancer Res 1989; 49:2554–60.

29. Mullen BJ, Harris RBS, Patton JS, Martin RJ. Recombinant tumor necrosis factor-alpha chronically administered in rats: lack of cachectic effect. Proc Soc Exp Biol Med 1990; 193:318–25.

30. Feingold KR, Grunfeld C. Tumor necrosis factor alpha stimulates hepatic lipogenesis in the rat *in vivo*. J Clin Invest 1987; 80:184–90.

31. Semb H, Peterson J, Tavernier J, Olivecrona T. Multiple effects of tumor necrosis factor on lipoprotein lipase *in vivo*. J Biol Chem 1987; 62:8390–4.

32. Grunfeld C, Gulli R, Moser AH, Gavin LA, Feingold KR. The effect of tumor necrosis factor administration *in vivo* on lipoprotein lipase activity in various tissues of the rat. J Lipid Res 1989; 30:579–85.

33. Chajek-Shaul T, Friendman G, Stein I, Shiloni E, Etienne J, Stein Y. Mechanisms of the hypertriglyceridemia induced by tumor necrosis factor administration to rats. Biochim Biophys Acta 1989; 1001:316–432.

34. Krauss RM, Feingold KR, Grunfeld C. Tumor necrosis factor acutely increases plasma levels of very low density lipoproteins of normal size and composition. Endocrinology 1990; 127:1016–21.

35. Feingold KR, Soued M, Staprans I, Gavin LA, Donahue ME, Huang BJ, Moser AH, Gulli R, Grunfeld C. The effect of TNF on lipid metabolism in the diabetic rat: Evidence that inhibition of adipose tissue lipoprotein lipase activity is not required for TNF induced hyperlipidemia. J Clin Invest 1989; 83:1116–21.

36. Feingold KR, Adi S, Staprans I, Moser AH, Neese R, Verdier JA, Doerrler W, Grunfeld C. Diet affects the mechanisms by which TNF stimulates hepatic triglyceride production. Am J Physiol 1990; 259:E177–84.

37. Feingold KR, Soued M, Adi S, Staprans I, Neese R, Shigenaga J, Doerrler W, Moser AH, Dinarello CA, Grunfeld C. The effect of interleukin-1 on lipid metabolism in the rat: Similarities to and differences from tumor necrosis factor. Arteriosclerosis Thromb 1991; 11:495–500.

38. Feingold KR, Serio MK, Adi S, Moser AH, Grunfeld C. Tumor necrosis factor stimulates hepatic lipid synthesis and secretion. Endocrinology 1989; 124:1336–42.

39. Feingold KR, Soued M, Serio MK, Moser AH, Dinarello CA, Grunfeld C. Multiple cytokines stimulate hepatic lipid synthesis in vivo. Endocrinology 1989; 125:267–74.

40. Grunfeld C, Adi S, Soued M, Moser AH, Fiers W, Feingold KR. Search for mediators of the lipogenic effects of tumor necrosis factor: Potential role for interleukin-6. Cancer Res 1990; 50:4233–8.

41. Wolfe RR, Shaw JHF, Durkot MJ. Effect of sepsis on VLDL kinetics: responses in basal state and during glucose infusion. Am Physiol 1985; 248:E732–40.

42. Grunfeld C, Verdier JA, Neese RA, Moser AH, Feingold KR. Mechanisms by which tumor necrosis factor stimulates hepatic fatty acid synthesis in vivo. J Lipid Res 1988; 29:1327–35.

43. Wilmore DW, Long JM, Mason AD, Skreen RW, Pruitt BA. Catecholamines: mediators of the hypermetabolic response to thermal injury. Ann Surg 1974; 180:653–69.

44. Long CL, Schaffel N, Geiger JW, et al. Metabolic response to injury and illness: estimation of energy and protein needs from indirect calorimetry and nitrogen balance. JPEN 1979; 3:452–6.

45. Arbeit JM, Lees DE, Corsey R, Brennan MF. Resting energy expenditure in controls and cancer patients with localized and diffuse disease. Ann Surg 1984; 199:292–8.

46. Nixon DW, Kutner M, Heymsfield S, Foltz AT, Carty C, Seitz S, Caspter K, Evans WK, Jeejeebhoy KN, Daly JM, Heber D, Poppendiek H, Hoffman FA. Resting energy expenditure in lung and colon cancer. Metabolism 1988; 37:1059–64.

47. Feingold KR, Soued M, Serio MK, Adi S, Moser AH, Grunfeld C. The effect of diet on tumor necrosis factor stimulation of hepatic lipogenesis. Metabolism 1990; 39:623–32.

48. Fujii T, Sato K, Ozawa M, Kasono K, Imamura H, Kanaji Y, Tsushima T, Shizume K. Effect of interleukin-1 (IL-1) on thyroid hormone metabolism in mice: Stimulation by IL-1 of iodothyronine 5′-deiodinating activity (Type I) in the liver. Endocrinology 1989; 124:167–74.

49. Hellerstein MK, Meydani SN, Meydani M, Wu K, Dinarello CA. Interleukin-1 induced anorexia in the rat. J Clin Invest 1989; 84:228–35.

50. Sherwin SA, Knost JA, Fein S, Abrans PG, Foon KA, Ochs JJ, Schoenberger C, Maluish AE, Oldham RK. A multiple-dose phase I trial of recombinant leukocyte A interferon in cancer patients. JAMA 1982; 248:2461–6.

51. Vadhan-Raj S, Al-Katib A, Bhalla R, Pelus L, Nathan CF, Sherwin SA, Oettgen HF, Krown SE. Phase I trial of recombinant interferon gamma in cancer patients. J Clin Oncol 1986; 4:137–46.

52. DiBisceglie AM, Martin P, Kassianides C, Lisker-Melman M, Murray L, Waggoner J, Goodman Z, Banks SM, Hoofnagle JH. Recombinant interferon alpha therapy for chronic hepatitis C: a randomized, double-blind, placebo-controlled trial. N Engl J Med 1989; 321:1506–20.

53. Michie HR, Sherman ML, Spriggs DR, Rounds J, Christies M, Wilmore DW. Chronic TNF infusion causes anorexia but not accelerated nitrogen loss. Ann Surg 1989; 209:19–24.

54. Oliff A, Defeo-Jones D, Boyer M, Martinez D, Kiefer D, Vuocolo G, Wolfe A, Socher SH. Tumor secreting human TNF/cachectin induce cachexia in mice. Cell 1987; 50:555–63.

55. Teng MN, Park BH, Koeppen HKW, Tracey KJ, Fendly BM, Schreiber H. Long-term inhibition of tumor growth by tumor necrosis factor in the absence of cachexia or T-cell immunity. Proc Natl Acad Sci USA 1991; 88:3535–9.

56. Langstein HN, Doherty GM, Fraker DL, Buresh CM, Norton JA. The roles of interferon gamma and tumor necrosis alpha in an experimental rat model of cancer cachexia. Cancer Res 1991; 51:2302–6.

57. Waage A, Espevik T, Lamvik J. Detection of tumor necrosis factor-like cytotoxicity in serum from patients with septicaemia but not from untreated cancer patients. Scand J Immunol 1986; 24:739–43.

58. Socher SH, Martinez D, Craig JB, Kuhn JG, Oliff A. Tumor necrosis factor not detectable in patients with clinical cancer cachexia. J Leuk Biol 1988; 43:436–44.

59. Mulligan HD, Tisdale MJ. Lipogenesis in tumour and host tissues in mice bearing colonic adenocarcinomas. Br J Cancer 1991; 63(5):719–22.

60. Hommes M, Romijn JA, Godfried MH, Eeftinck Schattenkerk JKM, Buurman WA, Endert E, Sauerwein HP. Increased resting energy expenditure in human immunodeficiency virus-infected men. Metabolism 1990; 39:1186–90.

61. Melchior JD, Salmon D, Rigaud D, Leport C, Bouvet E, Detruchis P, Vilde J-L, Vachon R, Coulaud J-P, Apfelbaum M. Resting energy expenditure is increased in stable, malnourished HIV-infected patients. Am J Clin Nutr 1991; 53:437–41.

62. Hommes MJT, Romjin JA, Endert E, Sauerwein HP. Resting energy expenditure and substrate oxidation in human immunodeficiency virus (HIV)-infected asymptomatic men: HIV affects host metabolism in the early asymptomatic stage. Am J Clin Nutr 1991; 54:311–5.

63. Grunfeld C, Pang M, Shimizu L, Shigenaga JK, Jensen P, Feingold KR. Resting energy expenditure, caloric intake and short-term weight change in human immunodeficiency virus infection and the acquired immunodeficiency syndrome. Am J Clin Nutr 1992; 55:455–60.

64. Melchior JC, Raguin G, Rigaud D, Bouvet E, Matheron S, Boulier A, Vilde JL, Vachon F, Apfelbaum M. Proceedings VII Intl. Conf. on AIDS, Florence, Italy, June 16-21, 1991, V.2, p. 293 (Abstract).

65. Kotler DP, Tierney AR, Brenner SK, Couture S, Wang J, Pierson JR RN. Preservation of short-term energy balance in clinically stable patients with AIDS. Am J Clin Nutr 1990; 51:7–13.

66. Lahdevirta J, Maury CPJ, Teppo AM, Repo H. Elevated levels of circulating cachectin/tumor necrosis factor in patients with acquired immunodeficiency syndrome. Am J Med 1988; 85:289–91.

67. Beutler B. The presence of cachectin/tumor necrosis factor in human disease states. Am J Med 1988; 85:287–8.

68. Tracey KJ, Cerami A. The role of cachectin/tumor necrosis factor in AIDS. Cancer Cells 1989; 1:62–3.

69. Reddy MM, Sorrell SJ, Lange M, Grieco MH. Tumor necrosis factor and HIV P24 antigen in the serum of HIV-infected population. J AIDS 1988; 1:436–40.

70. Grunfeld C, Kotler DP, Shigenaga JK, Doerrler W, Tierney A, Wang J, Pierson Jr RN, Feingold KR. Circulating interferon alpha levels and hypertriglyceridemia in the acquired immunodeficiency syndrome. Am J Med 1991; 90:154–62.

71. Grunfeld C, Pang M, Doerrler W, Shigenaga JK, Jensen P, Feingold KR. Lipids, lipoproteins, triglyceride clearance and cytokines in human immunodeficiency virus infection and the acquired immunodeficiency syndrome. J Clin Endo Met (in press).

72. Dworkin BM, Seaton T, Wormser G. The role of tumor necrosis factor (TNF) and altered metabolic rate in weight loss in AIDS. VI Int Conf on AIDS, San Francisco, June 21, 1990, Vol. 1, p. 218 (Abstract).

73. Hellerstein MK, Grunfeld C, Wu K, Christiansen M, Kaempfer S, Kletke C, Shackleton CHL. Increased de novo hepatic lipogenesis in HIV-infected humans. J Clin Endo Met (in press).

74. Waage A, Halstensen A, Espevik T. Association between tumor necrosis factor in serum and fatal outcome in patients with meningococcal disease. Lancet 1987; i:355-7.

75. Girardin E, Grau GE, Dayer J-M, Roux-Lombard P, the J5 Study Group, Lambert P-H. Tumor necrosis factor and interleukin-1 in the serum of children with severe infectious purpura. N Engl J Med 1988; 319:397-400.

76. Scuderi P, Lam KS, Ryan KJ, Petersen E, Sterling KE, Finely PR, Rag CG, Slyneu DJ, Salzman SE. Raised serum levels of tumor necrosis factor in parasitic infections. Lancet 1986; ii: 1364-5.

77. Grunfeld C, Kotler DP, Hamadeh R, Tierney A, Wang J, Pierson Jr RN. Hypertriglyceridemia in the acquired immunodeficiency syndrome. Am J Med 1989; 86:27-31.

78. Grunfeld C, Doerrler W, Pang M, Jensen P, Weisgraber KH, Feingold KR. Abnormalities of apolipoprotein E in the acquired immunodeficiency syndrome. Submitted.

79. Stein TP, Nutinsky C, Condoluci D, Schluter MD, Leskiw MJ. Protein and energy substrate metabolism in AIDS patients. Metabolism 1990; 39:876-81.

80. Grunfeld C, Pang M, Doerrler W, Jensen P, Shimizu L, Feingold KR, Cavalieri R. Indices of thyroid function and weight loss in human immunodeficiency virus infection and the acquired immunodeficiency syndrome. Submitted.

81. Kotler DP, Francisco A, Clayton F, Scholes JV, Orenstein JM. Small intestinal injury and parasitic disease in the acquired immunodeficiency syndrome (AIDS). Ann Intern Med 1990; 113:444-9.

82. Gillin S, Shike M, Alcock N, Urmacher O, Krown S, Kurtz R, Lightdale C, Winawer S. Malabsorption and mucosal abnormalities of the small intestine in the acquired immunodeficiency syndrome. Ann Intern Med 1985; 102: 618-22.

83. Boyle JT, Celano P, Koldovsky O. Demonstration of a difference in expression of maximal lactase and sucrase activity along the villus in the adult rat jejunum. Gastroenterology 1980; 79:503-7.

84. Shiau UF, Kotler DP, Levine GM. Can normal small bowel morphology be equated with normal function? Gastroenterology 1979; 76:1246A.

85. Batman PA, Miller AR, Forster SM, Harris JR, Pinching AJ, Griffin GE. Jejunal enteropathy associated with immunodeficiency virus infection: quantitative histology. J Clin Pathol 1989; 42:275-81.

86. Ullrich R, Zeitz M, Heise M, L 'age M, Hoffken G, Rieken EO. Small intestinal structure and function in patients infected with human immunodeficiency virus (HIV): evidence for HIV-induced enteropathy. Ann Intern Med 1989; 111:15–21.

87. Heise C, Dandekar S, Donovan R, Kumar P, Halstead CH. HIV infection of jejunal mucosa in AIDS and ARC: association with intestinal function. FASEB J 1989; 3:757A.

88. Shiau YF, Kotler DP, Levine GM. Can normal small bowel morphology be equated with normal function? Gastroenterology 1979; 76:1264A.

89. Boyle JT, Celano P, Koldovsky O. Demonstration of a difference in expression of maximal lactase and sucrase activity along with villus in the adult rat jejunum. Gastroenterology 1980; 79:503–7.

90. Soave R, Johnson WD. Cryptosporidium and isospora belli infections. J Infect Dis 1988; 157:225–9.

91. Soave R. Cryptosporidiosis and isosporiasis in patients with AIDS. Infect Dis Clin North Am 1989; 2:485–93.

92. Shadduck JA. Human microsporidiosis and AIDS. Rev Infect Dis 1989; 11: 203–7.

93. Desportes I, Le Charpentier Y, Galain A, et al. Occurrence of a new microsporidan: *Enterocytozoon bieneusi* in the enterocytes of a human patient with AIDS. J Protozol 1985; 32:250–4.

94. Orenstein JM, Chiang J, Steinberg W, Smith P, Rotterdam H, Kotler DP. Intestinal microsporidiosis as a cause of diarrhea in HIV-infected patients: a report of 20 cases. Hum Pathol 1990; 21:475–81.

95. Roth RI, Owen RL, Keren DF, Volberding PA. Intestinal infection with *Mycobacterium avium* in acquired immunodeficiency syndrome (AIDS): histological and clinical comparison with Whipple's disease. Dig Dis Sci 1985; 30:497–504.

96. Chiu J, Nussbaum J, Bozzette S, et al. Treatment of disseminated *Mycobacterium avium* complex infection in AIDS with amikacin, ethambutol, rifampin and ciprofloxacin. Ann Intern Med 1990; 113:358–61.

97. Nelson JA, Wiley CA, Reynolds-Kohler C, et al. Human immunodeficiency virus detected in bowel epithelium from patients with gastrointestinal symptoms. Lancet 1988; 2:259–62.

98. Mathijs JM, Hing M, Grierson J, Dwyer DE, et al. HIV infection of rectal mucosa. Lancet 1988; 1:1111.

99. Fox CH, Kotler DP, Tierney AR, Wilson CS, Fauci AS. Detection of HIV-1 RNA in intestinal lamina propria of patients with AIDS and gastrointestinal disease. J Infect Dis 1989; 159:467–71.

100. Rene E, Jarry A, Brousse N, et al. Demonstration of HIV infection of the gut in AIDS patients: Relation with symptoms and other digestive infection. Gastroenterology 1988; 94:373A.

101. Hoover EA, Mullin JI, Quackenbush SL, Gasper PW. Experimental transmission and pathogenesis of immunodeficiency syndrome in cats. Blood 1987; 70:1880–92.

102. Miller TL, Orav EJ, Martin SR, Cooper ER, McIntosh K, Winter HS. Malnutrition and carbohydrate malabsorption in children with vertically transmitted human immunodeficiency virus 1 infection. Gastroenterology 1991; 100:1296–302.

103. Zeitz M, Ullrich R, Heise W, Bergs C, L 'age M, Riecken EO. Malabsorption is found in early stages of HIV infection and independent of secondary infections. Proc. VII Int. Conf. on AIDS, Florence, Italy, June 16–21, 1991, V.2, p. 46 (Abstract).

104. Harriman GR, Smith PD, McDonald KH, Cecil HF, Koenig S, Lack EE, Lane HC, Fauci AS. Vitamin B_{12} malabsorption in patients with the acquired immunodeficiency syndrome. Arch Intern Med 1989; 149:2039–41.

105. Burkes RL, Cohen E, Kralo M, Sinow RM, Carmel R. Low serum cobalamin levels occur frequently in the acquired immunodeficiency syndrome and related disorders. Eur J Hematol 1987; 38:141–7.

106. Kotler DP, Haroutiounian G, Greenberg R, Setchell K, Balistieri WF. Increased bile salt deconjugation in AIDS. Gastroenterology 1985; 88:1455A.

107. Kapembwa M, Bridges C, Joseph AEA, Fleming SC, Griffin GE. Ileal absorptive function in acquired immunodeficiency syndrome. Proceedings: V. International Conference on AIDS 1989; 218A.

108. Mitchell NH, Hamilton TS, Steggerda FR, Bean HW. Chemical composition of the adult human body and its bearing on the biochemistry of growth. J Biol Chem 1945; 158:625–32.

109. Kapembwa MS, Fleming SC, Griffin GE, Caun K, Pinching AJ, Harris JRW. Fat absorption and exocrine pancreatic function in human immunodeficiency virus infection. Q J Med 1990; 74:49–56.

110. Cuff PA. Acquired immunodeficiency syndrome and malnutrition: Role of gastrointestinal pathology. Nutr Clin Prac 1990; 5:43–58.

111. Wartofsky L and Burman KD. Alterations in thyroid function in patients with systemic illness: the "euthyroid sick syndrome." Endocr Rev 1982; 3:164–217.

112. Grunfeld C, Soued M, Adi S, Moser AH, Dinarello CA, Feingold KR. Evidence for two classes of cytokines that stimulate hepatic lipogenesis: Relationships among tumor necrosis factor, interleukin-1 and interferon-alpha. Endocrinology 1990; 127:46–54.

113. Okusawa S, Gelfand JA, Ikejima T, Connolly RJ, Dinarello CA. Interleukin-1 induces a shock-like state in rabbits. Synergism with tumor necrosis factor and the effect of cyclooxygenase inhibition. J Clin Invest 1988; 81:1162–72.

114. Bartholeyns J, Freudenberg MD, Galanos C. Growing tumors induce hypersensitivity to endotoxin and tumor necrosis factor. Infect Immunol 1987; 55:2230–3.

115. Black K, Garrett IR, Mundy GR. Chinese hamster ovarian cells transfected with the murine interleukin-6 gene cause hypercalcemia as well as cachexia, leukocytosis and thrombocytosis in tumor-bearing nude mice. Endocrinology 1991; 128:2657–9.

116. Kotler DP, Culpepper-Morgan J, Tierney AR, Klein EB. Treatment of disseminated cytomegalovirus infection with 9-(1,3dihydroxy-2-propoxymethyl)guanine: evidence of prolonged survival in patients with the acquired immunodeficiency syndrome. AIDS Res 1987; 2:299–308.

117. Kotler DP, Tierney AR, Altilio D, Wang J, Pierson Jr RN. Body mass repletion during ganciclovir therapy of cytomegalovirus infections in patients with the acquired immunodeficiency syndrome. Arch Int Med 1989; 149: 901–5.

118. Yarchoan R, Weinhold KJ, Lyerly HK, Gelmann E, Blum RM, Shearer GM, Mitsuya H, Collins JM, Myers CE, Klecker RW, Markham PD, Durack DT, Lehrman SN, Barry DW, Fischl MA, Gallo RC, Bolognesi DP, Broder S. Administration of 3′-azido- 3′deoxythymidine, an inhibitor of HTLV-III/LAV replication, to patients with AIDS or AIDS-related complex. Lancet 1986; i:575–80.

119. American College of Physicians. Position paper. Parenteral nutrition in patients receiving cancer chemotherapy. 1989; 110:734–6.

120. Faviglione MC, Battan R, Pablos-Mendez A, Aceves-Casillas P, Mullen M, Taranta A. Infections associated with Hickman catheters in patients with acquired immunodeficiency syndrome. Am J Med 1988; 36:781–6.

121. Altilo D, Tierney A, Kotler D. Bacteremias associated with chronic indwelling venous catheters in patients with acquired immunodeficiency syndrome. Nutr Clin Pract (in press).

122. Popp MB, Fisher RI, Wesley R, Aamodt R, Brennan MF. A prospective randomized study of adjuvant parenteral nutrition in the treatment of advanced diffuse lymphoma: influence on survival. Surgery 1981; 90:195–202.

123. Burt ME, Stein TP, Brennan MF. A controlled, randomized trial evaluating the effects of enteral and parenteral nutrition on protein metabolism in cancer-bearing man. J Surg Res 1983; 34:303–14.

124. Kotler D, Tierney A, Ferraro R, Cuff P, Wang J, Pierson R, Heymsfield S. Effect of enteral alimentation upon body cell mass in patients with the acquired immunodeficiency syndrome. Am J Clin Nutr 1991; 53:149–54.

125. Kotler DP, Tierney AR, Culpepper-Morgan JA, Wang J, Pierson Jr RN. Effect of home total parenteral nutrition upon body composition in patients with AIDS. J Parenter Enter Nutr 1990; 14:454–458.

126. Kelson K, Malcolm J, Brantsma A, Sutherland DC. Percutaneous endoscopic gastrostomy feeding in AIDS. Proc. VII Intl. Conf. on AIDS. June 16–21, 1991, Florence, Italy, V.1, p. 285 (Abstract).

127. Von Roenn JH, Murphy RL, Weber KM, Williams LM, Weitzman SA. Megestrol acetate for treatment of cachexia associated with human immunodeficiency virus (HIV) infection. Ann Int Med 1988; 109:840–1.

128. Tierney AR, Cuff P, Kotler DP. The effect of megestrol acetate (megace) on appetite, nutritional repletion and quality of life in AIDS cachexia. Proc. VII Intl. Conf. on AIDS. June 16–21, 1991, Florence, Italy, V.1, p. 247 (Abstract).

129. Dickmeyer MS, Brown S, Pursell K, Thaler H, Armstrong D. Improved appetite and weight gain in patients with acquired immunodeficiency syndrome treated with megestrol acetate. Proc. VII Intl. Conf. on AIDS. June 16–21, 1991, Florence, Italy, V. 1, p. 231 (Abstract).

9

Oral Lesions of HIV Infection: Features and Therapy

Deborah Greenspan and John S. Greenspan
University of California–San Francisco, San Francisco, California

The oral lesions of HIV infection are important for several reasons. First, they often, but not always, represent a relatively early stage of HIV disease. Thus, their prompt and accurate diagnosis is important in staging and may be a determining factor in the initiation of preventive therapy such a prophylactic pentamidine and/or zidovudine. Many of the oral lesions of HIV disease can produce significant pain and discomfort, and their early recognition and therapy may prevent significant morbidity (1).

Oral lesions become increasingly prevalent as the CD4 count drops. In one recent major study, in three cohorts of homosexual and bisexual men in San Francisco, one or another of the oral lesions was found in approximately 30% of otherwise asymptomatic men (2). With the onset of significant HIV disease and AIDS, the frequency of oral lesions becomes much higher (3). In the Netherlands, oral examinations of a group of homosexual men attending a hospital clinic resulted in change of CDC disease classification in a significant number (4). A recent study showed that oral lesions and CD4 counts was an effective staging system for progression of HIV disease (5).

I. NEOPLASMS

A. Kaposi's Sarcoma

Kaposi's sarcoma (KS) can occur in the oral cavity before skin lesions appear. Clinically, the lesion may appear as red or purplish macules, papules, or nodules. These do not blanch on pressure, and there may be a yellowish tinge to the surrounding mucosa. The lesions are usually symptomless, unless infected or ulcerated, when there may be pain, tenderness, or bleeding.

The lesions may occur anywhere in the mucosa, but the palate and gingiva are the most common locations (6). Some tongue and gingival lesions may be of normal color, probably because they are deeper lesions and covered with normal-appearing mucosa. In a recent study of an AIDS clinic patient population, oral KS lesions were the first KS lesions in 42% of the patients (7). Of those with oral lesions, 22% had this as their first AIDS diagnosis. Although KS is most commonly seen in homosexual men in the United States, the lesion is occasionally seen in women (8).

Oral KS lesions often respond well to appropriate local therapy, such as radiation therapy, surgery, or chemotherapy. Intralesional vinblastine has been used with some success, resulting in significant regression of the oral lesions with minimal systemic side effects (9). Some success has also been reported with the use of the carbon dioxide laser. Thirty-six patients with oral lesions were treated with external radiation therapy, and the lesions regressed (10).

B. AIDS-Associated Lymphoma

AIDS-associated lymphoma can present in the mouth as a solitary or multiple ulcers or swellings. These may be of sudden onset, are usually painful, and grow rapidly. They may frequently be the first evidence of this malignancy. They can present diagnostic challenges, particularly in the absence of disseminated disease, and can be confused clinically with inflammatory disease such as periodontal disease. Diagnosis is made on biopsy and in our experience often requires plastic embedding and lymphocyte marker studies. In common with AIDS lymphomas in general, the oral lesions are usually large B cell in phenotype, and about half the cases contain Epstein-Barr virus (11).

C. Other Malignancies

At this time there is no convincing evidence for an association between HIV infection and other oral malignancies such as squamous cell carcinoma.

II. OPPORTUNISTIC INFECTIONS

A. Bacterial Infections

1. *Periodontal Disease*

Periodontal disease in HIV-infected individuals has some of the features seen in that disease in the general population. Thus, there is progressive inflammation-mediated destruction of the periodontal tissues caused by bacterial infection due to organisms found in dental plaque. However, in HIV infection the disease has a more rapid onset, is more destructive, progresses more rapidly, and can become much more severe, even life-threatening. At the Oral AIDS Center at ICSF, we have seen this severe form of periodontal disease in HIV-positive homosexual men, intravenous drug–using women, hemophiliacs, and children (12). Other centers have also reported HIV-associated periodontal disease (13).

HIV-associated disease of the tissues supporting the teeth ranges from marginal inflammation (HIV-gingivitis, HIV-G) through a severe form of acute necrotizing ulcerative gingivitis (ANUG) and a severe, often localized periodontitis (HIV-periodontitis, HIV-P) to a severe spreading destructive infection of gingiva, soft palate, and associated bone (necrotizing stomatitis, NS) resembling noma or cancrum oris (14). HIV-G presents as a thin red line involving the gingival margin, often in the absence of accumulations of plaque and often in the presence of good oral hygiene. ANUG may present with pain, spontaneous bleeding, and halitosis, accompanying ulcerating necrotizing lesions of the gingival papillae. In HIV-P, there is also severe pain and bleeding associated with rapidly progressive destruction of the periodontal tissues supporting the teeth. The loss of bone and soft tissue as well as of periodontal attachment can result in loosening and even loss of teeth, often in the absence of periodontal pocketing. In this respect, HIV-P is quite different from the common form of chronic inflammatory periodontal disease seen in the general population. The organisms involved in HIV-P probably include such pathogens as *Porphyromonas gingivalis, B. intermedius, Fusobacterium nucleatum, Actinobacillus actinomycetemcomitans, Eikenella corrodens,* and *Wolinella* sp. In addition, *Candida albicans* may also be involved. In general, and with the exception of *C. albicans*, these organisms are similar to those found in classical periodontitis (15). Neutrophil functional defects may also be involved (16). In the most severe form of HIV-associated periodontal disease, NS, the lesion may involve rapid destruction extending well beyond the teeth, with an osteomyelitis component causing sequestration. This may be severe and potentially life-threatening if not recognized and treated promptly (17).

Several recent studies indicate that HIV periodontitis is rare in those with asymptomatic HIV disease but is seen in over one third of those with falling CD4 count and with significant HIV disease (18). In a recent study involving the Walter Reed cohort, HIV periodontitis was more common in smokers than in those with the same CD4 counts who did not smoke (19).

Treatment of this group of conditions is directed towards relief of pain, elimination of putative causative agents, prevention of further tissue destruction, and promotion of healing. An essential first step is a thorough cleaning and debridement, utilizing local anesthesia when necessary. This painstaking procedure is best performed by a periodontist or by a dental hygienist under the supervision of a periodontist. It should be followed by the use of chlorhexidine mouth rinses in the case of HIV-G and, where there is more extensive loss, in HIV-P, by irrigation of severely affected sites with povidone-iodine (Betadine[R]). Povidone-iodine acts as an obtundant and is a powerful antiseptic. Chlorhexidine gluconate (Peridex[R]) rinses used in people with HIV-associated periodontal disease have been shown to improve and maintain the clinical response. ANUG and NS may require the use of an antibiotic, as the major pathogens appear to be gram-negative organisms; in such cases we have used metronidazole (Flagyl[R]) in addition to the other measures described above (20). Oral lesions associated with *Mycobacterium avium-intercellulare* have been reported (21).

B. Viral Infections

1. Herpes Simplex Virus

In the HIV-positive population, recurrent herpes simplex can present as herpes labialis or as intraoral lesions. Herpes labialis can be of prolonged duration, and there recently have been reported cases of severe orofacial herpes that have been shown to be caused by acyclovir-resistant strains (22). Recurrent intraoral lesions usually occur on keratinized mucosa, such as the hard palate and gingiva. They begin as small vesicles, which often rupture and coalesce to form areas of ulceration. However, in this population these lesions may be seen in atypical locations such as the dorsal surface of the tongue. Treatment with acyclovir is recommended only for persistent lesions.

2. Varicella-Zoster Virus

Orofacial herpes zoster is not uncommon in association with HIV infection. Pain, sometimes referred to the teeth, may precede visible lesions. The latter follow the distribution of one or more branches of the trigeminal nerve and start as crops of vesicles. These become ulcerated and crusted over with eventual healing, sometimes with residual scarring. Rare cases have been seen of Ramsay Hunt syndrome, in which there is accompanying facial paralysis due to involvement of the facial nerve. It has been suggested that orofacial herpes zoster may presage imminent development of AIDS in those who are HIV-infected (23).

3. Cytomegalovirus

Isolated reports have implicated cytomegalovirus in some of the prolonged oral ulcers seen in HIV-infected individuals (24). However, no series have been reported other than in patients with disseminated CMV infection, and it seems unlikely that CMV is a common cause of oral ulceration in HIV disease. In our experience when CMV ulcers do occur, the clinical appearance differs from that of aphthous ulcers and recurrent herpes simplex. CMV lesions may be seen at any mucosal site but may present as periodontal disease, with areas of soft tissue necrosis, exposing bone. Diagnosis is made by biopsy and immunohistochemistry.

4. Human Papillomavirus (HPV)

Oral warts have been reported with increasing frequency in association with HIV infection. These warts may be of varying clinical and histological appearance and include three types. These may be cauliflowerlike, spiky, or flat (resembling focal epithelial hyperplasia). Unusual HPV types have been identified in these HIV-associated warts, notably HPV 7, which has previously been seen only in butchers' warts of the skin (25). The flat warts resembling focal epithelial hyperplasia are associated with HPV types 13 and 32. Warts may be removed surgically, sometimes using the CO_2 laser, but recurrence is common. It is important to emphasize that the HPV types seen in anogenital warts (HPV 6, 11, 16, 18) are rarely seen in HIV-associated oral warts, and thus it must not be assumed that these oral lesions are due to sexually transmitted virus.

5. Hairy Leukoplakia

In association with HIV infection, Epstein-Barr virus (EBV) causes a thickening of the epithelial cells of the tongue and less commonly of other parts of the oral mucosa. We named the lesion hairy leukoplakia because of its characteristic appearance. The lesion appears as white corrugations or projections on the lateral margin of the tongue or as smoother white patches on the ventral surface of the tongue and rarely of the buccal mucosa or other parts of oral mucosa (26).

The lesions are usually painless but may give rise to a feeling of discomfort. There is often superinfection with *C. albicans*, but that yeast does not appear to be an etiological factor. EBV, however, is readily demonstrated by a variety of techniques (27,28). The EBV in HL is both unusual and interesting in that deletions in the EBNA 2 gene and genomic rearrangements, both previously regarded as rare, are often found (29,30). Hairy leukoplakia was discovered as a result of the AIDS epidemic, and it probably represents opportunistic EBV infection at a fairly late stage in the course of HIV infection. The pathogenesis appears to involve loss of Langerhans cells, which are either absent or greatly reduced in number in the HL lesion, although present in normal numbers in nonlesional mucosa from the same individual (31). HL is only very rarely seen in HIV-negative individuals (32). People with hairy leukoplakia who are HIV-seropositive but do not have AIDS subsequently develop AIDS fairly rapidly, with 47% of a group of 199 individuals doing so within 2 years (33). However, not all patients with hairy leukoplakia develop AIDS rapidly. We have studied a small population who have not developed the full syndrome within 3 years. The most valid predictor of this long-term nonconversion was normal skin-test reactivity to challenge with *Candida* antigen (34). Although usually asymptomatic, the lesion of HL can occasionally provoke soreness and feelings of discomfort, often called a "cotton-wool" feeling. Patients may also complain of the unsightly appearance of the white lesions. In such cases, treatment may be indicated. A course of acyclovir will usually result in total elimination of the lesion, but recurrence of the lesion is common (35,36). Although initial reports suggested that HL resolved with AZT therapy, a more recent and extensive study has shown that the lesion resolves spontaneously with about the same frequency in those not taking AZT as it does in those receiving AZT, while subsequent recurrence was also equally common in both groups (37).

C. Fungal Infections

Although a number of fungi are commonly present in the environment and many cause oral disease in patients with severe immunodeficiency, for example, leukemia, candidiasis is the only oral fungal disease seen with any frequency in association with HIV infection. Rare cases of histoplasmosis, cryptococcosis, and geotrichosis have been seen (1,38). By contrast, a very large percentage of those with otherwise asymptomatic HIV infection and HIV disease, including AIDS, experience oral candidiasis in one form or another (39,40).

1. Oral Candidiasis

Typically, oral candidiasis presents either in a pseudomembranous form (thrush) or in the erythematous form (41). Occasionally both are seen together. More rarely, epithelial hyperplasia associated with *Candida* (candidal leukoplakia) occurs. The infection may also occur at the corners of the mouth, producing angular cheilitis. Pseudomembranous candidiasis appears as removable white plaques, which can be found on any oral mucosal surface. Erythematous candidiasis occurs as red patches, which appear most commonly on the palate and dorsal surface of the tongue, which may appear depapillated. Angular cheilitis may appear as cracking, redness, or ulceration at the corners of the mouth. This may occur unilaterally or bilaterally and may be found in the absence of intraoral candidiasis.

Diagnosis is made from smears from the lesions demonstrating the presence of hyphae and blastopores, indicating active infection. These smears may be examined using a gram-stained preparation or a potassium hydroxide preparation. The advantage of the latter technique is that it is quick and inexpensive to prepare and screen. The presence of *Candida* on culture may indicate the carrier state and not necessarily infection.

One study of homosexual men showed a point prevalence of oral candidiasis of about 12% among people who were HIV-seropositive (42). Another study of patients with AIDS found candidiasis in over 90% (43), while we have found that patients with pseudomembranous and the more subtle erythematous form are equally likely to progress to AIDS (median 25 months) and to death (44). Oral candidiasis usually responds to treatment with either systemic or topical preparations. Ketoconazole (Nizoral[R]) 200 mg tablets, taken once or twice a day with food is a useful systemic medication, although there are reports of elevation of liver function tests following long-term administration. Fluconazole (Diflucan[R]) 100 mg tablets taken once daily for 7 days is an effective oral systemic agent. Useful topical agents include clotrimazole oral troche (Mycelex[R]) 10 mg, one tablet dissolved slowly in the mouth five times a day, nystatin oral pastille 200,000 units, one or two pastilles dissolved slowly four to five times a day, and nystatin vaginal tablets, 100,000 units, to be dissolved slowly in the mouth three times a day. There is an argument for maintaining individuals who have had one episode of oral candidiasis on antifungal therapy. There is little or no data on the most effective agent or dose. The same strain of *C. albicans* has been found before and after treatment by DNA probe analysis, suggesting unique adaptation of the yeast to each host (45).

D. Salivary Gland Disease

Salivary gland enlargement and xerostomia have been recognized for some time in the pediatric AIDS population (46). More recently, these salivary gland problems have been seen with increasing frequency among adult HIV-positive patients. The etiology of HIV salivary gland disease (SGD) is unknown and attempts to seek viral factors have been unsuccessful thus far (47). The histopathology of the major glands in HIV SGD and of labial salivary gland biopsies from such patients resemble those seen in Sjogren's syndrome (48). A recent study showed an increase in circulating CD8 lymphocytes and an increase in HLA DR5 in HIV-positive individuals with a sicca syndrome involving parotid gland enlargement, pulmonary problems, and lymphadenopathy (49). This probably represents the same entity.

E. Oral Ulcers

Although oral ulcers of the recurrent aphthous type do not appear to be more common in the HIV-infected population, such lesions, when they occur, seem to be of increased severity and follow a more prolonged course with slower healing than in the general population. Again, no specific viral or other pathogen has been identified in these oral ulcers, and, like HIV SGD, they may represent an autoimmune or other form of immune dysregulation.

These ulcers, like those seen in the general population, appear to fall into three distinct types: minor, major, and herpetiform (50). All appear on nonkeratinized mucosa such as buccal mucosa, soft palate, oropharynx, and ventral tongue. The minor ulcers (<1 cm) can be solitary or occur in small groups. The major ulcers (>1 cm) are usually solitary and can be of long duration and present a diagnostic problem, often mimicking malignancy. Herpetiform ulcers occur as crops of large numbers of small ulcers (1–3 cm), which may coalesce. The ulcers appear most commonly on the soft palate and often pose a diagnostic dilemma. However, they usually respond well to topical therapy with any of a variety of steroids. These include decadron elixir used as a mouthwash and expectorated, and Lidex[R] ointment (0.05%) mixed 50% with Orabase[R] and applied to the ulcers several times a day.

There are reports of patients having similar ulcers of the gastrointestinal tract. When these ulcers occur in the esophagus, systemic therapy may be indicated (51).

F. Oral Lesions in Pediatric HIV Disease

Some of the lesions discussed above may be seen in the pediatric population (52). The most common lesions include oral candidiasis, parotid enlargement, and herpes simplex. Hairy leukoplakia and periodontal disease are seen rarely. A recent study showed that oral candidiasis and herpes simplex were markers of poor prognosis, whereas children with parotid enlargement tended to fare better.

REFERENCES

1. Greenspan D, Greenspan JS, Pindborg JJ, Schiodt M. AIDS and the mouth. Copenhagen: Munksgaard, 1990.

2. Feigal DW, Katz MH, Greenspan D, Westenhouse J, Winkelstein W, Lang W, Samuel M, Buchbinder SP, Hessol NA, Lifson AR, Rutherford GW, Moss A, Osmond D, Shiboski S, Greenspan JS. The prevalence of oral lesions in HIV-infected homosexual and bisexual men: three San Francisco epidemiologic cohorts. AIDS 1991; 5:519-25.

3. Tukutuku K, Muyembe-Tramfun L, Kayembe K, Ntumba M. Oral Manifestations of AIDS in a heterosexual population in a Zaire hospital. J Oral Path Med 1990; 19:232-4.

4. Schulten EA, ten Kate RW, van der Waal I. The impact of oral examination on the Centers for Disease Control classification of subjects with human immunodeficiency virus infection. Arch Intern Med 1990; 150(6):1259-61.

5. Royce R, Luckmann RS, Fusaro RE, Winkelstein Jr. The natural history of HIV-1 infection: staging classifications of disease. AIDS 1991; 5:355-64.

6. Lummerman H, Freedman PD, Kerpel SM, Phelan JA. Oral Kaposi's sarcoma: a clinicopathologic study of 23 homosexual and bisexual men from the New York metropolitan area. Oral Surg Oral Med Oral Pathol 1988; 65: 711-6.

7. Dodd C, Greenspan D, Overby G, Feigal DW, Hollander H, Schiodt M, MacPahil L, Greenspan JS. Oral Kaposi's sarcoma: The sequence of appearance with respect to other AIDS complications. Vth International Conference on AIDS, Montreal, June 1989. Abstract # Th.B.P. 340.

8. Dodd CA, Greenspan D, Greenspan JS. Oral Kaposi's sarcoma in a woman as a first indication of infection with the human immunodeficiency virus. JADA 1991; 122:61-3.

9. Epstein JB, Scully C. Intralesional vinblastine for oral Kaposi's sarcoma in HIV infection. Lancet 1989; 2:1100-1.

10. Ficarra G, Person AM, Silverman S, et al. Kaposi's sarcoma of the oral cavity: a study of 134 patients with a review of the pathogenesis, epidemiology,

clinical aspects, and treatment. Oral Surg Oral Med Oral Pathol 1988; 66: 543–50.

11. Green TL, Eversole LR. Oral lymphomas in HIV-infected patients: association with Epstein-Barr virus DNA. Oral Surg Oral Pathol 1989; 67:437–42.

12. Winkler JR, Grassi M, Murray PA. Clinical description and etiology of HIV-associated periodontal diseases. In: Robertson PB, Greenspan JS, eds. Perspectives on oral manifestations of AIDS. Littleton, MA: PSG Publishing Co. Inc., 1988: 49–70.

13. Quart AM, Small CB, Klein RS. Periodontal disease in heterosexual patients with AIDS. Vth International Conference on AIDS, Montreal, June 1989. Abstract ThBP 352.

14. Williams CA, Winkler JR, Grassi M, Murray PA. HIV-associated periodontitis complicated by necrotizing stomatitis. Oral Surg Oral Med Oral Pathol 1990; 69:351–5.

15. Murray PA, Grassi M, Winkler JR. The microbiology of HIV-associated periodontal lesions. J Clin Periodontol 1989; 16:636–42.

16. Ryder MI, Winkler JR, Weintreb RN. Elevated phagocytosis, oxidative burst and F action formation in PMNs from individuals with intraoral manifestations of HIV infection. J AIDS 1988; 1:346–53.

17. Winkler JR, Murray PA, Hammerle C. Gangrenous stomatitis in AIDS (letter). Lancet 1989; 2 (8554):108.

18. Masouredis CM, Winkler JR, Katz M, et al. Prevalence of HIV-associated periodontitis and gingivitis in HIV-infected patients attending an AIDS clinic. Submitted.

19. Swango PA, Kleinman DV, Konzelman JL. HIV and periodontal health. A study of military personnel with HIV. J Am Dent Assoc 1991; 122(8):49–54.

20. Winkler JR, Murray PA, Grassi M, Hammerle C. Diagnosis and management of HIV-associated periodontal lesions. J Am Dent Assoc 1989; 119 (Suppl.):S25–34.

21. Volpe F, Schimmer A, Barr C. Oral manifestations of disseminated *Mycobacterium avium intracellulare* in a patient with AIDS. Oral Surg 1985; 5:567.

22. MacPhail LA, Greenspan D, Schiodt M, Drennan D, Mills J. Acyclovir-resistant, foscarnet-sensitive oral herpes simplex type 2 lesion in a patient with AIDS. Oral Surg Oral Med Oral Pathol 1989; 67:427–32.

23. Melbye M, Grossman RJ, Goedert JJ, Eyster ME, Biggar RJ, Risk of AIDS after herpes zoster. Lancet 1987; 1(8535):728–31.

24. Langford A, Ruf B, Groth A, Pohle HD, Reichart P. Cytomegalovirus associated oral ulcerations in HIV-infected patients. J Oral Pathol Med 1990; 19(2):71–6.

25. Greenspan D, de Villiers EM, DeSouza Y, Greenspan JS. Unusual HPV types in oral warts in association with HIV infection. J Oral Pathol 1989; 17:482–7.

26. Greenspan D, Greenspan JS, Conant M, et al. Oral "hairy" leucoplakia in male homosexuals: evidence of association with papillomaviruses and a herpes-group virus. Lancet 1984; 2:831.

27. Greenspan JS, Greenspan D, Lennette ET, et al. Replication of Epstein-Barr virus within the epithelial cells of oral "hairy" leukoplakia, an AIDS-associated lesion. N Engl J Med 1985; 313:1564-71.

28. DeSouza YG, Greenspan D, Felton JR, Hartzog GA, Hammer M, Greenspan JS. Localization of Epstein-Barr virus DNA in the epithelial cells of oral hairy leukoplakia by in situ hybridization of tissue sections [letter]. N Engl J Med 1989; 320:1559–60.

29. Sixbey JW, Shirley P, Chesney PJ, Buntin DM, Resnick L. Detection of a second widespread strain of Epstein-Barr virus. Lancet 1989; 2:761–5.

30. Patton DF, Shirley P, Raab-Traub N, Resnick L, Sixbey JW. Defective viral DNA in Epstein-Barr virus-associated oral hairy leukoplakia. J Virol 1990; 64:397–400.

31. Daniels TE, Greenspan D, Greenspan JS, et al. Absence of Langerhans cells in oral hairy leukoplakia, an AIDS-associated lesion. J Invest Dermatol 1987; 89:178.

32. Greenspan D, Greenspan JS, DeSouza Y, Levy JA, Unger AM. Oral hairy leukoplakia in an HIV-negative renal transplant recipient. J Oral Pathol Med 1989; 18:32–4.

33. Greenspan D, Greenspan JS, Hearst N, et al. Relation of oral hairy leuko-plakia to infection with the human immunodeficiency virus and the risk of developing AIDS. J Infect Dis 1987; 155:475.

34. Greenspan D, Greenspan JS, Overby G, Hollander H, Abrams DI, Macphail LA, Borowsky C, Feigal DW. Risk factors for rapid progression from hairy leukoplakia to AIDS: a nested case control study. J AIDS 1991; 4:652–8.

35. Resnick L, Herbst JS, Ablashi DV, Atherton S, Frank B, Rosen L, Horwitz SN. Regression of oral hairy leukoplakia after orally administered acyclovir therapy. JAMA 1988; 259(3):384–8.

36. Greenspan D, DeSouza Y, Conant MA, Hollander H, Chapman SK, Lennette ET, Petersen V, Greenspan JS. Efficacy of desciclovir in the treatment of Epstein-Barr virus infection in oral hairy leukoplakia. J AIDS 1990a; 3:571–8.

37. Katz MH, Greenspan D, Heinic GH, Chan AK, Hollander H, Chernoff D, Greenspan JS. Resolution of hairy leukoplakia: An observational trial of Zidovudine versus no treatment. J Infect Dis 1991; 164:1240–1.

38. Lynch DP, Naftolin LZ. Oral *Cryptococcal neoformans* in AIDS. Oral Surg Oral Med Oral Pathol 1987; 64:449–53.

39. Klein RS, Harris CA, Small CR, et al: Oral candidiasis in high-risk patients as the initial manifestation of the acquired immunodeficiency syndrome. N Engl J Med 1984; 311:354.

40. Tavitian A, Raufman JP, Rosenthal LE. Oral candidiasis as a marker for esophageal candidiasis in the acquired immunodeficiency syndrome. Ann Intern Med 1986; 104:54.

41. Pindborg JJ. Classification of oral lesions associated with HIV infection. Oral Surg Oral Med Oral Pathol 1989; 67:292–5.

42. Feigal DW, Katz MH, Greenspan D, Westenhouse J, Winkelstein W, Lang W, Samuel M, Buchbinder SP, Hessol NA, Lifson AR, Rutherford GW, Moss A, Osmond D, Shiboski S, Greenspan JS. The prevalence of oral lesions in HIV-infected homosexual and bisexual men: three San Francisco Epidemiologic Cohorts. AIDS 1991; 5:519–25.

43. Phelan JA, Saltzman BR, Friedland GH, Klein RS. Oral findings in patients with acquired immunodeficiency syndrome. Oral Surg Oral Med Oral Pathol 1987; 64:50–6.

44. Dodd CL, Greenspan D, Katz MH, Westenhouse JL, Feigal DW, Greenspan JS. Oral candidiasis in HIV infection: pseudomembranous and erythematous candidiasis show similar rates of progression to AIDS. AIDS 1991; 5:1339–43.

45. Miyasaki SH, Polacheck I, Hicks J, Greenspan D, Greenspan JS. The identification and tracking of *Candida albicans* isolates from oral lesions in HIV-seropositive individuals. 5th International Conference on Acquired Immunodeficiency Syndrome, Montreal, Canada. 1989, Abstract #ThBP323.

46. Couderc LJ, D'Agay MF, Danon F, Harzic XX, Brocheriou C, Clavel JP. Sicca complex and infection with human immunodeficiency virus. Arch Intern Med 1987; 147:898–901.

47. Schiodt M, Greenspan D, Daniels TE, Nelson J, Leggott PJ, Wara DW, Greenspan JS. Parotid gland enlargement and xerostomia associated with labial sialadenitis in HIV-infected patients. In 2nd Int. Symposium on Sjogren's Syndrome. J Autoimmun 1989; 2(4):415.

48. Schiodt M, Greenspan D, Levy J, et al. Does HIV cause salivary gland disease? AIDS 1989; 3:819–22.

49. Itescu S, Brancato LJ, Winchester R. A sicca syndrome in HIV infection: association with HLA DR5 and CD 8 lymphocytosis. Lancet 1989; 2:466–8.

50. Macphail LA, Greenspan D, Feigal DW, Lennette ET, Greenspan JS. Recurrent aphthous ulcers in association with HIV infection: description of ulcer types and analysis of T-lymphocyte subsets. Oral Surg Oral Med Oral Pathol 1991; 678–83.

51. Bach MC, Howell DA, Valenti AJ, Smith T, Dretler RH, Winslow DL. Aphthous ulcerations of the gastrointestinal tract in patients with AIDS. Ann Intern Med 1990; 112(6):465–52.

52. Leggott PJ, Robertson PB, Greenspan D, et al. Oral manifestations of primary and acquired immunodeficiency diseases in children. Pediatr Dent 1987; 9:89–104

10

Human Papillomavirus-Associated Anogenital Neoplasia in Persons with HIV Infection

Donald W. Northfelt
*University of California–San Francisco, and
San Francisco General Hospital, San Francisco, California*

Joel M. Palefsky
*University of California–San Francisco,
San Francisco, California*

I. INTRODUCTION

The association between human papillomavirus infection (HPV) and the development of anal and cervical cancers is widely appreciated. A number of recent investigations suggest that human immunodeficiency virus (HIV)–induced immunodeficiency promotes the development of neoplasia in HPV–infected cervical and anal mucosa. These observations imply that cervical and anal cancers may become increasingly common as the HIV epidemic matures. The incidence of HPV-associated malignancy has not yet increased dramatically among persons with HIV infection, but advances in the care of HIV disease may paradoxically cause this to occur. Patients with profound immunodeficiency who would have quickly succumbed to opportunistic infections earlier in the epidemic now survive longer because they receive more effective antiretroviral, prophylactic, and antimicrobial therapies. Prolonged survival with severe immunodeficiency provides the necessary milieu for the emergence of diseases that develop after longer periods of time, such as anogenital carcinomas. This chapter reviews the new understanding of the interaction of human papillomavirus (HPV) infection with HIV-induced immunodeficiency in the development of anogenital neoplasia.

II. BIOLOGY OF HPV

Papillomaviruses are nonenveloped icosahedral capsids, 45–55 μm in diameter, containing a genome of circular double-stranded DNA comprised of approximately 8000 base pairs (1). Papillomaviruses are classified into genotypes and subtypes on the basis of DNA homology: different genotypes share less than 50% homology, and different subtypes share more than 50% homology (2). More than 60 HPV genotypes have been characterized.

Different HPV genotypes are associated with different disease states. Types 1, 2, and 4 cause common warts and plantar warts; types 5 and 8 are associated with epidermodysplasia verruciformis, a rare skin disorder in which HPV infection and a cell-mediated immunodeficiency lead to the development of squamous cell skin cancers (3). Types 6 and 11 are primarily associated with anogenital condyloma and laryngeal papilloma, and frank neoplastic changes are uncommon when only these types are present. Types 16 and 18 are generally believed to confer a high risk of invasive anogenital cancer, whereas types 31, 33, and 35 are associated with an intermediate risk of progression to malignancy (4–9).

Venereal transmission of condyloma acuminata was first demonstrated in the 1950s, when it was found that as servicemen returned from Korea with genital condyloma, their wives soon developed similar lesions (10). By the early 1970s, HPV had been implicated as the etiological agent responsible for this process (11). Cervical cancer was also suspected, on epidemiological grounds, to be caused by a sexually transmitted agent for some time prior to the identification of HPV in neoplastic anogenital lesions. For example, the risk of developing cervical cancer has been correlated with lifetime number of sexual partners, early age at first intercourse, and history of sexually transmitted diseases (12–14). Genital infection with HPV shares many of these associations (15).

III. HPV-ASSOCIATED ANOGENITAL NEOPLASIA

There is a considerable body of evidence linking HPV infection to the development of both benign and neoplastic anogenital lesions. Between 80 and 90% of exophytic cervical condyloma acuminata have been found to contain HPV DNA (16–18). As noted above, HPV genotypes 6 and 11 are most commonly detected in these benign lesions. The so-called oncogenic HPV genotypes (HPV 16, 18, and 31) have been detected in 80–90% of cervical intraepithelial neoplasia (CIN) grade 3 lesions and invasive cervical cancers (19). HPV DNA has also been found in lymph node metastases of invasive cervical cancer, with the genotype of HPV in the metastatic site matching that found in the primary tumor (20). Additional observations suggesting a role for HPV 16, 18, and 31 in the development of anogenital neoplasia have come from prospective natural history studies of asymptomatic women infected with various HPV genotypes. For example, in a cohort of HPV DNA-positive women with normal cervical Papanicolaou (Pap) smears on initial evaluation, progression to high-grade intraepithelial neoplasia during 2 years of follow-up occurred in 42% of HPV 16/18/31-positive women, 29% of HPV 6/11-positive women, and 6% of HPV DNA-negative controls (21).

HPV infection is presumed to play a similar etiological role in the development of anal neoplasia. Epidemiological investigations of anal cancer incidence have identified many of the same risk factors associated with cervical neoplasia and HPV infection, including history of genital or anal condyloma and history of other sexually transmitted diseases. In addition, male homosexuality and the practice of receptive anal intercourse have been associated with anal cancer risk, emphasizing this mode of acquisition of HPV (22,23). In a manner similar to investigations performed on cervical cancer specimens, HPV antigens, DNA, and mRNA have been detected by in situ hybridization in anal cancer specimens (24,25). These observations have been confirmed by amplification of HPV DNA from anal cancer specimens using the polymerase chain reaction (26).

The mechanisms by which HPV contributes to the development of anogenital neoplasia are not well understood. However, the actions of several HPV gene products and their possible roles in the process of malignant transformation have recently been described. In particular, the E6 and E7 genes of HPV 16 appear to be critical in the development of neoplasia. These genes are transcriptionally active in cervical cancers and derived cell lines in which the viral genome is integrated into the host genome; it is speculated that integration disrupts normal control of E6 and E7 gene expression (27). Further work has established that E6 and E7 bind to p53 and the Rb protein, respectively (28,29). These cellular proteins, products of so-called tumor suppressor genes or antioncogenes, are believed to function as essential growth regulators in the normal cell. Loss or mutation of these genes has been associated with malignant transformation and the development of retinoblastoma, colorectal cancer, and other tumors. It had been hypothesized that binding of p53 and/or Rb protein by E6 and E7 inactivates their tumor suppressor function, leading to transformation.

IV. HPV-ASSOCIATED ANOGENITAL NEOPLASIA AND IMMUNODEFICIENCY

Cell-mediated immunity is believed to play an important role in the control of HPV infection and associated neoplasia. Most of the investigations of cell-mediated immunity and HPV infection have been performed on patients with epidermodysplasia verruciformis. Impairment of cell-mediated cytotoxicity and decreased numbers of T-helper cells have been found in such patients (30–32). Other investigators have reported positive evidence of cell-mediated immune response to HPV; lymphocyte proliferative responses, lymphokine release, and cytotoxic responses to challenge with papillomavirus virions or peptides have all been observed in vitro (33–35).

In the realm of clinical investigation, anogenital neoplasia has a recognized association with chronic immunodeficiency. Studies of cohorts of immunosuppressed organ transplant recipients have demonstrated a 100-fold increase in incidence of vulvar and anal carcinomas and a 14-fold increase in the incidence of cervical carcinoma as compared with controls (36,37). The high incidence of anogenital cancer in immunosuppressed transplant recipients is believed to be a consequence of their high prevalence of detectable anogenital HPV infection. The prevalence of detectable HPV infection is 5–17 times greater in immunosuppressed transplant recipients than in the general population (38).

It is becoming increasingly clear that patients with HIV-induced immunodeficiency are also at risk for the development of cervical and anal neoplasia. A number of recent studies have added considerably to the understanding of this relationship. Several of these studies demonstrate that the role of HPV infection in HIV-related anogenital neoplasia may be analogous to that seen in other immunodeficiency states.

V. HIV INFECTION AND HPV-ASSOCIATED CERVICAL NEOPLASIA

Over the past few years, a number of anecdotal reports have appeared regarding the possible connection between HIV-induced immunodeficiency and cervical neoplasia (39–41). Such reports led Schrager et al. (42) to determine whether women with and without HIV infection differ in prevalence of cervicovaginal cellular changes suggesting lower genital tract neoplasia or HPV infection. Cytological preparations of cervicovaginal smears from 35 HIV-infected women and 23 uninfected women were examined by one cytologist who was blinded to the subjects' HIV status. The groups were demographically similar, but differed significantly in three important respects: among HIV-infected women, fewer used barrier contraception, more had histories of sexually transmitted diseases, and less time had elapsed since their most recent sexual encounters with HIV-infected men. Thirty-one percent of HIV-infected women had cytological squamous atypia, compared to 4% of HIV-seronegative women ($p = 0.019$). Twenty-six percent of HIV-infected women had cytological or histopathological findings suggestive of genital HPV infection, compared to 4% of HIV-seronegative women ($p = 0.072$). Molecular analyses for detection of HPV were not performed. The authors concluded that HIV-infected women have a high prevalence of cervicovaginal cytological abnormalities and evidence of genital HPV infection, although they acknowledged that the differences observed between groups may have been related in part to different sexual practices.

Feingold et al. (43) extended these observations by obtaining molecular evidence of HPV infection in the cervicovaginal epithelium of women with HIV infection. HPV DNA was detected in clinical specimens using Southern blot hybridization. They found that 49% of the HIV-infected women studied had HPV infection, compared with 25% of a group of non-HIV-infected women with similar sociodemographic and behavioral characteristics ($p < 0.05$). Forty percent of the HIV-infected women had squamous intraepithelial lesions on cervical cytology, compared with 9% of the noninfected women ($p < 0.01$). Women with concurrent HIV and HPV infection were 42 times more likely to have a cytological abnormality than were women without evidence of either virus. In addition, it was noted that 50% of women with symptomatic HIV infection (AIDS, persistent generalized lymphadenopathy, oral candidiasis) had a cytological abnormality, whereas only 23% with asymptomatic HIV infection were cytologically abnormal. These and other data (44,45) suggest that more prolonged and/or severe immunosuppression, reflected by symptomatic disease, may allow progression of HPV-mediated cytological abnormalities.

Maiman et al. (46) recently described their findings in 37 women under age 50 with histologically confirmed invasive cervical cancer seen during a 3-year period at their facility in New York. The seven women with HIV infection in the cohort all had relatively advanced clinically staged disease at presentation (bulky stage IB or greater); in contrast, only 50%

of the 30 non–HIV-infected women presented with such advanced disease (p = 0.05). Following primary therapy, all HIV-infected women had persistent or recurrent disease, whereas only 58% of non–HIV-infected women with advanced cancer and none of the non–HIV-infected women with early disease had this outcome. The median times to recurrence and death in the HIV-infected women were 1 and 9 months, respectively; comparable figures for the non–HIV-infected women were 10 and 23 months.

The same investigators also described 77 women with cervical intraepithelial neoplasia (CIN) of various grades (46); HIV infection was present in 25 of these women. The HIV-infected women were significantly more likely to have higher grade CIN and to have multifocal cervical involvement and multiple genital site involvement. Among the HIV-infected women, there was a tendency for those with symptomatic HIV disease to have higher grades of CIN than were present in those who were asymptomatic.

Reports from the VII International Conference on AIDS in June 1991 provided additional evidence regarding the relationship of HIV infection to the development of advanced or progressive cervical neoplasia associated with HPV infection (47–54). The results of studies described in these reports are summarized in Table 1. Two studies reported that cervical HPV infection is significantly more prevalent in HIV-infected women than in non–HIV-infected women (47,48). Two studies reported that CIN/SIL (squamous intraepithelial lesion) is significantly more prevalent in HIV-infected women than in non–HIV-infected women (48,49). Three studies suggested that women with more advanced HIV disease, i.e., those with symptoms or lower CD4 counts, are more likely to have CIN and detectable HPV infection (48,50,51), although the results of a fourth study contradict this finding (49). An important observation on the natural history of CIN in this setting was made by Agarossi et al. (52). They found that CIN is significantly more likely to progress to a higher grade over one year of observation in women co-infected with HPV and HIV than in women with neither infection. In summary, these reports from the 1991 Conference support the hypothesis that HIV-infected women are at increased risk for the development of HPV-associated cervical neoplasia.

Despite the apparent high prevalence of cervical neoplasia in HIV-infected women, only a few cases of invasive cervical cancer have been reported (40,45,46,55,56). In fact, one recent seroepidemiological study found an HIV seroprevalence of only 2% among Kenyan women with cervical cancer (57). However, experience with immunosuppressed transplant recipients suggests that a prolonged period of immunodeficiency (mean, 88 months) may be necessary to permit development of anogenital

Table 1 Studies of Cervical Neoplasia and HPV Infection Presented at the VII
International Conference on AIDS, 1991

Objective	Conclusion	Ref.
Examine relationship between HIV infection, cervical/anal cytological abnormalities, and HPV infection in female IV drug users	1) Observed trend toward an association between cervical cytological abnormalities and HIV infection 2) Significant association of detectable HPV-DNA and HIV infection	47
Examine and compare the frequency of HPV infection and and CIN in women with symptomatic HIV infection, asymptomatic HIV infection, or without HIV infection	1) Detectable HPV infection and CIN are more frequent in symptomatic HIV-infected women than in asymptomatic HIV-infected women or non-HIV-infected women	50
Evaluate the clinical course of HPV infection and CIN in women with HIV infection (IV drug users)	1) Over 12 months of observation, regression of CIN is significantly more likely in HIV-negative, women than in HIV-positive, HPV-positive women 2) Over 12 months of observation, progression of CIN is significantly more likely in IIIV-positive, HPV-positive women than in HIV negative, HPV-negative women.	52
Evaluate the role of HIV infection on the risk of genital HPV infection and CIN in women (IV drug users)	1) HPV infection is significantly more prevalent in HIV-infected women 2) CIN is significantly more prevalent in HIV-infected women than in non-HIV-infected women 3) CD4 cell counts are significantly lower in HIV-infected women with HPV infection and CIN than in HIV-infected women without these findings.	48
Investigate the natural history of HPV infection (time interval not specified), comparing symp-	1) HPV infection is significantly more likely to be present, and tends to persist, in HIV-infected,	53

(continues)

Table 1   (Continued)

Objective	Conclusion	Ref.
tomatic, HIV-infected women with asymptomatic women with/ without HIV infection	symptomatic women compared to asymptomatic women 2) Cervical SIL is significantly more likely to be found in women with persistent HPV infection	
Determine whether the changing immune competence in HIV infection alters the process of HPV cervical infection	1) Within the cohort studied, 21% have detectable HPV infection and 38% have cervical SIL 2) Mean CD4 count is lower in the subgroup with detectable HPV, and in the subgroup with SIL, than in the subgroup without detectable HPV	51
Examine the relationship of CD4 status, prevalence on CIN, and prevalence of HPV infection in HIV-infected women	1) CIN III is significantly more prevalent in women with CD4 <200 than in those with CD4 >200 2) Eleven of 12 cases of histologically confirmed HPV infection occurred in women with CIN, but no association of HPV infection and immune status was seen	54
Assess the association between cervical SIL and heterosexually transmitted HIV infection	1) In comparison to non-HIV-infected post-partum women, HIV-infected post-partum women are significantly more likely to have SIL 2) No difference in prevalence of SIL among HIV-infected women with >400 CD4 cells versus <400 CD4 cells	49

Abbreviations:
CIN = cervical intraepithelial neoplasia; HIV = human immunodeficiency virus; HPV = human papillomavirus; SIL = squamous intraepithelial lesion.

cancer (36). Most patients with HIV infection die of opportunistic infections much earlier in the course of symptomatic HIV disease, and therefore may not survive long enough to develop cervical cancer and be identified in a study such as the one performed in Kenya. Improvements in survival are currently being achieved through the use of effective antiretroviral, prophylactic, and antimicrobial therapies (58,59). These successes may permit the emergence of cervical carcinoma among HIV-infected women with a high prevalence of HPV infection and cervical intraepithelial neoplasia.

VI. HIV INFECTION AND HPV-ASSOCIATED ANAL NEOPLASIA

The relationship of HIV infection, HPV infection, and anal neoplasia has also been described in a number of recently published reports. Although an association of anal neoplasia and HPV infection in homosexual men has been recognized for some time (22,23), it is now apparent that HIV-infected, immunodeficient men are particularly at risk for the development of HPV-related anal neoplasia.

Several investigations have provided preliminary evidence of the relationship of HIV infection, HPV infection, and anal neoplasia. Lorenz et al. (60) reviewed the surgical experience with anal carcinoma in HIV-infected men at the University of California, San Francisco, noting poor treatment outcome and short survival in these patients. Evaluation for HPV infection was not performed. Two small studies (24,61) demonstrated HPV in neoplastic anal lesions of homosexual men by histopathological and/or immunohistochemical techniques. One subject in each study had a diagnosis of AIDS at the time that anal neoplasia was found. Frazer et al. (62) examined a larger cohort of homosexual men, using anorectal cytological smears, HIV antibody testing, and T-lymphocyte phenotyping. They found that HIV seropositivity, lower CD4+ T-lymphocyte counts, and lower CD4+/CD8+ ratios were significantly associated with more pronounced cytological atypia.

These preliminary findings led Palefsky et al. (63) to assess the prevalence of anal HPV infection and precancerous abnormalities of the anal epithelium in 97 severely immunodeficient, HIV-infected homosexual men. Thirty-nine percent of subjects were found to have abnormal anal cytology, and 54% had HPV DNA in their anal cytological specimens. Abnormalities on anal cytological smear were significantly associated with presence of HPV DNA (risk ratio, 4.6), and median CD4+ T-lymphocyte counts of subjects with abnormal cytological findings were significantly lower than those of subjects with normal findings ($p = 0.05$).

Another cohort of 105 homosexual men, including subjects with and without HIV infection, took part in a similar study conducted by Caussy et al. (64). HPV DNA was found in anal cytological specimens from 53% of HIV-infected subjects, compared to 29% of non–HIV-infected subjects ($p = 0.012$). Anal neoplasia was also present more frequently in HIV-infected men (24% vs. 7%; $p = 0.03$). Multivariate logistic regression analysis of data from the HIV-infected subjects showed low CD4+ T-lymphocyte count to be an independent risk factor for detection of HPV DNA ($p = 0.04$). Similar findings have been reported from a study of 120 Danish homosexual men (65) and from a study of 101 homosexual men attending a sexually transmitted diseases clinic in Seattle (66).

A study of anal condyloma and anal intraepithelial neoplasia in HIV-infected homosexual and bisexual men was described at the VII International Conference on AIDS (67). Half of the men studied had anal condyloma, and half of these had histological evidence of AIN, including four with AIN-3. The degree of immunodeficiency and prevalence of detectable HPV infection in the cohort were not described. However, this study does confirm the findings of others noted above with respect to the high prevalence of anal condyloma and AIN in HIV-infected homosexual and bisexual men.

Caussy et al. (64) proposed a model to explain the role of HIV-induced immunodeficiency in promoting HPV-induced anal neoplasia. They hypothesized that normal immune mechanisms prevent latent anal HPV infection from causing neoplasia. When these mechanisms are impaired as a consequence of HIV infection, HPV can become active in promoting the development of premalignant and malignant epithelial lesions. The progression of cervical neoplasia in HIV-infected women can be presumed to occur by the same mechanism. It follows that the rationale cited earlier in predicting an increase in the incidence of cervical carcinoma also applies in predicting a greater future incidence of anal carcinoma in HIV-infected patients (63).

VII. CLINICAL IMPLICATIONS OF HPV-ASSOCIATED ANOGENITAL NEOPLASIA IN PERSONS WITH HIV INFECTION

The studies cited above demonstrate that anogenital HPV infection and neoplasia are common in persons with HIV infection. Information on the natural history of these conditions is limited, but it should be presumed that these lesions are precancerous and likely to evolve into invasive cancer over time. Early detection or preinvasive or minimally invasive cancers of the anogenital region can provide the opportunity to cure these diseases, as has been demonstrated by the successful use of cervical Pap smears in screening programs in the general population. It therefore seems reasonable to assume that some patients with HIV infection, particularly those with relatively better prognosis (higher CD4+ lymphocyte count, no prior opportunistic infections or malignancies), would benefit from early detection and treatment of anogenital neoplasia. Proposed guidelines for management of cervical and anal neoplasia in HIV-infected persons are shown in Table 2 (68).

Table 2 Proposed Guidelines for Management of HIV-Associated Anogenital Neoplasia

Screening for cervical neoplasia:
  for all HIV-infected women
    annual Pap smear
    consider baseline colposcopic examination
  for HIV-infected women at high risk for HPV infection[a]
    Pap smear every 6 months
    careful inspection of vulvar, vaginal, and anal epithelium
    consider routine colposcopic examination
Treatment for cervical neoplasia:
  (follow established standard treatment guidelines)
Screening for anal neoplasia: for HIV-infected men with history of anal intercourse
  ? anal Pap smear (see text)
  anoscopy on a routine basis (annually?)
  biopsy of any abnormality identified on anoscopy
  frequent anoscopic follow-up if abnormalities previously identified (every 3–6 months?)
Treatment for anal neoplasia:
  for anal intraepithelial neoplasia
    electrocautery or cryotherapy
  for invasive cancer
    surgical excision ± radiotherapy

[a]History of multiple sexual partners, sexual partners with HIV infection.
Source: Adapted from Ref. 68.

Table 3 Anal Pap Smear Technique

1. Moisten a Dacron swab with saline or tap water.
2. Insert swab into distal rectum, at least 2 cm from anal verge.
3. Rotate swab while withdrawing through anal canal.
4. Smear swab onto glass slide and fix with spray-fixative or by immersion in alcohol within 10 seconds of withdrawal.
5. Stain fixed smear by routine Papanicolaou method for interpretation by cytopathologist.

Source: Adapted from Ref. 68.

The anal Pap smear (Table 3) may be useful as a screening tool for use in patients with HIV infection who are at high risk for anal HPV infection and anal neoplasia (23,68). Preliminary studies have suggested that anal Pap smears have a sensitivity of approximately 70%, similar to that of cervical Pap smears. However, the grading of anal Pap smears has not correlated well with the histopathological grade of simultaneously biopsied lesions, with the Pap smear generally underestimating the degree of dysplasia.

A study is currently underway in which a large cohort of HIV-infected men will be examined with anal Pap smears and biopsies in order to validate the use of the Pap smear as a screening tool in this setting. Recommendations regarding the widespread use of the anal Pap smear for population screening must await the result of this or similar studies.

VIII. CONCLUSION

The studies cited in this review suggest that cervical cancer and anal cancer are likely to become more common problems in the setting of HIV-induced immunodeficiency as the epidemic progresses. This shift in the spectrum of HIV-related disease may occur in response to ongoing improvements in therapy and overall prognosis for patients with HIV infection. Observations regarding the development of malignancies in other states of immunodeficiency suggest that these cancers will become more frequent as therapeutic interventions prolong survival. Strategies for prevention, detection, and treatment of HIV-associated anogenital malignancies will be needed.

ACKNOWLEDGMENT

The authors thank Nadine Lurie for her editorial assistance.

REFERENCES

1. Pfister H. Papillomaviruses: general description, taxonomy, and classification. In: Salzman NP, Howley PM, eds. The papovaviridae. Vol 2. New York: Plenum Press, 1987:1–38.

2. Coggin JR, zur Hausen H. Workshop on papillomaviruses and cancer. Cancer Res 1979; 39:545–6.

3. Jablonska S, Dabrowski J, Jakubowicz K. Epidermodysplasia verruciformis as a model in studies on the role of papillomaviruses in oncogenesis. Cancer Res 1972; 32:583–9.

4. Crum C, Mitao M, Levine R, Silverstein S. Cervical papillomaviruses segregate within morphologically distinct precancerous lesions. J Virol 1985; 54: 675–81.

5. Beaudenon S, Kremsdorf D, Croissant O, et al. A novel type of human papillomavirus associated with genital neoplasias. Nature 1986; 321:246–9.

6. Gissmann L. Papillomaviruses and their association with cancer in animals and man. Cancer Surv 1984; 3:161–81.

7. Lorincz AT, Lancaster W, Temple G. Cloning and characterization of a new human papillomavirus from a woman with dysplasia of the uterine cervix. J Virol 1986; 58:225–9.

8. Lorincz AT, Quinn A, Lancaster W, Temple GF. A new type of papillomavirus associated with cancer of the uterine cervix. Virology 1987; 159:187–90.

9. Koutsky LA, Galloway DA, Holmes KK. Epidemiology of genital human papillomavirus infection. Epidemiol Rev 1988; 10:122–63.

10. Barrett TJ, Silber JD, McGinley JP. Genital warts: a venereal disease. JAMA 1954; 154:333–4.

11. Oriel JD. Natural history of genital warts. Br J Vener Dis 1971; 47:1–13.

12. Brinton LA, Hamman RF, Huggins GR, et al. Sexual and reproductive risk factors for invasive squamous cell cervical cancer. JNCI 1987; 79:23–30.

13. Slattery ML, Overall JC, Abbott TM, et al. Sexual activity, contraception, genital infection, and cervical cancer: support for a sexually transmitted disease hypothesis. Am J Epidemiol 1989; 130:248–58.

14. Jones CJ, Brinton JA, Hamman RF, et al. Risk factors for in situ cervical cancer: results from a case-control study. Cancer Res 1990; 50:3657–62.

15. Levy C, Bauer HM, Reingold A, et al. Determinants of genital human papillomavirus infection in young women. JNCI 1991; 83:997–1003.

16. Gissmann L, Wolnik L, Ikenberg H, et al. Human papillomavirus type 6 and 11 DNA sequences in genital and laryngeal papillomas and in some cervical cancers. Proc Natl Acad Sci USA 1983; 80:560–3.

17. Reid R, Greenberg M, Jenson AB, et al. Sexually transmitted papillomaviral infections. I. The anatomic distribution and pathologic grade of neoplastic lesions associated with different viral types. Am J Obstet Gynecol 1987; 156:212–22.

18. Willet GD, Kurman RJ, Reid R, et al. Correlation of the histologic appearance of intraepithelial neoplasia of the cervix with human papillomavirus types. Int J Gynecol Pathol 1989; 8:18–25.

19. Pfister H. Relationship of papillomaviruses to anogenital cancer. Obstet Gynecol Clin North Am 1987; 14:349–61.

20. Lancaster WD, Castellano C, Santos C, et al. Human papillomavirus deoxyribonucleic acid in cervical carcinoma from primary and metastatic sites. Am J Obstet Gynecol 1986; 154:115–9.

21. Koutsky L, Kiviat N, Paarvonen J, et al. Development of high grade cervical intraepithelial neoplasia (CIN 2-3) among women tested for human papillomavirus (HPV) DNA: life table analysis. International Society of Sexually Transmitted Disease Research, 8th Meeting, Copenhagen, Denmark, Sept 10–13, 1989. Abstract #58.

22. Daling JR, Weiss NS, Hislop TG, et al. Sexual practices, sexually transmitted diseases, and the incidence of anal cancer. N Engl J Med 1987; 317:973–7.

23. Holly EA, Whittemore AS, Aston DA, et al. Anal cancer incidence: genital warts, anal fissure or fistula, hemorrhoids, and smoking. JNCI 1989; 81: 1726–31.

24. Gal AA, Meyer PR, Taylor CR. Papillomavirus antigens in anorectal condyloma and carcinoma in homosexual men. JAMA 1987; 257:337–40.

25. Gal AA, Saul SH, Stoler MH. In situ hybridization analysis of human papillomavirus in anal squamous cell carcinoma. Mod Pathol 1989; 2:439–43.

26. Palefsky JM, Holly EA, Gonzales J, et al. Detection of human papillomavirus DNA in anal intraepithelial neoplasia and anal cancer. Cancer Res 1991; 51:1014–9.

27. Munger K, Phelps WC, Budd V, Howley PM, Schlegel R. The E6 and E7 genes of the human papillomavirus type 16 together are necessary and sufficient for transformation of primary human keratinocytes. J Virol 1989; 63: 4417–21.

28. Dyson N, Howley PM, Munger K, Harlow E. The human papilloma virus-16 E7 oncoprotein is able to bind to the retinoblastoma gene product. Science 1989; 243:934–7.

29. Werness BA, Levine AJ, Howley PM. Association of human papillomavirus types 16 and 18 E6 proteins with p53. Science 1990; 248:76–9.

30. Kaminski M, Pawinska M, Jablonska S, et al. Increased natural killer cell activity in patients with epidermodysplasia verruciformis. Arch Dermatol 1985; 121:84–6.

31. Majewski S, Skopinska-Rozewska E, Jablonska S, et al. Partial defects of cell-mediated immunity in patients with epidermodysplasia verruciformis. J Am Acad Dermatol 1986; 15:966–73.

32. Majewski S, Malejczyk J, Jablonska S, et al. Natural cell-mediated cytoxicity against various target cells in patients with epidermodysplasia verruciformis. J Am Acad Dermatol 1990; 22:423–7.

33. Haftek M, Jablonska S, Orth G. Specific cell-mediated immunity in patients with epidermodysplasia verruciformis and plane warts. Dermatologica 1985; 170:213–20.

34. Strang G, Hickling JK, McIndoe JK, et al. Human T cell responses to human papillomavirus type 16 L1 and E6 synthetic peptides: identification of T cell determinants, HLA-DR restriction and virus type-specificity. J Gen Virol 1990; 71:423–31.

35. Walter M, Gissmann L, Zentgraf H, Kirchner H. Measurement of cell-mediated immunity against bovine papillomavirus by lymphoproliferative reactions. Immunobiology 1987; 174:244–50.

36. Penn I. Cancers of the anogenital region in renal transplant recipients: analysis of 65 cases. Cancer 1986; 58:611–6.

37. Penn I. Tumors of the immunocompromised patient. Ann Rev Med 1988; 39:63–73.

38. Sillman FH, Sedlis A. Anogenital papillomavirus infection and neoplasia in immunodeficient women. Obstet Gynecol Clin North Am 1987; 14:537–58.

39. Byrne MA, Taylor-Robinson D, Munday PE, et al. The common occurrences of human papillomavirus infection and intraepithelial neoplasia in women infected by HIV. AIDS 1989; 3:379–82.

40. Henry MJ, Stanley MW, Cruikshauk S, Carson L. Association of human immunodeficiency virus-induced immunosuppression with human papillomavirus infection and cervical intraepithelial neoplasia. Am J Obstet Gynecol 1989; 160:352–3.

41. Brandbeer C. Is infection with HIV a risk factor for cervical intraepithelial neoplasia. lancet 1987; 2:1277–88.

42. Schrager LK, Friedland GH, Maude D, et al. Cervical and vaginal squamous abnormalities in women infected with human immunodeficiency virus. J Acq Immun Def Synd 1989; 2:570–5.

43. Feingold AR, Vermund SH, Burk RD, et al. Cervical cytologic abnormalities and papillomavirus in women infected with human immunodeficiency virus. J Acq Immun Def Synd 1990; 3:896–903.

44. Vermund SH, Kelley KF, Burk RD, et al. Risk of human papillomavirus (HPV) and cervical squamous intraepithelial lesions (SIL) is highest among

women with advanced HIV disease. Abstracts, Volume 3, VI International Conference on AIDS 1990; S.B.517:215.

45. Schafer A, Friedmann W, Mielke M, Schwartlander B, Koch MA. The increased frequency of cervical dysplasia-neoplasia in women infected with the human immunodeficiency virus is related to the degree of immunosuppression. Am J Obstet Gynecol 1991; 164:593–9.

46. Maiman M, Fruchter RG, Serur E, et al. Human immunodeficiency virus infection and cervical neoplasia. Gynecol Oncol 1990; 38:377–82.

47. Williams A, Palefsky J, Padian N, et al. Association of HIV-1, cervical/anal cytologic abnormalities, and human papillomavirus in female injection drug users in San Francisco, California, USA. Abstracts, VII International Conference on AIDS 1991; M.C.3116:327.

48. Conti M, Agarossi A, Muggiasca L, Casolati E, Ravasi L. Risk of genital HPV and CIN in HIV positive women. Abstracts VII International Conference on AIDS 1991; M.B.2408:284.

49. Chiphaugwa J, Dallabetta G, Miotti P, et al. Cervical squamous intraepithelial lesions (CSIL) and HIV-I infection in Malawian women. Abstracts, VII International Conference on AIDS 1991; M.C.98:47.

50. Zorilla C, Romaguera J, Corrada R, et al. Increased incidence of cervical intraepithelial neoplasia (CIN) and human papillomavirus (HPV) infection in cervical smears of HIV seropositive women in Puerto Rico. Abstracts, VII International Conference on AIDS 1991; M.C.3170:340.

51. Lombardo J, Klosner P, Chung R, Jenson A, Raska K. Cervical human papillomavirus (HPV)-infection in HIV-positive females. Abstracts, VII International Conference on AIDS 1991; M.B.2403:282.

52. Agarossi A, Casolati E, Muggiasca L, et al. Natural history of cervical HPVi and CIN in HIV positive women. Abstracts, VII International Conference on AIDS 1991; M.B.2425:288.

53. Burk RD, Fleming I, Ho GYF, Klein RS. Cervical squamous intraepithelial lesions (SIL) in women with HIV: relationship to persistent human papillomavirus (HPV) infection of the cervix. Abstracts, VII International Conference on AIDS 1991; M.A.1246:153.

54. Laguardia K, McGuinness K, Hunter D. Cervical disease among HIV-infected women by immune status. Abstracts, VII International Conference on AIDS 1991; M.C.97:47.

55. Rellihan MA, Dooley DP, Burke TW, Berkland ME, Longfield RN. Rapidly progressing cervical cancer in a patient with human immunodeficiency virus infection. Gynecol Oncol 1990; 36:435–8.

56. Monfardini S, Vaccher E, Pizzocaro G, et al. Unusual malignant tumors in 49 patients with HIV infection. AIDS 1989; 3:449–52.

57. Rogo KO, Kavoo-Linge. Human immunodeficiency virus seroprevalence among cervical cancer patients. Gynecol Oncol 1990; 37:87–92.

58. Lemp GF, Payne SF, Neal D, Temelso T, Rutherford GW. Survival trends for patients with AIDS. JAMA 1990; 263:402–6.

59. Gail MH, Rosenberg PS, Goedert JJ. Therapy may explain recent deficits in AIDS incidence. J Acq Immun Def Synd 1990; 3:296–306.

60. Lorenz HP, Wilson W, Leigh B, Crombleholme T, Schecter W. Squamous cell carcinoma of the anus and HIV infection. Dis Colon Rectum 1991; 34: 336–8.

61. Croxson T, Chabon AB, Rorat E, Barash IM. Intraepithelial carcinoma of the anus in homosexual men. Dis Colon Rectum 1984; 27:325–30.

62. Frazer IH, Crapper RM, Medley G, Brown TC, MacKay IR. Association between anorectal dysplasia, human papillomavirus, and human immuno-deficiency virus infection in homosexual men. Lancet 1986; 2:657–60.

63. Palefsky JM, Gonzales J, Greenblatt RM, Ahn DK, Hollander H. Anal intra-epithelial neoplasia and anal papillomavirus infection among homosexual males with group IV HIV disease. JAMA 1990; 263:2911–6.

64. Caussy D, Goedert JJ, Palefsky J, et al. Interaction of human immunodefi-ciency and papilloma viruses: association with anal intraepithelial abnor-mality in homosexual men. Int J Cancer 1990; 46:214–9.

65. Melbye M, Palefsky J, Gonzales J, et al. Immune status as a determinant of human papillomavirus detection and its association with anal epithelial ab-normalities. Int J Cancer 1990; 46:203–6.

66. Kiviat N, Rompalo A, Bowden R, et al. Anal human papillomavirus infec-tion among human immunodeficiency virus-seropositive and -seronegative men. J Infect Dis 1990; 162:358–61.

67. de Ruiter A, Carter P, Katz D, et al. HIV, anal condylomata, and anal intra-epithelial neoplasia. Abstracts, VII International Conference on AIDS 1991; TU.B.86:79.

68. Palefsky J. Human papillomavirus infection among HIV-infected individuals. Hematol Oncol Clin North Am 1991; 5:357–70.

11

AIDS-Associated Kaposi's Sarcoma

James O. Kahn and Donald W. Northfelt
University of California—San Francisco, and San Francisco General Hospital, San Francisco, California

Steven A. Miles
University of California—Los Angeles, Los Angeles, California

I. INTRODUCTION

Kaposi's sarcoma (KS) was one of the first clinical manifestations of the AIDS epidemic (1,2). Initially, AIDS-KS appeared in 40–45% of AIDS patients, but as an index AIDS diagnosis, its incidence has declined to 10% among all risk groups and to 18% in homosexual men (3–5). The changing incidence of AIDS-KS has raised questions regarding its etiology and pathogenesis. The ability to culture AIDS-KS cells, the critical nature of growth factors influencing cellular growth and kinetics, and the influence of HIV proteins on the development of AIDS-KS have substantially affected our understanding of the etiology and pathogenesis of AIDS-KS. Improvements in the clinical care of patients will ultimately depend on an understanding of the etiology and pathogenesis of AIDS-KS. Presently, treatment of AIDS-KS is based on the clinical requirement to control visceral involvement, edema, or cosmetically intolerable lesions. A comparison of different treatment modalities has suffered from the lack of a standard prospectively defined clinical staging system that permits an accurate comparison of subjects at study entry. Consequently, response criteria have varied between studies, making comparisons difficult. Nevertheless, therapy directed to the clinical needs of the patients can be rationally planned. The enumeration of CD4 + T lymphocytes and an understanding of the extent of the clinical problems caused by AIDS-KS for the individual patient aids in the planning of the immunological, antiviral, and antitumor treatments for the patient afflicted with AIDS-KS.

II. ETIOLOGY AND PATHOGENESIS

The reason for the marked increased incidence of AIDS-KS in patients with HIV infection is unknown. However, recent laboratory studies have provided important clues to its pathogenesis that may provide new avenues of therapy. Both angiogenic growth factors and an altered progenitor cell appear to be key factors in the development of Kaposi's sarcoma.

A. In Vitro Studies of KS Cells

Kaposi's sarcoma–derived cells were first grown in long-term culture with conditioned media from retrovirally infected T-cell lines (6). Confirming earlier immunohistochemical studies of skin lesions, the immunohistochemical stains of isolated AIDS-KS cells suggested that they were derived from mesenchymal tissue with characteristics of both endothelial and smooth muscle cells. Southern analysis of DNA failed to detect any sequences that were homologous to HIV or other human retroviruses. In other studies, transfection of DNA from human AIDS-KS lesions identified the presence of an oncogene (an acutely transforming DNA sequence) called ks-FGF. Unfortunately, subsequent studies have shown that this gene was most important in other epithelial tumors but not in epidemic Kaposi's sarcoma (7).

B. Angiogenic Growth Factors

Factors in the conditioned media from the retrovirus-infected T cells promote the growth of AIDS-KS cells and, to a lesser extent, normal human endothelial cells. Moreover, both the media and protein extracts from AIDS-KS cells support the growth and proliferation of newly derived AIDS-KS cells (8). This suggests that both retrovirus-infected T cells and AIDS-KS cells produce angiogenic factors that could increase the progress of KS. The angioblastic reaction observed at the site of inoculation of AIDS-KS cells in nude mice confirms that AIDS-KS cells produce substances that are angiogenic (9).

Additional studies of potential angiogenic factors show that AIDS-KS cells express basic fibroblast growth factor (bFGF), interleukin-1α (IL-1α) (8), and IL-6 (10). AIDS-KS cells also appear to be more responsive to platelet-derived growth factor (PDGF) than their normal counterparts (11). This may provide a growth advantage. High affinity receptors for several cytokines, including IL-1, IL-2, IL-6, IL-8, tumor necrosis factor (TNF), and PDGF, are present on AIDS-KS cells (12). These receptors may be functional, as suggested by the fact that antibodies to IL-1, basic fibroblast growth factor (bFGF), or PDGF and antisense oligonucleotides to IL-6 inhibit AIDS-KS cells. Since AIDS-KS cells make and respond to several of these cytokines, AIDS-KS cells could participate in both paracrine and autocrine growth loops in vitro and in vivo.

Production of several of these factors by mesenchymal cells is normal and does not necessarily indicate an altered cell phenotype. For example, expression of IL-6 by mesenchymal tissues is normal (13). However, it is remarkable that AIDS-KS cells, but not endothelial or smooth muscle cells, respond to IL-6 (10,13). This also appears to be the case with Oncostatin-M, a T-cell– and monocyte–produced cytokine that selectively increases IL-6 expression in endothelial cells (14,21). The unique proliferative response of these cells to these cytokines may distinguish KS cells from their normal mesenchymal counterparts. In addition, since both IL-6 and IL-6 receptor mRNA are found in AIDS-KS lesions, this autocrine growth loop may be functional in vivo (15).

IL-6 may also be important because of its central role in modulating the response of cells to other cytokines known to be perturbed in HIV-infected individuals. Because multiple cytokines can modulate IL-6 in vivo and in vitro (15), it is possible that increases in the level of other cytokines such as Oncostatin-M could increase IL-6 and thereby increase the growth of KS lesions. This could account for some of the variation in the clinical course of patients. For example, both TNF-α and IL-1β are often increased in patients with HIV (16,17). This expression is transient and usually occurs coincident with opportunistic infections. It is interesting to speculate that increases in one or several of these cytokines during opportunistic infections could increase IL-6 within AIDS-KS cells and increase tumor cell growth. This could explain the explosive growth of AIDS-KS lesions seen at times of opportunistic infections.

C. Role of HIV in the Development of KS

An additional factor, the transactivating protein of HIV (HIV-*tat*), may be a mitogen for AIDS-KS cells (18). HIV-*tat* increases the proliferation of AIDS-KS cells but has no effect on smooth muscle or endothelial cell cultures. However, the mitogenic effects of HIV-*tat* are modest (less than twofold) and are not of the magnitude seen with cytokines such as Oncostatin-M, TNF, or IL-1β. Nonetheless, the demonstration that HIV-*tat* could contribute to the development of AIDS-KS is important for several reasons. First, it confirms earlier animal data that demonstrated that HIV-*tat*, under the control of the HIV LTR, could produce KS-like lesions in transgenic mice (19). Second, it is the first demonstration that HIV could directly induce angiogenesis and may be the sole factor necessary for the development of HIV-associated KS. Finally, it provides a rationale for the use of *tat* inhibitors as primary therapy for KS (20). However, additional work in this area is required before a clear role for *tat* in the etiology of KS is accepted.

D. Other Growth Factors

Recent studies identified Oncostatin-M as a major growth factor for AIDS-KS cells (21). Oncostatin-M is a potent mitogen for KS and induces IL-6 in AIDS-KS cells (15,19). Oncostatin-M may be a transforming agent as it alters the histological characteristics of KS cells in culture and supports the growth of these cells in soft agar (14). It also is the principal T-cell–derived growth factor from retrovirally infected T cells (22).

E. New Directions of Research

The very nature of the AIDS-KS progenitor cells has also recently come into question. Work from two groups suggests that adherent cells, with immunological and phenotypical characteristics similar to mesenchymal AIDS-KS progenitor cells, can be found in the peripheral blood of patients with HIV-associated KS (23). If true, this finding would completely alter our understanding of the nature of the multifocal KS tumors. For example, rather than postulating that local production of growth factors such as Oncostatin-M, TNF-alpha, IL-1β, or PDGF would result in the formation of AIDS-KS cells, it is postulated that circulating AIDS-KS progenitor cells could implant into tissues and proliferate locally. Infection with HIV and the immune disturbances associated with HIV infection could increase the frequency of these circulating cells and could give rise to spontaneous production of tumors at multiple sites. This provocative hypothesis is currently under study in several laboratories.

F. New Therapeutic Agents

The large number of laboratory studies and the information derived from these investigations have significantly altered our concept and understanding of the pathogenesis and etiology of KS. These studies also provide the basis for new therapeutic interventions, which may potentially have activity in modulating the growth of AIDS-KS in vivo. For example, IL-4 is a potent inhibitor of IL-6 expression in monocytes and inhibits IL-6 production and proliferation of AIDS-KS cells (15). Recombinant platelet factor-4 also inhibits the proliferation of AIDS-KS cells in vitro (15). The effects of bFGF on AIDS-KS cells suggest that anionic surfactants such as pentosan polysulfate or the newly described polysulfated polysaccharide (SPPG) that binds bFGF could inhibit AIDS-KS cell growth. Finally, a variety of inhibitors of IL-6 and Oncostatin-M have been described (14). It is possible that inhibitors of these cytokines or receptor-mediated inhibitors of IL-1 or TNF-α could have biological activity in patients with HIV-associated KS. Thus, the in vitro study of the growth of AIDS-KS cells has led to a wide variety of potential therapeutic interventions.

III. EVALUATION OF AIDS-KS

Progression of AIDS-KS and survival are probably related to the degree of immunological deficiency (24,25). The Oncology Committee of the AIDS Clinical Trials Group (ACTG) supported by the National Institute of Allergy and Infectious Disease (NIAID) has developed uniform and precise criteria for disease evaluation, response to treatment, and clinical staging of KS in individuals with HIV infection (26). The initial extent of disease evaluation is based on a complete physical examination. A biopsy confirming the diagnosis of AIDS-KS is required. A chest roentgenogram, complete blood count, serum chemistries, and enumeration of CD4+ T lymphocytes subsets should be performed. Additional studies are performed only as indicated by the patient's symptoms and findings on physical examination or laboratory studies. Three to five indicator lesions that have not been treated locally with either intralesional chemotherapy or external beam radiation are selected for response to the planned intervention and are noted on a standard body diagram. Cross-sectional vectors of the indicator lesions are measured at the greatest perpendicular diameter. The character of the AIDS-KS lesions—color, degree of nodularity, and the presence or absence of lesional edema—is also noted. Visceral involvement and edema including a checklist of anatomical areas (legs, genitalia, periorbital regions) are important elements to define extent of disease.

IV. STAGING OF AIDS-KS

The ACTG has also recommended a staging system that classifies patients according to the extent of tumor (T), the status of the immune system

Table 1 Kaposi's Sarcoma Assessment

Limited disease	Extensive disease
No previous OI	Previous OI
No "B" symptoms	"B" symptoms
No edema	Edema of face or extremities
CD4+ T lymphocytes > 200	CD4+ T lymphocytes < 200
AIDS-KS lesions < 25	AIDS-KS lesions > 25
Slow-appearing AIDS-KS < 10/month	Rapidly progressive > 10/month
No pulmonary AIDS-KS	Pulmonary involvement with AIDS-KS
Tolerates zidovudine	Intolerant of zidovudine
Serum p24 < 35 pg/ml	Serum p24 > 35 pg/ml

Table 2 Therapy for AIDS-Associated Kaposi's Sarcoma

Local therapy	Chemotherapy
Radiation	Single agents
Liquid nitrogen	Doxorubicin 10 mg/m^2 once a week
Intralesional vinblastine	Vinblastine 0.1 mg/kg once a week
Surgery	Vincristine 2.0 mg/week
Interferon-alpha + AZT	Combination chemotherapy
	Vincristine 2.0 mg + bleomycin 15 U/m^2 every 2 weeks
	Vincristine 2.0 mg alternating weekly with vinblastine 0.1 mg/kg
	Vincristine 2.0 mg + bleomycin 10 U/m^2 + doxorubicin 15 mg/m^2
	Chemotherapy + zidovudine 500 mg/day
	Chemotherapy + zidovudine + G-CSF or GM-CSF
	Chemotherapy + ddI or ddC

Table 3 General Guidelines for Chemotherapy Administration

CD4+ cells	Antiretroviral	Immuno-modulator	Local control	Systemic chemotherapy
>500	Unknown	Unknown	Yes	If clinically indicated
200–500	Yes	Yes	Yes	If clinically indicated
<200	Yes	Limited value	Yes	If clinically indicated

as measured by CD4+ T lymphocyte cell numbers (I), and concomitant or antecedent systemic illness (S). Subjects with AIDS-KS are divided into good risk and poor risk categories based on the proposed TIS classification. It is hoped that the TIS staging classification, like the TNM system for nonhematological malignancies, will be effective in predicting the outcome of treatment and, ultimately, patient survival.

The TIS staging system proposed by the ACTG combined with the uniform response criteria will enable clinicians to evaluate different therapeutic options and help plan rational therapy for individual patients. At San Francisco General Hospital we utilize a model similar to the TIS staging system to help direct therapeutic choices (27). This assessment scale (Table 1) divides patients into limited disease and extensive disease categories. Definition of the two different categories utilizes an assessment of immunological function, clinical presentation, patient tolerance of antiretroviral medications, and an evaluation of tumor-associated complications, including edema. Most patients do not satisfy all the criteria for limited or extensive disease. In those circumstances where it is not clear whether a patient has limited or extensive disease, a decision is made based on the most relevant individual clinical criteria. The separation of AIDS-KS into two categories is useful since therapy can also be divided into local and systemic interventions (Table 2). The interventions apply to the categorization of disease: limited disease usually requires local therapy and extensive disease usually requires systemic therapy. Table 3 illustrates our approach to therapy for AIDS-KS.

V. RESPONSE CRITERIA FOR AIDS-KS

It is difficult to compare studies of therapy for AIDS-KS in part due to heterogeneity of recruited subjects and in part due to the lack of consistent response criteria. The ACTG has recommended a uniform response definition that should be incorporated into all AIDS-KS protocols. In general, this system proposes the following criteria: a *complete response* (CR) is the absence of any detectable residual disease, including tumor-associated edema, persisting for at least 4 weeks. Remaining pigmented macular lesions require a biopsy to document the absence of malignant cells. Medically appropriate restaging of visceral disease is encouraged. A *partial response* (PR) is a 50% or greater decrease in the number and or size of previously existing lesions lasting for at least 4 weeks without the appearance of new skin or oral lesions or new visceral sites of involvement or the appearance or worsening of tumor-associated edema or effusions. In those patients with predominantly nodular lesions, flattening to an indurated plaque of 75% or more of the nodules will also be considered a PR. *Stable disease* is any response not meeting the criteria for CR, PR, or progressive disease. *Progressive disease* is an increase of 25% or more in the size of previously existing lesions and/or the appearance of new lesions or new sites of disease or a 25% or more change in the character of lesions from macular to nodular or the development of new or increasing AIDS-KS-associated edema or effusions.

VI. LOCAL INTERVENTIONS

The major clinical objective for local therapy is cosmetic control of lesions on visible skin. The unifying affect of local therapies is the induction of an inflammatory response leading to the clinical resolution of the AIDS-KS lesion. Other therapies that also provide a limited but effective inflammatory reaction would doubtless have a similar clinical effect. Further research will attempt to define the most effective, least locally toxic, and most economically sensible approach to local AIDS-KS therapy.

Radiation therapy, directed to the AIDS-KS lesion and administered either as a single dose or on a daily fractional basis, is a useful treatment option (28). Facial AIDS-KS, lymphatic obstruction secondary to tumor involvement, painful lesions on the soles of feet, and palatal tumors are often effectively palliated by radiation therapy.

We have recently completed a study of topically applied liquid nitrogen (LN_2) for AIDS-KS. LN_2 is easily applied directly from an applicator or with a cotton-tipped applicator dipped into a LN_2 bath. LN_2 often provides an excellent clinical response, especially with plaquelike facial lesions. Biopsies of LN_2-treated AIDS-KS lesions demonstrate resolution of the spindle cells characteristic of AIDS-KS. LN_2 is relatively safe, inexpensive, and easy to apply, making it useful as treatment in the ambulatory setting (29).

Vinblastine (0.2 mg/ml) injected directly into AIDS-KS lesions (intralesional) has produced acceptable clinical results without significant hematological or immunological toxicities. The major problem associated with intralesional vinblastine is the pain associated with the injection of this caustic material (30–32).

Surgical excisin of lesions on the foot, skinfolds, in areas of flexion/extension, or the conjunctiva is relatively safe, easy to perform, and produces an adequate clinical result. Unfortunately the clinical result is often quite transient, and incomplete excision may lead to problems with wound healing and infection.

VII. SYSTEMIC INTERVENTIONS

A. Single Agents

1. Interferon Therapy

Recombinant interferon-α has demonstrated anti-HIV activity (33) and has been used successfully to treat AIDS-KS in a multi-institution study (34). In general, patients with more limited disease responded better than do those with extensive disease. As a single agent, interferon-α at doses of 30–36 million units per day administered subcutaneously appears to induce the maximal response. This dose is associated with hepatic, hematological, and significant systemic toxicities. Lower doses of interferon-α, 5×10^6 units/day, combined with standard doses of zidovudine seem to be well tolerated (35). In patients with HIV infection, the combination of interferon-α and zidovudine has elicited antitumor and antiviral responses. Two independent ACTG investigations have demonstrated that lowered doses of interferon-α combined with zidovudine may have clinical utility against AIDS-KS (36). At San Francisco General Hospital, we use interferon-α in combination with zidovudine in subjects with CD4+ T lymphocytes > 200 cells/mm^3. The role for interferon-α in stabilizing AIDS-KS following effective chemotherapy is unclear (37). A preliminary study of interferon-β treatment reported activity similar to interferon-α. The toxicity was less than with interferon-α. Other investigators have not observed significant clinical response with interferon-β.

2. Chemotherapy

Single-agent vinblastine was one of the first agents used to treat AIDS-KS. In one study, vinblastine was administered once weekly starting at a dose of 4 mg, with an increase in the dose each week such that total leukocytes remain above 2500 cells/μl (38). The median dose was 6 mg. Thirty-eight subjects were studied; one sustained a complete response, nine subjects had a partial response, and 19 subjects had stable disease. The median time to response was 5 weeks. The median duration of response for all patients was more than 13 weeks. Toxicity was minimal with the median nadir of total leukocytes being 2.6×10^3 cells/μl.

Single-agent etoposide has been used intravenously at a dose of 150 mg/m^2 for 3 consecutive days every 4 weeks for AIDS-KS (39). Using this regimen in 41 subjects with no B symptoms and no previous opportunistic infection, 12 patients had a complete response and 19 patients had a partial response. The median duration of response was approximately 9 months. Alopecia, neutropenia, and gastrointestinal toxicities were common.

Sixty subjects with AIDS-KS and either B symptoms, systemic disease, or CD4+ T lymphocytes less than 400 cells/mm^3 were treated with single-agent bleomycin (40). Thirty subjects were treated with 5 mg/day bleomycin administered intramuscularly for 3 days every 2 or 3 weeks, and 30 subjects were administered bleomycin by slow continuous intravenous infusion (6 mg/m^2/day for 4 days every 4 weeks). Forty patients received zidovudine in association with bleomycin within a dose range of 200–1200 mg/day with a mean daily dose of 900 mg. Twenty-nine (48.3%) patients had a partial response; 18 subjects (30%) had disease stabilization. There was no significant difference in response rate comparing the intramuscular and intravenous routes of administration. Toxicity was minimal consisting of fevers, cutaneous toxicity, Raynaud's phenomenon, and mild myelo-suppression. Twenty-three patients died (38.3%). In a second study of single agent bleomycin, 18 of 50 subjects had cutaneous side effects (41).

Single-agent vincristine has been administered by weekly intravenous injection to 23 patients with AIDS-KS (42). Eighteen subjects were evaluated for a response; 11 had a partial response, while a minor response was observed in seven subjects. The median duration for the subjects achieving a partial response was more than 4 months. The major toxicity was peripheral neuropathy. Small studies of single-agent ICRF-187, oral vinzolidine and oral idarubicin, mitoxantrone, epirubicin, and doxo-rubicin have been performed (42–46). Response rates have varied from 0 to 42% with toxicities that are agent-specific.

The ACTG has begun a study of single-agent oral etoposide. This phase 1 dose escalation study was begun to define the clinical response, toxicity, and maximally tolerated dose of weekly administered oral etoposide. Etoposide was selected based on previous studies demonstrating clinical effectiveness, the availability of an orally administered dosage form suitable for outpatient use, and its relatively low immediate toxicity. Six dose levels were studied, beginning at 150 mg/week. Etoposide was administered in a single day, and escalated by 50 mg increments to a total dose of 400 mg/week. Four subjects were entered at each dose level. The study has been completed, and the results are undergoing analysis.

B. Multiagent Chemotherapy

Most of the single chemotherapeutic agents mentioned above have been used in combination to treat AIDS-KS. The basis for combining agents in treating AIDS-KS is the desire to enhance efficacy while minimizing toxicity. Utilizing agents with different mechanisms of action reduces the development of cross-resistance, whereas combining clinically manageable doses of drugs limits the toxicity associated with effective single-agent chemotherapy doses.

Thirty-one subjects with AIDS-KS received combination chemotherapy consisting of doxorubicin 40 mg/m^2 day 1, bleomycin 15 U days 1 and 15, and vinblastine 6 mg/m^2 day 1 (37). All chemotherapy was administered intravenously. Seven subjects achieved a complete response, 19 subjects achieved a partial response, five patients had no response. The median response duration for those subjects with a complete response was 8.5 months. Dose reductions of 25–50% were necessitated by hematological toxicity in 18 patients. Two patients with fevers and neutropenia were hospitalized. Nineteen subjects developed an opportunistic infection or had an opportunistic infection diagnosed within 2 months of terminating therapy.

Eighteen subjects were treated with a six-drug regimen of doxorubicin 20 mg, vinblastine 4 mg, and bleomycin 15 U on day 1, followed by actinomycin D 1 mg, vincristine 1.4 mg, and dacarbazine 375 mg on day 8 (47). Three subjects had a complete response, 11 had a partial response, and one a minor response. The median duration of complete response was 1 month, and the median duration of partial response was 5 months. Twelve subjects died of opportunstic infections, and five subjects died of progressive KS. Myelosuppression was common. It was suggested that aggressive chemotherapy did not prolong survival of patients with advanced stage disease. Patients who had an improved performance status shortly after initiating chemotherapy had a 6-month median survival as compared with 2 months for those whose performance did not improve.

Twenty-four subjects with AIDS-KS were treated with a regimen consisting of vincristine 2 mg, alternating with vinblastine 0.1 mg/kg, on a weekly basis (48). Doses were modified for myelosuppression or paresthesias. Twenty-one subjects were evaluable: one achieved a complete response, eight achieved a partial response, seven had stable disease, and five had progressive disease. The median time to response was 13 weeks. After 35 weeks of observation, neither a median duration of response nor a median survival had been determined. The major toxicity was peripheral neuropathy. Three subjects had therapy discontinued due to moderate muscle weakness. Six subjects developed mild paresthesias not requiring dose modification. Hematological toxicities were minimal. Six subjects died while on study.

In another study, 33 patients were nonrandomly assigned to one of two treatment regimens (49). Group 1 (21 patients) was treated with doxorubicin 10 mg/m^2, vincristine 2 mg, and bleomycin 10 U/m^2. Group 2 (12 patients) was treated with doxorubicin 20 mg/m^2, vincristine 2 mg, and bleomycin 10 U/m^2. Chemotherapy was administered by intravenous infusion every 2 weeks. In groups 1 and 2 there were five and three subjects with complete responses, respectively, and 14 and four subjects with partial responses, respectively. In this study patient characteristics that predicted a shorter survival included Karnofsky performance status below 70%, hemoglobin less than 10 g/dl, and history of weight loss. One third of all subjects developed neutrophil counts below 1000 cells/mm^3, and five subjects developed bacterial infections on therapy. Mild to moderate paresthesias were observed in 60% of subjects, with seven patients requiring dose reductions and two subjects requiring discontinuation of vincristine. Three subjects had bleomycin toxicities though dose adjustment was not described. Twenty-three subjects developed an opportunistic infection, 17 of which were *Pneumocystis carinii* pneumonia (PCP). PCP prophylaxis was not required in this study.

Bleomycin and vincristine were administered to a group of 18 subjects with some degree of pretreatment hematological cytopenia (50). In this bimonthly regimen, vincristine at 2.0 mg and bleomycin at 10 U/m^2 were administered intravenously. PCP prophylaxis was prescribed for all subjects. Two subjects achieved a complete response; 11 sustained a partial response; two had a minimal response; and three had progressive disease. The median response for subjects with a complete or partial response ranged from 3 to 39 weeks. The median survival for the group was 6 months from initiation of therapy. Seventeen of the eighteen subjects had a nadir granulocyte count ≤ 1500/mm^3. Minimal to moderate nausea and vomiting were recorded in nine cases and partial alopecia in 12 cases. Ten subjects developed a vincristine-related sensory peripheral neuropathy, and six subjects had their vincristine dose delayed or reduced. Four subjects developed bleomycin-associated skin changes requiring discontinuation of therapy in two subjects. Overall, 16 subjects developed opportunistic infection, 11 with PCP. This study demonstrated that subjects with extensive disease or with compromised hematological function can be successfully treated with combination chemotherapy. Nevertheless, these subjects have profound limitations, and the underlying immune suppression often leads to a number of opportunistic infections and/or death.

A small study of 14 subjects evaluated the combination of monthly actinomycin D 1 mg/m^2 (day 1), vinblastine 6 mg/m^2 (day 1), bleomycin 10 mg/m^2 (days 1 and 8), and human lymphoblastoid alpha interferon 10 million U/m^2 subcutaneously three times a week beginning day 14 (51).

One subject had a complete response and four had a partial response. The median length of survival was 48 weeks; 11 subjects died of progressive AIDS-KS. The authors suggested that this therapy is not appropriate for subjects with AIDS-KS. Alternatively, recombinant interferon-α2b was used as maintenance therapy following cytotoxic chemotherapy in 21 subjects (35). Six subjects with a complete response and 15 subjects with a partial response to doxorubicin (20 mg/m^2), bleomycin 10 U/m^2, and vincristine 2 mg were then treated with recombinant interferon-α2b at three fixed dose levels: 5, 10, and 15 million units. Response was limited; the maximum tolerated dose was 10 million units with fatigue, fevers, and diarrhea being the most common toxicities.

In an attempt to evaluate the role of combination chemotherapy and antiretroviral therapy, 18 subjects were treated with vincristine and vinblastine as described above, and zidovudine was added at a daily dose of 1200 mg (52). All subjects tolerated full-dose therapy for at least 4 weeks, but by 12 weeks most subjects required dose reduction of zidovudine. When zidovudine was reduced to 400–800 mg/day, subjects tolerated combination chemotherapy and zidovudine without toxicity. One subject achieved a complete response, two a partial response, and four had no response. Four subjects had progressive disease, and five subjects were not evaluable. A second study evaluated the combination of chemotherapy and zidovudine. Fifteen subjects received weekly single-agent intravenous chemotherapy using bleomycin, vincristine, vinblastine, or etoposide, and one received combination bleomycin and vincristine every other week (53). Two subjects developed neutropenia and one died with staphylococcal septicemia. Five subjects required blood transfusions. Chemotherapy agents were changed five times secondary to disease progression. A mild sensory neuropathy was noted in two patients, and bleomycin-induced cutaneous toxicity was observed in one subject. Similar clinical results were reported with doxorubicin and zidovudine, dosed at 600 mg/day (54).

Future therapy will in part be based on previous studies and on the evolving care of the HIV-infected individual. It is clear that appropriate prophylaxis for opportunistic infections must be a cornerstone to therapy for all HIV-infected individuals. Therapies for AIDS-KS will need to be compatible with the prophylactic therapies chosen. HIV infection is the mechanism underlying immune suppression and proliferation of AIDS-KS lesions; therefore, treatment for lesions will ultimately need to include antiretroviral medications. Zidovudine has been studied in combination with a few chemotherapy agents in limited studies. These small studies suggest that the hematological toxicity profile of zidovudine may limit its utility with many chemotherapeutic agents. The role of other antiretrovirals combined with chemotherapy is yet to be determined. In order to better define the role of newer antiretroviral agents, the ACTG has initiated a study of doxorubicin, vincristine, and bleomycin in combination with ddI or ddC. Another strategy being actively evaluated involves the use of combination chemotherapy with antiretrovirals and the hematopoietins GM-CSF and G-CSF. The logic in these trials is to eliminate the often dose-limiting problem of bone marrow suppression induced by the cytotoxic agents and zidovudine.

VIII. SUMMARY

The underlying degree of immune suppression is an important consideration in the selection of treatment for AIDS-KS. In general, subjects with CD4+ T lymphocytes > $500/mm^3$ require only local therapy unless there is some specific disability caused by the AIDS-KS lesions. Subjects with CD4+ T lymphocytes between 200 and $500/mm^3$ may respond to recombinant interferon. This therapy is effective in controlling AIDS-KS, can be combined with zidovudine, and has anti-HIV properties. If interferon-α with zidovudine is clinically ineffective, systemic chemotherapy may then be required. Subjects with AIDS-KS and CD4+ T lymphocytes < $200/mm^3$ should receive PCP prophylaxis, may require systemic chemotherapy, and should be maintained on antiretroviral therapy.

Therapy of AIDS-KS is not curative, and a treatment plan of the underlying immune deficiency is essential for planning and implementing rational therapy. AIDS-KS is rarely life threatening but often cosmetically and functionally disabling. Treatment plans remain focused on palliative goals and include reduction of extremity or facial edema, elimination of painful lesions, relief of gastrointestinal disturbances induced by AIDS-KS lesions (including symptoms of outlet obstruction, diarrhea, and rarely blood loss), and reduction of the pulmonary burden of AIDS-KS to improve oxygenation and relieve obstructive pneumonias.

REFERENCES

1. Friedman-Kein A, Laubenstein L, Marmor M, et al. Kaposi's sarcoma and *Pneumocystis* pneumonia among homosexual men-New York City and California. MMWR 1981; 30:305–8.

2. Hymes KB, Cheung TL, Greene JB, et al. Kaposi's sarcoma in homosexual men: a report of eight cases. Lancet 1981; 2:598–600.

3. Des Jarlais DC, Stoneburner R, Thomas P. Declines in proportion of Kaposi's sarcoma among cases of AIDS in multiple risk groups in New York City. Lancet 1987; 2:1024–5.

4. Drew WL, Mills J, Hauer LB, et al. Declining prevalence of Kaposi's sarcoma in homosexual AIDS patients paralleled by fall in cytomegalovirus transmission. Lancet 1988; 1:66.

5. Rutherford GW, Schwarcz SK, Lemp GF, et al. The epidemiology of AIDS-related Kaposi's sarcoma in San Francisco. J Inf Dis 1989; 159:569–72.

6. Nakamura S, Salahuddin SZ, Biberfeld P, Ensoli B, Markham PD, Wong-Staal F, Gallo RC. Kaposi's sarcoma cells: long-term culture with growth factor from retrovirus-infected CD4+ T cells. Science 1988; 242:426–30.

7. Delli Bovi P, Donti E, Knowles DM, Friedman-Kien A, Luciw PA, Dina D, Dalla-Favera R, Basilico C. Presence of chromosomal abnormalities and lack of AIDS retrovirus DNA sequences in AIDS-associated Kaposi's sarcoma. Cancer Res 1986; 46:6333.

8. Ensoli B, Nakamura S, Salahuddin SZ, Biberfeld P, Larsson L, Beaver B, Wong-Staal F, Gallo RC. AIDS-Kaposi's sarcoma-derived cells express cytokines with autocrine and paracrine growth effects. Science 1989; 243:223–6.

9. Salahuddin SZ, Nakamura S, Biberfeld P, Kaplan MH, Markham PD, Larsson L, Gallo RC. Angiogenic properties of Kaposi's sarcoma-derived cells after long-term culture in vitro. Science 1988; 242:430–3.

10. Miles SA, Rezai AR, Salazar-González JF, Meyden MV, Stevens RH, Logan DM, Mitsuyasu RT, Taga T, Hirano T, Kishimoto T, Martínez-Maza O. AIDS Kaposi sarcoma-derived cells produce and respond to interleukin 6. Proc Natl Acad Sci USA 1990; 87:4068.

11. Sturzl M, Roth WK, Zietz C, Brockmeyer NH, Speiser B, Hofschneider PH. Kaposi's sarcoma is sustained by paracrine and autocrine mechanisms of growth factor action in vivo [Abstract]. Meeting of the Laboratory of Tumor Cell Biology, Bethesda, MD, 1991:T.10.

12. Lunardi-Iskandar Y, Lam HH, Judde JG, Gallo RC. Cytokine and hormone receptors on AIDS-Kaposi's sarcoma (KS)-derived cells [Abstract]. Meeting of the Laboratory of Tumor Cell Biology, Bethesda, MD, 1991:T.7.

13. Podor TJ, Jirik FR, Loskutoff DJ, Carson DA, Lotz M. Human endothelial cells produce IL-6. Lack of responses to exogenous IL-6. Ann NY Acad Sci 1989; 557:374–85.

14. Miles SA, Martínez-Maza O, Rezai A, Magpantay L, Salahuddin S, Nakamura S, Radka S, Linsley P. Oncostatin-M as a potent mitogen for AIDS-Kaposi sarcoma derived cells. 1992 submitted.

15. Miles SA, Rezai A, Kishimoto T, Mitsuyasu RT, Martínez-Maza O. Multiple cytokines simultaneously alter secretion of interleukin-6 and growth of AIDS Kaposi sarcoma cells. 1992 submitted.

16. Ammann AJ, Palladino MA, Volberding P, Abrams D, Martin NL, Conant M. Tumor necrosis factors alpha and beta in acquired immunodeficiency syndrome (AIDS) and AIDS-related complex. J Clin Immunol 1987; 7:481.

17. Berman MA, Sandborg CI, Calabia BS, Andrews BS, Friou GJ. Interleukin 1 inhibitor masks high interleukin 1 production in acquired immunodeficiency syndrome (AIDS). Clin Immunol Immunopath 1987; 42:133–40.

18. Ensoli B, Barillari G, Salahuddin SZ, Gallo RC, Wong-Staal F. Tat protein of HIV-1 stimulates growth of cells derived from Kaposi's sarcoma lesions of AIDS patients. Nature 1990; 345:84.

19. Vogel J, Hinrichs SH, Reynolds RK, Luciw PA, Jay G. The HIV tat gene induces dermal lesions resembling Kaposi's sarcoma in transgenic mice. Nature 1988; 335:606.

20. Hsu M, Schutt A, Holley M, Slice L, Sherman MI, Richman DD, Potash MJ, Volsky DJ. Inhibition of HIV replication in acute and chronic infections in vitro by a tat antagonist. Science 1992; 254:1799–1801.

21. Brown TJ, Rowe J, Jingwen L, Shoyab M. Regulation of IL-6 expression by Oncostatin-M. J Immunol 1991; 147:2175–80.

22. Sarngadharan MG, DeVico AL, Nair BC, Nakamura S, Copeland TD, Oroszlan S, Patel A, Gallo RC. Purification and partial characterization of the 30 kD factor that supports the growth of Kaposi's sarcoma-derived cells [Abstract]. Meeting of the Laboratory of Tumor Cell Biology, Bethesda, MD, 1991 (T.5).

23. Looney DJ, Poeschla E, Fiegal E, Badel P, Rappaport J, Wong-Staal F. Spindle like cells derived from the peripheral blood of patients with Kaposi's sarcoma [Abstract]. Meeting of the Laboratory of Tumor Cell Biology, Bethesda, MD, 1991 (T.9).

24. Vadhan-Raj S, Wong G, Genecco C, et al. Immunological variables as predicators of prognosis in patients with Kaposi's sarcoma and the acquired immunodeficiency syndrome. Cancer Res 1986; 46:417–25.

25. Taylor J, Afrasiabi R, Fahey JL, et al. Prognostically significant classification of immune changes in AIDS with Kaposi's sarcoma. Blood 1986; 67: 666–71.

26. Krown SE, Metroka C, Wernz JC. Kaposi's sarcoma in the acquired immune deficiency syndrome: a proposal for uniform evaluation, response, and staging criteria. J Clin Oncol 1989; 7:1201–7.

27. Kahn JO, et al. New insights into the pathogenesis and treatment of AIDS-associated Kaposi's sarcoma. In: Human retroviruses. Groopman, Chen, Essex, Weiss, eds. UCLA Symposia on Molecular and Cellular Biology. New York: Wiley-Liss, 1989.

28. Hill DR. The role of radiotherapy for epidemic Kaposi's sarcoma. Semin Oncol 1987; 14 (suppl 3):1207.

29. Tappero J, Berger TG, Kaplan LD, Volberding PA, Kahn JO. Cryotherapy for cutaneous Kaposi's sarcoma associated with AIDS: a phase 2 trial. J Acquir Immune Defic Syndr 1991; 4:839–46.

30. Newman SB. Treatment of epidemic Kaposi's sarcoma (KS) with intralesional vinblastine injection (IL-VLB) [Abstract]. Proc American Society of Clinical Oncology, New Orleans, 1988; 7:5.

31. Epstein J. Oral Kaposi's sarcoma in AIDS: management with intralesional chemotherapy [Abstract]. Fifth International Conference on AIDS, Montreal, M.B.O., 1989, Vol. 21, p. 190.

32. Conant MA, et al. Intralesional vinblastine (Velban) treatment of lesions of Kaposi's sarcoma [Abstract]. Fifth International Conference on AIDS, Montreal, T.B.P., 1989, Vol. 290, p. 335.

33. Ho DD, Hartshorn KS, Rota TR, et al. Recombinant human interferon alpha-A suppresses HTLV-III replication in vitro. Lancet 1985; 1:602–4.

34. Abrams DI, Volberding PA. Alpha interferon therapy of AIDS-associated Kaposi's sarcoma. Semin Oncol 1987; 14:43–7.

35. Kovacs JA, Deyton L, Davey R, et al. Combined zidovudine and interferon-alpha therapy in patients with Kaposi sarcoma and the acquired immunodeficiency syndrome (AIDS). Ann Intern Med 1989; 111:280–7.

36. Krown SE, Gold JWM, Niedzwiecki, et al. Interferon-alpha with zidovudine: safety, tolerance and clinical and virologic effects in patients with Kaposi sarcoma associated with the acquired immunodeficiency syndrome. Ann Intern Med 1990; 112:812–21.

37. Gill PS, et al. Interferon-alpha maintenance therapy after cytotoxic chemotherapy for treatment of acquired immunodeficiency syndrome-related Kaposi's sarcoma. J Biol Resp Mod 1990; 9:512.

38. Volberding PA, Abrams DI, Conant MA, et al. Vinblastine therapy for Kaposi's sarcoma in the acquired immunodeficiency syndrome. Ann Int Med 1985; 103:335–8.

39. Laubenstein LJ, Krigel RL, Odajnyk CM, et al. Treatment of epidemic Kaposi's sarcoma with etoposide or a combination of doxorubicin, bleomycin and vinblastine. J Clin Oncol 1984; 2:1115–20.

40. Lassoued K, et al. Treatment of the acquired immune deficiency syndrome-related Kaposi's sarcoma with bleomycin as a single agent. Cancer 1990; 66:1869.

41. Caumes E, et al. Cutaneous side-effects of bleomycin in AIDS patients with Kaposi's sarcoma. Lancet 1990; 336:1553.

42. Mintzer DM, Real FX, Jovino L, Krown SE, et al. Treatment of Kaposi's sarcoma and thrombocytopenia with vincristine in patients with the acquired immunodeficiency syndrome. Ann Int Med 1985; 102:200–2.

42a. Chachoua A, et al. Phase II trial of ICRF-187 in patients with acquired immune deficiency related Kaposi's sarcoma (AIDS-KS). Invest New Drugs 1989; 7:327.

43. Sarna G, et al. Oral vinzolidine as therapy for Kaposi's sarcoma and carcinomas of lung, breast and colon/rectum. Can Chemother Pharmacol 1985; 14:12.

44. Chachoua A, et al. Phase II study of oral idarubicin in patients with AIDS-associated Kaposi's sarcoma. Can Treat Rep 1987; 71:775.

45. Kaplan L, et al. Failure (and danger) of mitozantrone in AIDS-related Kaposi's sarcoma. Lancet 1985; 2:396.

46. Goss PE, Shepherd FA, Burkes R, Paul K. Phase II study of epirubicin in the treatment of Kaposi's sarcoma and AIDS. Proc ASCO 1989; 8:2.

47. Gelmann EP, et al. Combination chemotherapy of disseminated Kaposi's sarcoma patients with the acquired immune deficiency syndrome. Am J Med 1987; 82:456.

48. Kaplan L, et al. Treatment of Kaposi's sarcoma in acquired immunodeficiency syndrome with an alternating vincristine-vinblastine regimen. Cancer Treat Report 1986; 70:1121.

49. Gill PS, et al. Advanced acquired immune deficiency syndrome-related Kaposi's sarcoma. Cancer 1989; 65:1074.

50. Gill PS, et al. Treatment of advanced Kaposi's sarcoma using a combination of bleomycin and vincristine. Am J Clin Oncol 1990; 13:315.

51. Shepherd FA, et al. Combination chemotherapy and alpha-interferon in the treatment of Kaposi's sarcoma associated with acquired immune deficiency syndrome. CMAJ 1988; 139:635.

52. Kahn J, Kaplan LD, Volberding PA. Phase II study of weekly alternating vincristine and vinblastine for AIDS-associated KS. Proc ASCO 1990; 9:2.

53. Brunt AM, et al. The safety of intravenous chemotherapy and zidovudine when treating epidemic Kaposi's sarcoma. AIDS 1989; 3:457.

54. Hochester H, et al. Phase 1 study and pharmacokinetics of weekly doxorubicin and AZT in KS [Abstract]. IV International Conference on AIDS, Stockholm, June 1988:7550.

12

Burnout Among HIV/AIDS Health Care Providers
Helping the People on the Frontlines

Judy A. Macks
JKRAssociates, San Francisco, California

Donald I. Abrams
*San Francisco General Hospital and
University of California—San Francisco,
San Francisco, California*

Eleven years into the epidemic of human immunodeficiency virus (HIV) and acquired immune deficiency syndrome (AIDS) that has claimed more than 100,000 lives, the emotional and psychological demands of working in the field has taken its toll on health care providers and their organizations. Faced daily with the pain of caring for individuals who may experience profound physical and mental deterioration, inadequate resources, lack of treatment and cure, a floundering health care system, complex ethical and legal issues, as well as feelings of hopelessness., helplessness, anger, and inadequacy, many health care professionals are finding it increasingly difficult to sustain their commitment to and energy in their work. More and more are experiencing a constellation of signs and symptoms popularly referred to as *burnout*.

Research has clearly documented that health care practitioners are generally more susceptible to burnout than professionals in other areas of endeavor. For those health care practitioners who care for people with HIV disease, this vulnerability is heightened. In addition, they experience the stressor of working in an epidemic that places them at greater risk of exposure than other health care practitioners. Weary providers, particularly those working in high-incidence urban areas, describe their experiences on the front lines as "combat fatigue" as they witness extensive and cumulative losses, battle their own stress-inducing attitudes, combat the stigma and hypocritical morality associated with the epidemic, face their personal and profession's limitations in providing care and cure, and, for many, deal daily in their personal lives with their own HIV status and their friends', partners', and communities' illnesses and deaths.

Burnout is costly to the individual, the organization, and the population served. Clearly, depleted individuals have difficulty functioning both in the workplace and in their personal lives, and are at risk for increasingly poor health and psychological distress. Organizations suffer when their employees suffer. Typically, where burnout is high, organizations experience increased staff conflict, tardiness, absenteeism, higher turnover rates, and lower productivity. Most significantly, in professions whose primary mission is to help and care for people, the patients or client groups suffer. When staff members suffering from burnout withdraw from patient contact, erect walls of self-defense, become cynical, and begin to feel dehumanized themselves, the quality of care they can provide to their patients diminishes vastly.

As health care professionals and organizations grapple with finding the means to sustain themselves in the years to come, their response to burnout from an individual, work group, and organizational perspective will be key to providing optimal care to patients with HIV disease.

I. OVERVIEW OF STRESS AND BURNOUT

Stress can be defined in terms of demands (stressors) and resources (1,2). When an individual lacks adequate internal or external resources to meet a demand, he or she experiences stress. External resources, which might include economic, social, or tangible responses, are more easily identifiable. However, internal resources are equally important in responding to demands and decreasing stress. More specifically, external resources can include finding support among colleagues, family, and friends, exercising regularly, or engaging in relaxing activities. Internal resources refer to an individual's abilities, skills, knowledge, attitudes, and values, which can help to ameliorate stress. A health care provider may need to develop a new professional skill or modify certain beliefs and attitudes that create stress by adopting new ones. One such belief might be: "I can feel successful and good about work, even if I cannot cure my patient."

Demands, or stressors, can be both internally or externally based. External demands—such as changes, events, or others' needs or expectations—are more obvious. These might include diagnosing a patient with a life-threatening illness, the death of a patient, or terminating life supports. Internal demands, while less obvious, can create enormous amounts of stress for the practitioner. These stressors are based upon personal needs, expectations, standards, beliefs, attitudes, and history. For example, an individual who believes that curing a patient is the only measure of successful care, or that there is no place for personal needs or feelings as a professional, is more likely to experience stress as a result of his or her internal demands.

Burnout describes an individual's response to work-related stressors that have not been successfully managed or resolved. Although a number of researchers have explored this field, burnout is described somewhat differently by each of them. Edelwich describes burnout as "the progressive loss of idealism, energy and purpose experienced by people in the helping professions as the result of the conditions of their work" (3). Pines and Aronson describe it as "a state of physical, emotional and mental exhaustion caused by long-term involvement in situations that are emotionally demanding." The emotional demands are most often caused by a combination of very high expectations and chronic situational stresses (4). Scott and Jaffe concisely summarize the literature by describing burnout as "the end-stage result of the inability to manage work stress" (5).

According to Pines and Aronson, individuals who are highly motivated, idealistic and energetic, and expect their work to give their lives a sense of meaning—especially those who have viewed their work as a "calling"—are most vulnerable to burnout. With often unattainable altruistic goals, some people become disillusioned, questioning the meaning of life and their work. Unfortunately, burnout often strikes just those individuals with the highest level of commitment to their work. Pines and Aronson conclude that "we have found, over and over again, that in order to burn out, a person needs to have been on fire at one time" (4).

Specific individual physical, psychological, and behavioral symptoms can indicate burnout (Table 1). Many of these symptoms are also associated with stress, both personal and work-related. However, they indicate burnout when the stressors are work-related, and the number, duration, severity, and chronicity of symptoms are more extreme.

As the number of individuals suffering from burnout increases, the syndrome can also be manifested as a group and organizational phenomenon, thereby seriously impairing organizational functioning. It is not

Table 1 Physical, Psychological, and Behavioral Symptoms That
Indicate Burnout

Physical symptoms can include:
- chronic fatigue
- significant changes in appetite
- muscular tension
- somatic complaints
- vulnerability to illness
- sleep disturbance
- gastrointestinal problems
- headaches
- ulcers

Psychological, emotional, and spiritual symptoms can include
- depression
- anxiety
- feel helpless, hopeless, trapped
- repression of feeling
- anger and resentment
- obsessions, phobias
- suicidal ideation and attempts
- negative about self, work, life, others
- apathy
- alienation
- disillusionment
- unrealistic expectations
- sense of omnipotence
- paranoia
- cynicism
- loss of meaning

Behavioral symptoms can include:
- increased alcohol or drug use
- interpersonal conflict
- withdrawal and isolation
- decreased contact with clients
- criticism of coworkers
- overreaction
- irritation, resentfulness and antagonism
- overeating
- avoiding responsibilities
- decreased productivity
- missed appointments
- chronical tardiness for work
- lethargy
- distraction
- disorganization

uncommon for organizations suffering from burnout to experience low staff morale, communication breakdown, increased staff conflict, decreased productivity, organizational stagnation, inflexibility and rigidity, resistance to change, increased absenteeism, high turnover, scapegoating, and displaced anger.

II. BURNOUT AMONG HIV/AIDS HEALTH CARE PROFESSIONALS

A significant body of research documents the high incidence of burnout among health care professionals (6–9) and specifically for practitioners working with the terminally ill (10–12). Various stressors specifically related to the HIV epidemic further distinguish it from other life-threatening illnesses and, as such, pose greater burnout risk to health care professionals working in this arena. The historical context of health care in industrialized nations, the specific nature of the HIV epidemic, traits characteristic of many HIV providers, and factors affecting the workplace all contribute to this increasing sense of combat fatigue and potential AIDS-related burnout (ARB).

A. Contextual Stressors

The HIV epidemic has emerged at a time in the development of Western medicine during which the general population and medical professions have grown to believe in and expect that a cure exists or can be found for illnesses. Lulled by the illusion and expectation that answers can be found in science and technology, professionals and consumers of health care have felt both impotent and angry that HIV is a reality for now and years to come. Similarly, the HIV epidemic highlights other inadequacies about health care in the United States. It has further highlighted the inaccessibility of health care services for people of color, women, and the poor, and increasingly for the middle class as well.

The HIV epidemic itself has carried with it enormous stigma and issues of morality, which has set it apart from most other life-threatening illnesses. This has been a result of the transmissible nature of the illness, the populations most affected by the epidemic, and the necessity for openly addressing sexuality and sexual behavior as a part of treatment and prevention. The epidemic has aroused moral condemnation and prejudice toward homosexuals and intravenous drug users. Many health care professionals have maintained strong negative feelings about a disease that they perceive to be self-inflicted and avoidable, and one that some also perceive puts them at risk for becoming infected with HIV in the work setting. This stigma associated with HIV affects patients, individuals, and communities at risk for HIV, their health care providers, and the general public.

Health care providers who have been working in the epidemic for a number of years have had to confront the stress posed by the prejudices, negative attitudes, and often unrealistic fears of contagion of their colleagues. In their survey of caregivers' stress and coping in working with HIV, Vachon and Dennis noted that young physicians working with people with HIV whose parents were once proud of their son's or daughter's work were now ashamed to discuss their careers with others because of the association with HIV (13). This was particularly true for gay physicians whose parents had not discussed their child's sexual orientation within their social milieu.

The youth of HIV patients profoundly alters the experience of health care professionals in providing care to people with HIV, who frequently experience severe physical and mental deterioration. Because many HIV practitioners are young themselves, identification with the patient and his or her traumatic and vulnerable experience becomes more pronounced, raising issues of his or her own mortality and vulnerability. In this regard, stressful issues and decisions are magnified, such as initiation and termination of life supports, heroic measures, rational suicide, and others.

The typical stressors involved in working with people with catastrophic illness are compounded in AIDS caregiving not only by the youth of the patients, but also by the complexities of HIV and its therapies. The rapidly changing and expanding knowledge-base demands that providers find ways to stay up to date in a work environment already filled with overflowing case loads. Not only is the level of care required by a person with HIV highly demanding, but resources needed to meet the medical and psychosocial needs of people with HIV are rarely available. As a result, physicians and other health care providers are expected to fulfill multiple roles for which they have not generally been trained such as research scientist, patient advocate, hospice counselor, educator, academician, grant writer, financial manager, media persona, and politician. In addition, physicians have come under increasing community and public scrutiny to become more accountable to the communities they serve. Many physicians feel caught in the middle between communities to which they are committed (and are often affiliated with) and a profession that does not have a history of community accountability.

The sociocultural and political context in which the HIV epidemic exists creates yet additional stressors for health care professionals. The epidemic dramatically exposes preexisting inadequacies and social inequities of society. For example, the need to serve diverse communities has frequently led to sharp conflicts between staff, volunteers, and community leaders. Health organizations representing different client populations often find themselves refereeing struggles that can pit gay, white men against communities of color; men against women; middle-class against the poor. Instead of building successful coalitions and alliances, AIDS agencies find themselves constantly on the defensive. The increased competition for funding has also pitted the needs of people with HIV against those with other health care needs and life-threatening illnesses.

B. Individual and Internal Stressors

In addition to the external demands of the HIV epidemic on health care professionals, researchers have identified a number of commonly shared beliefs and personal characteristics among these providers which contribute to burnout. Maslach identified three key causes of burnout including: 1) the desire to make a difference and the inability to achieve real results, 2) working close to pain and suffering, and 3) negative relationships with colleagues (7). Jaffe (14,15) identifies three key internalized attitudes and expectations that he believes are counterproductive and stress-producing. These include: 1) health professionals should have no personal needs or feelings, 2) providers should always be immediately available to patients, and 3) practitioners should be able to make the patient healthy or at least make a significant difference. In their 1979 study of health care providers working with catastrophic illness, Eisendrach and Dunkel (16) reported a common profile among these caregivers, which included the following qualities: high self-expectations, low tolerance for disappointment, need for excellence and perfection, low self-esteem when not achieving, omnipotence, need for control, and the need to save. Eisendrach and Dunkel identify these shared characteristics as contributing to the "medical culture."

A large proportion of practitioners, especially those who became involved early in the HIV epidemic, share many of these characteristics. Many of these providers were individuals who had been personally affected by the epidemic. They were extremely committed, energetic, altruistic, determined to make a difference, and worked long hours. In the short run, these qualities resulted in creativity, hard work, initiation of new services, and programmatic and organizational growth. However, over time these same qualities, and the underlying attitudes and belief that they reflect, can and have contributed to increasing burnout amount HIV health care professionals.

On the other hand, many practitioners began working with people with HIV out of circumstance and professional role, rather than by seeking it out. Certainly, many family practitioners and general internists in private practice did not expect to be working in a profession in which many of their patients would be young and dying. Experience suggests that residents at large teaching hospitals where AIDS cases are concentrated are highly vulnerable to burnout. Ward nurses, nurses in HIV units, and psychosocial support staff are also at higher risk of developing burnout.

A study of 82 primary care physicians caring for AIDS patients in San Francisco by Horstman and McKusick (17) found that the majority reported an increase in stress, and a significant minority experienced increased anxiety and fear of death since they began working with AIDS patients. They found that while the years of involvement with AIDS patients did not correlate with these deleterious effects, the percentage of time physicians spent caring for AIDS patients did increase the likelihood of the above-mentioned distress symptoms. On the other hand, nearly half of the respondents also reported an increased experience of intellectual stimulation and career satisfaction as well since beginning to work with AIDS patients. Among these respondents, gay physicians were more likely to experience psychological distress than their heterosexual counterparts.

Most significantly, health care professionals working in any setting with HIV disease must face the daily stressors of their work, as well as the physical and emotional stress posed by their own health status. This practitioner is likely to be homosexual or bisexual and must deal not only with his own health but also possibly the declining health of a partner and certainly many friends as a result of HIV. At the same time, other practitioners who are members of at-risk communities, especially gay and bisexual men, but who are not infected with HIV are also inundated with cumulative loss. Many will be acting not only as professional caregivers, but as caregivers to friends and partners at home. Not uncommonly, many HIV-negative gay and bisexual men also experience survivor guilt, questioning why they are healthy when so many around them are sick and dying. Regardless of personal health status, many gay and bisexual practitioners may find it difficult professionally to empathize with their patients without having such contact also trigger feelings and reactions about their own health and those for whom they are caring. These stressors are on-going and difficult to resolve, leaving the practitioners and their organizations vulnerable to burnout.

Health care providers working with HIV on a daily basis have likened their experience of working with the constant onslaught of loss and grief to combat fatigue. Living with loss and grief on a daily basis, providers must contend with fluctuating feelings of sadness, anger, helplessness, despair, rage, uncertainty, and fear. Multiple loss frequently leads to "bereavement overload" in which people cannot complete grieving one loss before confronting the next one. Unresolved grief exacerbates the grief process and can result in difficulties in coping and managing one's own life and work, staff conflict, resistance to change, loss of vitality, and other problems for the individual and the organization.

C. Organizational Stressors

In addition to personal characteristics and situations, many health care professionals, including those working in the field of HIV/AIDS, share common role-related and institutional stressors. Scott and Jaffe (5) identified making decisions under pressure, working in a technical environment where mistakes can have deadly consequences, and enduring long hours as key role-related stressors. In addition, they reported that practitioners working with AIDS patients frequently deal with life and death issues, witness pain and suffering, and face the limits of what they can do for their patients. Vachon et al. (18) reported key physician stressors to include role conflict, workload, patients demanding a voice in their treatment, and meeting the psychosocial needs of patients, families, and staff. In her research of occupational stress in the care of the critically ill, the dying, and the bereaved, Vachon concluded that caregiver stress resulted more frequently from the work environment and professional role issues, rather than from the care of dying patients and their families (10). Some of the significant organizational variables caregivers identified as stressors included: team communication problems, nature of the system and/or unit, inadequate resources and staffing, communication problems with others in the organization or outside the system, unrealistic expectations of the organization, communication problems with administration, professional role ambiguity, role conflict, lack of control, role overload, and proximity to stressors.

In response to the rapid spread of the HIV epidemic and the spiraling medical and psychosocial needs of people with HIV, AIDS health care services and organizations have grown very rapidly over a very short period of time. The growth has, until recently, usually been a response to a crisis rather than planned growth based upon a long-term strategy. The growth has frequently meant a change from a participatory decision-making process to a more bureaucratic and hierarchical decision-making structure. As a result of the shift in structure and increasing staff size, communication problems arise because staff have less access to managers and each other. Rapid growth has also meant that many volunteers and frontline staff have moved into management positions, sometimes lacking training and experience for these positions. In addition, the increasing needs for health care combined with shrinking resources, struggling health care institutions, and an inadequate system places immense stress on health care professionals who are frequently caught in the middle between enormous patient physical and psychosocial needs and the limited care they can offer. Individuals working in urban, public hospitals, in particular, experience this stress of increasing need, workload, and shrinking resources. Other institutional stressors vary widely but can include management style, decision-making structure, communication systems, workload, patient population, and other factors.

III. STRATEGIES FOR PREVENTING BURNOUT

Managing stress and minimizing AIDS-related burnout requires a collaborative effort between the individual and the organization. Most solutions to managing stress and preventing burnout described in the literature focus on the individual and include such strategies as stress management skills development, relaxation strategies, counseling, support groups, and other individually focused interventions. These strategies are extremely useful in helping the individual to cope with ongoing stressors. However, they are most effective when offered in the context of a comprehensive organizational effort to address the organizational and environmental stressors that contribute to burnout in the workplace.

Research indicates that personal variables mediate an individual's response to environmental and occupational stressors, although this arena is still not fully understood. Elliot and Eisdorfer (19) identify two types of mediators: 1) individual qualities that make the person more resistant or vulnerable to stressors and 2) environmental contexts that intensify the stress or help to buffer the individual from the stress. Mediators might include demographics, personality and coping styles, cultural, religious and personal values, previous experience, family life and social support, health behaviors, ability to balance work and home life, and economic status.

According to Kobasa and Maddi (20), certain personality styles and coping abilities help to buffer individuals from stress and burnout. In their research they found that individuals with a personality style described as "personality hardiness" are better equipped to respond to stressors in a positive manner. The three significant characteristics of the "hardy" personality include: 1) commitment, 2) control, and 3) challenge. Commitment refers to individuals who feel engaged and involved in their work. Individuals who feel a sense of control are those who believe that they can influence and affect what occurs in their lives. They are also able to discriminate between those events that they do and do not have control over, and do not attempt to control those events or stressors that cannot be controlled. Challenge is a quality that certain people bring to the experience of change, viewing change as a positive experience. These individuals are flexible and able to tolerate uncertainty.

A. Individual Interventions

Based upon this and other research, practitioners have identified specific individually focused strategies that can help to ameliorate burnout. Among the measures successfully utilized by physicians surveyed by Horstman and McKusick (19), respondents identified talking with a friend, lover, or family member, teaching others about AIDS, remaining objective, and getting support from other physicians as most effective. Skills development is also an important strategy to respond to stressors. Stress management skills development offers practitioners a variety of ways to cope with stress more effectively. These skills can include relaxation strategies, cognitive restructuring, setting short and long-term goals for behavioral change, developing and maintaining healthy behavioral habits, and a variety of skills that focus on identifying and altering stress-inducing attitudes and beliefs. Developing additional skills in the areas of communication and conflict resolution, managing grief and loss, time management, and managing change can also help in ameliorating stress and burnout.

As with other occupations, it is imperative in dealing with the AIDS crisis that the health care provider learn to separate work from the rest of his or her life as much as possible. This strategy is difficult, especially for providers whose friends and acquaintances may be calling at home with requests for information and advice similar to those that are dealt with during the course of a normal work day. If, however, any insulation is to be found as a protection from developing AIDS-related burnout, attempts must be made to separate the work from homelife. One effective technique is to punctuate the work day with an activity that separates it from returning to one's home. For example, one could participate in physical exercise activities, thus giving the mind time to disengage from the details of the work day while promoting a sense of well-being in the often weary health care worker. In addition, periodic getaways have been reported to be rejuvenating to those working on the AIDS front lines. Horstman and McKusick (17) felt that the benefits were threefold: a change of scenery through such getaways tend to break the insulating effect of working in an epidemic, it diverts the practitioner with extramural mental stimulation, and it ultimately freshens the emotional resources.

Providers working in group practices and clinic situations may have an advantage over solo practitioners. They often have the option of being able to air their stressors and concerns with fellow colleagues informally in the corridor or over lunch. When such informal opportunities for sharing are not available, or even when they are, formal support groups also serve a useful purpose in combatting AIDS-related burnout. Support groups offer another strategy focused on the individual prevention of burnout through social support and skills development. In group settings, providers can explore and ventilate feelings associated with their work, decrease isolation, give and receive feedback and insight from their peers, and enhance mutual support in a structured setting. Support groups are most effective when they are facilitated by a trained professional from outside the organization and are offered during working hours or with compensatory time. One of the pitfalls of support groups is that they can turn into a gripe session focusing on organizational problems. It is extremely important to keep the group focused on individual issues related to stress, burnout, grief, and loss.

Other professional training, development, and growth opportunities can help diminish stress and burnout by offering staff opportunities for professional challenge, growth, and skills development. These might include educational programs in new areas such as management, fund raising and development, or job swapping.

B. Organizational Interventions

Organizational interventions are extremely important not only to support the individual's attempts at managing stress effectively and self-care, but to alter the institutional causes of burnout.* In response to the individual and organizational stressors and high risk of burnout associated with working in the field of HIV, JKRAssociates developed a model to work with loss-saturated work environments.† The goal of this model is to help organizations and their employees identify and implement organizational and individual strategies to respond to the ongoing and cumulative stress and grief. It is based on the assumption that stress and grief in the workplace is experienced and expressed—overtly and subtly—at the personal, interpersonal/work group, and organizational levels. This model involves a number of steps including 1) organizational assessment, 2) task force planning, 3) an all staff meeting to review information gathered in the assessment, education and training, and problem solving, 4) implementation and intervention of identified strategies, 5) follow-up and evaluation, and 6) implementation of changes and additional interventions.

This model has been adapted to work with a wide variety of health care institutions, social service agencies, community-based organizations, smaller groups of private practitioners working in the same discipline, physicians working in solo practices, and for providers working in HIV who do not work in the same organization.

Several key factors are necessary to ensure the success of this type of endeavor. First, the process of involving all staff in the assessment, problem-solving, and implementation phases ensures that all employees are included, have a voice in the outcome and have helped to create the solution. Second, the support of management is key to the success of this type of intervention, which focuses not only on the individual, but on organizational interventions as well. Third, strategies should target the individual, work groups, and the organization as a whole. Fourth, strategies should address the following: 1) policies and benefits, 2) ongoing acknowledgment of losses, 3) role of management, 4) enhancing communication systems, 5) formal support, 6) informal communication, 7) appreciation mechanisms, 8) honoring of cultural diversity, 9) issues related to the different HIV statuses of staff, 10) job structure and workload, and 11) staff development.

An initial assessment of the problem is essential to developing an organizational strategy for intervention. At a minimum, an assessment must

---

*I am indebted to Gary Dexter, Ph.D., and Susan Colson for their contribution to my thinking in this area.

†JKRAssociates is a consulting firm providing assistance to organizations in managing grief, loss, stress, and burnout in the workplace.

focus on the impact of stress and burnout on the organization. Optimally, an organizational assessment can be conducted from a much broader prospective to identify problems in various aspects of the organization that ultimately contribute to burnout.

Based upon the organizational assessment, organizational interventions can be designed to respond to the identified stressors and problems. Implementing policies and benefits that help mitigate stress and burnout directly (and indirectly through giving messages to staff that self-care is encouraged) are crucial to an effective response to burnout. Policies should be consistent and allow for flexibility regarding vacation and sick leave, compensatory time, bereavement leave, educational leave, mental health days, reasonable accommodation, part-time options, leave without pay, and related benefits.

Since workload and limited resources are frequently cited as primary stressors in health care settings and HIV focused work settings, interventions to address AIDS-related burnout may need to focus on job structure, role-related tasks and responsibilities, work distribution, and time schedules. Some organizations have found it helpful to reorganize jobs to avoid repetition, vary tasks and caseloads, share jobs or tasks, and develop more flexible time schedules.

Enhancing communication systems, both formal and informal, is also important in addressing burnout. Poor communication in the work setting is frequently a key stressor. Ameliorating this problem by addressing communication between individuals, work groups, teams, and management and staff will help decrease the likelihood of staff burnout. In addition, informal communication needs to be encouraged by scheduling opportunities for staff to be together in fun, relaxing, and informal ways.

Managers play a key role in providing consistent supervision that encourages each staff person to recognize his or her signs and symptoms of burnout and help the individual to strengthen various coping skills to manage stress. Depending upon the needs of the individual, supervisors can help supervisees to ask for help, set reasonable limits, manage their time, recognize their strengths and weaknesses, accept their own and others' limitations, and set long- and short-term goals. In order to be most effective, managers may need additional training in supervisorial skills and assisting others in managing grief, loss, stress, and burnout.

Health care organizations and work groups caring for people with HIV need to develop systems to acknowledge losses on an ongoing basis. This can take a variety of forms but should address systems for informing colleagues about the deaths of co-workers and patients, acknowledging losses, and developing group rituals for remembering those who have died. In this area of grief and loss, in particular, cultural diversity must be recognized and interventions designed to accommodate individual and cultural responses to grief and loss. In addition, issues that arise as a result of working together as a mixed antibody status staff group similarly should be addressed.

The organization itself needs to design and implement mechanisms that systematically appreciate and honor staff members for their hard work and commitment. Additionally, celebrations need to be maintained for acknowledging significant life events such as birthdays, anniversaries, awards and other notable achievements.

IV. SUMMARY

Human immunodeficiency virus disease has presented the medical professional with many challenges over the past 10 years. In the decade ahead, one aspect of working in the field that is certainly becoming an increasingly formidable issue will be dealing with AIDS-related burnout among health care professionals.

The risks of AIDS-related burnout are multiple. If providers cannot find effective strategies for coping, it is possible that some of the most sensitive and compassionate workers in the field may leave to seek less stressful career opportunities. Those who focus on the negative impact that HIV disease has had on society will react with increased finger pointing to the risk of burning out as another negative consequence of working with HIV infection. Individual burnout will ultimately impact on the organization requiring interventions at that level as well.

Setting up mechanisms for both individuals and organizational systems to combat AIDS-related burnout will, in the short run, add to increased costs of care in a disease already noted for its high treatment expense. However, intervening to prevent AIDS-related burnout will ultimately be cost effective by minimizing its negative effects on individuals and institutions.

Learning how to cope with AIDS-related burnout may benefit the medical professional caring for patients with HIV disease as well as the profession as a whole. Facilitation of communication among individuals will certainly be fostered. Already we have seen a reorganization of delivery of health care that encourages the emphasis on integration of the patient into a true partnership with their provider. Becoming aware of the problem of AIDS-related burnout and attempting to prevent it can only serve to foster greater humanism in service professionals.

A report of the National Academy of Science Committee for the oversight of AIDS activities recommended in 1988 that "research funding be made available to examine the feasibility and effectiveness of programs to alleviate stress in health care workers who care for AIDS patients." Such funding is long overdue and should be made available immediately. As we enter the second decade of facing the complex challenges of the HIV epidemic, the stress could potentially become overwhelming. Dysfunctional health care providers need not become part of the problem. Now is the time to find solutions.

REFERENCES

1. Selye E. Stress without distress. Philadelphia: Lippincott, 1974.

2. Rabkin JG, Struening EL. Life events, stress and illness. Science 1976; 194: 1013-20.

3. Edelwich J. Burnout: stages of disillusionment in the helping professions. New York: Human Sciences Press, 1980.

4. Pines and Aronson. Career burnout. New York: The Free Press.

5. Scott CD, Jaffe DT. Managing occupational stress associated with HIV infection. Occup Med 1989; 4:85-93.

6. Maslach C. Burned out. Hum Behav 1976; 5(9):16-22.

7. Pines A, Aronson E, Kafry D. Burnout: from tedium to personal growth. New York: Free Press, 1981.

8. Cherniss C. Professional burnout in human service organizations. New York: Praeger, 1981.

9. Vachon M. Occupational stress in the care of the critically ill, the dying and the bereaved. New York: Hemisphere Publishing Corporation, 1987.

10. Pines A, Maslach C. Characteristics of staff burnout in mental health settings. Hosp Community Psychiatry, 1978; 29:233-7.

11. Shubin S. Rx for stress—your stress. Nursing 1979; 9(1):52-5.

12. Storlie FJ. Burnout: the elaboration of a concept. In: McConnell EA, ed. Burnout in the nursing profession: coping strategies, causes, and costs. St. Louis: CV Mosby, 1982:81-5.

13. Vachon LS, Dennis J. HIV, stress and the health care professional. In: Dilley JW, Pies C, Helquist M, eds. Face to face: a guide to AIDS counseling. San Francisco: AIDS Health Project of UCSF, Distributed by Celestial Arts Distributing, 1989:276-88.

14. Jaffe DT. The inner strains of healing work: therapy and self-renewal for health professionals. In Scott C, Hawk J, eds. Heal thyself: the health of health care professionals. New York: Brunner-Mazel, 1986.

15. Jaffe DT. Self-renewal: personal transformation following extreme trauma. J Humanistic Psychol 1985; 25.

16. Eisendrach SJ, Dunkel J. Psychological issues in intensive care unit staff. Heart and Lung 1979; 8(4):751-8.

17. Horstman W, McKusick L. The impact of AIDS on the physician. In: McKusick L, ed. What to do about AIDS. Berkeley: University of California Press, 1986.

18. Vachon MLS, Lysall WAL, Freeman SJJ. Measurement and management of stress in health professionals working with advanced cancer patients. Death Education 1978; 1:365-75.

19. Elliott GR, Eisdorfer C, eds. Stress and human health: analysis and implications of research. New York: Springer, 1982.

20. Kobasa SC, Maddi SR. Personality and constitution as mediators in the stress-illness relationship. J Health Soc Behav 1981; 22.

13

Management of HIV Disease in Women

Constance B. Wofsy, Nancy S. Padian, Judith B. Cohen, Ruth Greenblatt, and Rebecca Coleman
University of California—San Francisco, and San Francisco General Hospital, San Francisco, California

Joyce A. Korvick
National Institute of Allergy and Infectious Diseases, National Institutes of Health, Bethesda, Maryland

I. EPIDEMIOLOGY OF AIDS IN WOMEN AND HETEROSEXUALLY TRANSMITTED HIV

A. Current Statistics on AIDS in Women

AIDS and AIDS-related complications in women have now been reported as one of the five major leading causes of death in women in several major metropolitan cities on the East coast (1). As of the fall of 1991, 20,309 cases of AIDS in adult or adolescent women (10% of the total number of adult cases) have been reported to the Centers for Disease Control (CDC) (2). More than half of these cases have been reported since 1989 (3). The majority (approximately 62%) of these cases have occurred among women aged 25–39 years with the greatest number of cases reported among women aged 30–34 years (2). Ethnic minorities, particularly blacks (52% of female cases) and Hispanics (21% of female cases), are greatly overrepresented in these numbers with these groups having cumulative incidence rates that are 13 and 8 times, respectively, higher than that of white women

(4). Nonwhite women are especially conspicuous in the risk categories of intravenous drug use (76%), heterosexual contact with an intravenous drug user (81%), and among cases who were born in a Pattern-II country* (99%) (2).

Although more than half of all female cases occur among women who are injection drug users (IDUs), cases attributed to heterosexual contact with an infected partner or partner from a known risk group, especially an intravenous drug–using partner, have increased faster than cases from any other risk group (4). Three percent of all cases among women were attributed to heterosexual contact with a partner with unidentified risk in 1983–84, compared to 16% of female cases in 1989–90 (3). These changes herald the spread of HIV outside immediately identifiable risk groups. To identify high-risk exposure, careful questioning is critical; Lamb et al. (5) reported that after intensive reinterviewing, 42% of infected persons identified in a sexually transmitted disease (STD) clinic who were originally classified with no identifiable risk could be reclassified, and most were heterosexual partners of infected or at-risk individuals.

Sexually transmitted diseases, which may be markers for HIV risk behaviors and/or true cofactors for HIV transmission, presage future trends in the AIDS epidemic. Increased incidence of STDs in general, and in syphilis and PPNG (penicillinase-producing *Neisseria gonorrhoeae*) in particular, highlight the need for AIDS prevention and intervention programs (6,7). These upward trends have been associated with the use of crack cocaine and the concomitant practice of sex in exchange for drugs and have been most dramatic among young black women in urban centers throughout the United States (8).

B. Efficiency of Sexual Transmission Involving Women

Results from cross-sectional studies of couples consisting of one HIV-infected partner are fairly consistent in reporting an approximately 15–20% transmission rate from infected men to their female sexual partners (9). Results from studies of infected women to their male partners are far more erratic, with reports of equally efficient bidirectional heterosexual transmission rates that range from nonexistent to only one half the rate of male-to-female transmission (10). Factors that might influence transmission include the presence of other STDs (10,11), with low HIV trans-

---

*Areas in central Africa, southeast Asia, the Caribbean, or South America, where heterosexual transmission constitutes the major mode of spread.

mission rates where STD rates are low (10). For example, in a study of HIV-infected prostitutes in Nairobi, female-to-male transmission was independently associated with acquisition of genital ulcer disease (GUD), indicating that presence of GUD in the women might increase the infectiousness of HIV (11). More advanced HIV disease may be more prevalent as the epidemic in women progresses and risk of heterosexual transmission increases (12). Although in Pattern-I countries* women may acquire HIV, their role in further transmitting HIV is somewhat unclear.

Prospective heterosexual partner studies of couples discordant for HIV to evaluate seroincidence infections are greatly confounded by the fact that couples are encouraged to change to safer sex practices over the course of the study. Nonetheless, seroconversion rates from these studies ranged from no seroconversions (13) to approximately 17% (14) with an average time of follow-up of 1 year. Discrepancies in transmission according to gender of index case (first infected partner) ranged from no female-to-male transmission (15) to significant differences in gender-specific seroconversion rates (16).

Data on sexual transmission between women remain sparse. Cases reported to the CDC among lesbians represent less than 1% of all cases in women (4). Ninety-five percent of these cases occurred among IDUs, while the rest have been attributed to receipt of contaminated blood or blood products (4). There have been published case histories that suggest transmission between women in association with traumatic sex (17).

C. Risk Factors for Heterosexual Transmission

Risk factors that increase the likelihood that a random partner is infected (9), such as large number of sexual partners or sexual contact with an intravenous drug user, are best examined in surveys such as those done at STD clinics or among intravenous drug users. Risk factors for transmission between discordant couples are best evaluated from heterosexual partner studies and may be behavioral or biological, although these categories overlap (Table 1).

Behavioral risk factors mainly include sexual practices, which may be synergistic with drug use, or the independent effect of smoking. The strong protective effect of condoms has been consistently reported. Many prospective studies have reported no new seroconversions among couples who

---

*Areas such as the United States, Canada, and Europe, where transmission among homosexual men and intravenous drug users predominates.

Table 1 Factors Associated with Heterosexual Transmission of HIV

Factor	Male-to-female	Female-to-male
Lack of condoms	yes	yes
Anal intercourse	yes	no
Sex during menses	no	yes
Number of sexual contacts	yes	yes
Advanced disease state (as measured by CD4, p24 antigen, or AIDS diagnosis)	yes	yes
AZT[a]	possibly	unknown
Genital sores, infections or inflammations	yes	yes
Oral contraceptives[b]	yes	unknown
IUD use	possibly	unknown
Cervical ectopy	yes	unknown

[a]Possibly protective by decreased viral load.
[b]Whether oral contraceptives are protective or increase the likelihood of transmission is controversial.
Source: Reproduced from AIDSFILE with permission.

regularly report their use (16,18). In several studies anal intercourse has been reported as a risk for male-to-female transmission (19), while sexual intercourse during menses has been reported as a risk factor for female-to-male transmission (20). Number of sexual contacts has been associated with transmission regardless of the gender of the index case (21).

Biological risk factors relate to factors that may increase infectiousness or susceptibility to infection. CD4 counts, presence of p24 antigen, and AIDS diagnosis have all been used as surrogates for disease stage. The association between progression of HIV disease and increased infectiousness has not been found uniformly across studies. Laboratory studies indicate that it might be easier to isolate HIV from semen among men with advanced disease compared to asymptomatic men, and that males receiving zidovudine (AZT) are less likely to shed HIV, although AZT does not uniformly inhibit viral shedding (22).

Susceptibility has been measured in a variety of ways. Lack of circumcision in the male has been associated with female-to-male transmission in at least two studies (11,23). History of genital sores and genital infections have been associated with transmission with increased infectiousness in the HIV-infected individual and susceptibility in the partner. In a Uganda STD clinic, HIV-seropositive men and women were more than twice as likely to have a history of genital sores than HIV-negative clients

(24), and men who presumably acquired HIV from female partners were more than six times as likely to have a history of genital sores than men who remained uninfected (25). The effect of pregnancy and hysterectomy at the time of exposure have been examined, but as of yet, no studies report strong findings for these factors. Likewise, oral contraceptive use has variably been reported as protective (26), a risk factor (27) (correlated with cervical ectopy, which was independently associated with transmission), and unassociated with transmission (14). There have also been some reports of increased likelihood of transmission with IUD use (28). The effect of other contraceptive measures is an area that obviously merits further study.

II. BARRIERS TO PREVENTION STRATEGIES

Prevention strategies for women differ from those for men in two major ways. Women generally have less direct control of sexual behavior change, and prevention of HIV transmission for women must focus on both vertical and horizontal transmission. Most prevention efforts are primarily directed at injection drug use and sexual transmission. However, drug-related prevention messages may not be specific to women users. The best developed drug treatment programs are for heroin users, with fewer resources available for polydrug or crack users, who are more likely to be women who often exchange sex for drugs (8). Residential treatment programs that serve women without separating them from their families appear to have the highest success rates, both in terms of retention in treatment and low rates of relapse; however, many effective residential prevention/treatment programs do not accept women with children (29). Standard prevention messages for sexual transmission, when directed at women, have a higher potential for failure for several reasons (30). They may be seen as irrelevant: the messages of "abstain, be monogamous, or use condoms" may translate to "abstain and have no partner, hence no support; get your partner to be monogamous, or convince him to use condoms." This message denies the need for love and support and suggests that control of a man's sexual behavior is possible for women.

Efforts to promote condom use among women at risk often emphasize condom use skills. Reliance on women to introduce condoms into a sexual situation may require women to assume new roles in an intensely emotional and private situation. In many cultural contexts, negative connotations include presumptions of infidelity, disease, or trying to control a man's sexuality. The range of reactions from male partners can include sexual rejection, domestic violence, and termination of the relationship. Clearly, there is a strong need for developing prevention methods for women to use that are under their control and developing condom promotion strategies for both sexes (31).

At present, a widely used strategy to prevent the spread of HIV antenatally is HIV antibody testing of women in prenatal and family planning clinics. However, women at risk may not be eager to know their HIV status and may avoid programs that expect them to be tested because of discovery of drug use or the likelihood that their babies will be taken from them (32). Further, knowledge of HIV status appears to have little effect on decisions about pregnancy (33). The profound meaning of childbearing to women of many cultures is more central to their decision making than external factors like illness or economics.

Cultural and environmental factors may hamper prevention efforts in the new drug-using pattern of crack cocaine, particularly among young adults in inner city areas. The lifestyle associated with cract use, particularly unsafe sexual behavior with many partners, has a major impact on HIV risk behavior. This lifestyle has already been associated with epidemic increases in syphilis, and early evidence suggests that HIV infection will increase concomitantly (8,34).

Comparing successful and unsuccessful prevention strategies can guide more widespread prevention efforts as risk for women continues to increase. First, some of the most expensive efforts, directed at general audiences via the mass media and nonspecific educational materials like brochures, fail to reach those who are at most risk but do not perceive themselves to be at risk. Most women still do not personalize HIV risk, because they do not know anyone like themselves who has AIDS. Therefore, prevention efforts that are more personalized, and delivered by plausible interpersonal efforts, are the most likely to be heard and considered relevant. The most effective prevention programs to date are those presented in outreach efforts by women who are like those at risk, delivered in ways and locations that are part of women's everyday lives (35).

Important or pressing daily realities must be incorporated. Often, women who know that they are at risk of HIV infection from a spouse still need to stay with that spouse for many immediate reasons that outweigh the distant or vague risk of acquiring HIV infection. Finally, the reality that for many women major decisions about their own health-related sexual behavior are influenced or controlled by men necessitates the inclusion of men in prevention efforts to slow the spread of heterosexual transmission.

III. CLINICAL MANIFESTATIONS

A. Opportunistic Infections, HIV-Associated Infections, and Malignancies

By the current CDC definition of AIDS, *Pneumocystis carinii* pneumonia (PCP) remains the leading AIDS-defining diagnosis in women (36). Lack of access to care, inertia, attention to health care of the child in lieu of committed self-care, and the large proportion of disenfranchised women will all contribute to less early detection and intervention and thus a sustained high frequency of PCP. Other AIDS-defining diagnoses seen with particular frequency include esophageal candida, disseminated *Mycobacterium avium* complex infection, and mucocutaneous herpes simplex virus infection. Women are not protected from any of the other AIDS-defining opportunistic infections. Bacterial infections, especially respiratory infections with encapsulated organisms such as *Streptococcus pneumoniae* and *Hemophilus influenza*, are more frequent in intravenous drug users than in homosexual men (37).

Kaposi's sarcoma (KS), although seen frequently in homosexual men, is found in less than 2% of HIV-infected women as an initial AIDS diagnosis and is infrequent in heterosexual men. There may be a sexually transmitted cofactor associated with angiogenesis (38), and KS, when seen in women, has been associated with sex with a bisexual man (19). Non-Hodgkin's lymphoma, an AIDS-defining diagnosis, is too infrequently encountered in women to judge whether it is more frequent in HIV-infected women than in HIV-negative women (39); however, it would still constitute an AIDS-defining diagnosis. Growing evidence suggests both the increased occurrence and aggressiveness of cervical cancer in association with HIV. To date, no increased frequency of breast cancer, lung cancer, or other malignancies has been seen compared to the general population rates.

Non-AIDS-defining conditions may be quite nonspecific and frequently center on the gynecological system. In a cohort of 117 symptomatic HIV-infected Rhode Island women followed at regular intervals, the initial clinical manifestations of HIV infection were candida vaginitis (37%), lymphadenopathy (15%), bacterial pneumonia (13%), acute retroviral syndrome (7%), and constitutional symptoms such as unexplained weight loss or protracted diarrhea (7%) (40). The remaining 22 (21%) had more typical HIV-related syndromes such as thrush, idiopathic thrombocytopenia purpura, hairy leukoplakia, herpes zoster, PCP, AIDS encephalitis, and cytomegalovirus retinitis (40). The more frequent nonspecific presentations of vaginitis, pneumonia, and constitutional symptoms might prompt only the most suspicious to consider HIV disease, especially in smaller communities. As of December 1990, 73% of women with AIDS were residents of metropolitan cities with populations over one million, mostly on the Atlantic seaboard; only 26% were reported from smaller cities, making it harder to target a specific population and minimizing clinical suspicion by the physician. Since women frequently utilize the emergency room, family planning clinic, STD clinic, youth guidance center, jail clinic facilities, and drug treatment units, these are the sites at which to target early diagnosis and early intervention with antiviral and prophylactic therapies.

B. Treatment of HIV and Associated Illnesses in Women

Guidelines established for now licensed therapies, specifically zidovudine (AZT), didenosine (ddI), and prophylaxis against PCP, are derived from multicenter studies. Although subjects in these studies were predominantly men, the results led to licensure and established recommendations for persons of both genders. Data from two large national studies sponsored by the AIDS Clinical Trials Group (ACTG protocols 016 and 019) comparing AZT to placebo in mildly asymptomatic or asymptomatic HIV-infected patients have recently been analyzed and suggest no difference in the benefit or toxicity of AZT for women or persons of color compared to men or Caucasians, although the numbers were small (41–44).

In the absence of data to the contrary, women, like men, are advised to initiate AZT therapy at 500–600 mg/day when absolute CD4 lymphocyte counts fall below 500 and to start prophylaxis for PCP when CD4 counts fall below 200, particularly when ancillary symptoms such as fever, hairy leukoplakia, or thrush are present (45,46). Potential issues relevant to treatment with antiretrovirals or PCP prophylaxis include the mean lower body weight in women, mean lower hemoglobin with the potential for AZT or dapsone to worsen anemia, and absence of established controls for absolute CD4 counts in men versus women. The more recently licensed antiretroviral, ddI, has been evaluated using even smaller numbers of patients. The most frequent toxicities of ddI and/or the not yet licensed drug dideoxycytosine (ddC) are rash, pancreatitis, peripheral neuropathy, and diarrhea. None of these toxicities has a predictable or obvious female-related propensity.

Tuberculosis, bacterial endocarditis, and sepsis are all seen more frequently in intravenous drug users and the HIV-infected (37,47). Treatment guidelines do not differ by gender, and the clinical presentation is not expected to have gender-related differences exclusive of infection of the reproductive organs. Since half of HIV-infected women are injection drug users and tuberculosis is particularly prevalent among intravenous drug users many co-infected women are receiving methadone and TB therapy. Antituberculous treatment with rifampin alters the hepatic metabolism of many drugs including methadone and can result in wide swings of dose requirement even among those previously on a well-established methadone program. Other factors that may influence the response to therapy include differences in pharmacokinetic disposition of drugs or interactions with commonly used drugs such as methadone or oral contraceptive pills. Problems with access to care are compounded by the high prevalence of HIV infection and large numbers of uninsured women receiving care at municipal hospitals in large metropolitan cities with an increasingly re-ant and exhausted population of care providers. For example, in 1989, New York City medical training programs experienced a 28.2% decline in matches of U.S. graduating medical students and residency programs (48).

C. Gynecological Manifestations and Sexually Transmitted Diseases

Gynecological conditions such as cervicitis, salpingitis, vaginitis, genital ulceration, genital warts, and dysplastic epithelial changes may be more frequent, severe, and/or less responsive to treatment among women with HIV infection compared to women without HIV infection. Most of these conditions are STDs. The associations between these conditions and HIV infection are potentially confounded by sexual and drug use behaviors which are independently predictive of both HIV infection and the occurrence of most STDs. Very little information is available on the occurrence of other gynecological conditions such as menstrual irregularity and infertility in HIV-infected women.

1. Human Papilloma Viruses and Dysplastic Change

Genital warts are a sexually transmitted disease caused by several types of human papilloma virus (HPV). HPV can cause both flat condylomas and exophytic lesions (condyloma acuminatum) of the vulva, vagina, cervix, and anus. Several factors appear to increase the risk of clinically apparent genital HPV infection; these include use of oral contraceptives (49), smoking (49), immune abnormalities (50–52), and pregnancy (50, 52). Treatment of warts has been reported to be less effective among persons with abnormal immune function (52). In the AIDS era, the occurrence of anogenital warts and an incomplete response to treatment have been associated with HIV infection and CD4 cell depletion (53,54). Oral warts also have been associated with HIV infection and related immune abnormalities (55,56).

Many studies have linked genital and anal HPV infections with the development of dysplastic lesions and malignancies of squamous epithelium (52–64). Infections with HPV types 16, 18, and 31 have been most closely associated with malignant transformation (65). Malignancies associated with HPV occur more often among persons with immune dysfunction. Squamous cell carcinoma of the skin is frequently reported in persons with epidermodysplasia verruciformis, a disorder associated with deficiencies in cell-mediated immunity (66). Organ transplant recipients who receive immunosuppressive treatment also have a higher incidence of HPV-associated genital malignancies (67).

Individuals with HIV infection are also at increased risk for HPV-associated epithelial malignancies, and this risk correlates with the degree of immune compromise. Anal dysplasia and squamous cell carcinomas have been reported with increased frequency among HIV-infected homosexual men; the incidence appears to be highest among men with symptomatic disease and/or helper T-cell dysfunction (68–74).

In women HPV-related dysplastic lesions most frequently present on the cervix and can be detected with cytological examination of the cervical epithelium (PAP smears). The morphology of these cervical lesions extends from the relatively benign koilocytic atypia, which signifies HPV infection, to the much more poorly differentiated epithelium of high grade lesions (75). Cervical epithelial abnormalities appear more frequently in women with HIV infection than HIV-uninfected women. In one study, 40% of 35 HIV-infected women had squamous intraepithelial lesions (SIL) on cervical cytology compared with only 9% of 32 uninfected women; women with symptomatic HIV infection were more likely to have SIL than those with asymptomatic infection (76).

Invasive cervical carcinoma appears to be more common among women with HIV infection. Carpenter et al. (40) studied 65 women with documented HIV infection; high grade cervical lesions were present in 25%. In this cohort, 40% of the 35 women with a history of injection drug use had high grade SIL versus only 7% of the 30, who apparently were infected with HIV via heterosexual contact. Maiman and colleagues (77) studied 114 women; 7 of 37 women who had invasive cervical cancer were HIV-infected. After diagnosis the HIV-infected women fared worse than the uninfected; none of the HIV-infected women were cured of their disease compared with 63% of the uninfected. These findings demonstrate the value of early detection of cervical epithelial abnormalities in women with HIV infection and have resulted in suggestions of biannual cytological screening in this patient population.

Cytological screening may not be as sensitive among HIV-infected women. In a study of 32 HIV-infected women, Maiman and colleagues (78) found that only 1 in 13 women had intraepithelial neoplasia on PAP smear despite abnormal colposcopy and biopsy evidence of the condition. While these findings must be considered preliminary since a small number of women were examined, this study raises the possibility that cytological screening may fail to detect epithelial lesions in HIV-infected women. Routine colposcopy has been advocated by some experts to permit reliable detection of cervical lesions in the most treatable stage. Colposcopy is a cumbersome and expensive procedure; before implementation as a screening test, more documentation regarding the insensitivity of cervical cytology is needed (78).

2. Candida *Infections*

Candida vaginitis, a condition frequently seen among the general population, appears to be particularly prevalent among HIV-infected women (40,79,80). The CDC have proposed (in guidelines slated to become effective April 1992) that candidal vaginitis become designated as an HIV-associated disorder and evidence of symptomatic HIV-related illness (81). A prospective study of a large cohort of HIV-infected women in Rhode Island demonstrated that candida vaginitis developed in women with only mild immune abnormalities (40). Women with HIV infection and candida vaginitis were found to have a mean CD4 cell count of 506 in contrast to those with candida esophagitis in whom the mean CD4 cell count was 30. *Candida* vaginitis occurred in 44 of 200 women and was the most common symptomatic disorder that heralded a change in overall health and the occurrence of other HIV-related conditions (40). Despite this association, a history of new, recurrent, or refractory vaginitis did not appear to prompt a consideration of the possibility of HIV infection in the Rhode Island study cohort. Therapy with topical antifungals such as clotrimazole or miconazole is usually effective. Since these preparations are available without prescription for patient self-treatment, it is important to convey to patients that new onset, refractory, or frequent *Candida* infections can be signs of more serious medical conditions. It is similarly important that medical providers consider the possibility of HIV infection in women with vaginal candidiasis and that risk assessment, counseling, and screening be offered where appropriate. Refractory cases of candida vaginitis can be treated with systemic therapy such as ketoconazole (400 mg/day for 14 days followed by 5-day courses each month for 6 months with monitoring of liver function tests) or fluconazole, which can be extremely effective but are expensive and require a prescription (82).

3. Genital Ulceration and Salpingitis

In the Rhode Island study, severe genital herpes was the initial AIDS-defining diagnosis in 18% of the 44 women who developed AIDS during study follow-up (40). Herpes simplex virus type 2 infections are highly prevalent in the general population (83) and are even more prevalent among HIV-infected individuals (84). Symptomatic recurrences of genital herpes occur more frequently and are more severe among HIV-infected persons, especially those with low CD4 cell counts (85). During initial episodes oral acyclovir therapy is recommended as a means of reducing the duration and severity of symptoms (86). The recurrence rate in patients with frequent or severe episodes can be reduced with lower dose suppressive therapy (86). On occasion, acyclovir-resistant herpes has been identified in patients with refractory genital ulcerations and severe immune impairment. Infections due to strains with documented acyclovir resistance may be treated with foscarnet (87), a parenteral drug, though the potential teratogenicity of this agent mandates avoidance in pregnant women or those who plan pregnancy.

The occurrence of other genital ulcerative diseases (syphilis and chancroid) is associated with HIV infection (88–90), which may reflect enhanced viral transmission in persons with these STDs, altered clinical presentation of the STDs, or shared risk factors such as sexual behavior. Associations between cervicitis, salpingitis (pelvic inflammatory disease, PID), and HIV infection have also been described in several studies (88,91,92). Current studies, though limited in scope, suggest that the presentation of upper genital tract disease in PID may be altered or more severe in women with coincident HIV infection (91,92).

4. Progression of Disease

Studies of disease progression in women are limited and have been derived from three principal sources—large national data bases limited to the date of AIDS diagnosis and date of death; small to moderate size cohort studies of 50–200 women, often followed less than 3 years; and large cohort studies conducted in other countries, e.g., Africa, where economic, sociological, and medical and public health conditions differ so extremely from those in the United States that findings may not be applicable to the

United States or Western Europe. Reports from the CDC suggest that survival of women and heterosexual men is similar. Studies of cohorts in other cities suggest shortened survival for women (93). A recent study of survival in San Francisco suggests similar survival in men and women receiving antiretroviral therapy, but in those not receiving antiretroviral therapy, males survived longer than women (94). In the Bronx, impact of access to or adherence to follow-up care strongly influenced survival, with substantially shortened survival in women who had had no prior care before a severe HIV-related infection (93).

IV. TREATMENT OF HIV DISEASE AND OPPORTUNISTIC INFECTIONS IN PREGNANCY

Early studies suggested an adverse effect of pregnancy on progression of HIV disease. More recently, studies reported from cities in the United States and Europe suggest no difference in progression or immunological state or clinical endpoints after 2–3 years; however, immunosuppressed pregnant women are at risk for serious infections, especially pneumonias, both bacterial and pneumocystic (40,95). HIV-infected women are fertile; women IV drug users at a methadone clinic had had a mean of 2.5% live births, and 60% had had an abortion (96). When pregnancy termination choices were examined in 28 HIV-infected pregnant women compared to 36 HIV-seronegative pregnant women, all of whom were in drug treatment, 50% and 44%, respectively, chose abortion; their choice was dictated by previous experience with abortion, not by their HIV infection or other factors (97). Thus, many HIV-infected women will become pregnant and carry those pregnancies to term.

A. Considerations in the Decision to Treat During Pregnancy

The use of any drug during pregnancy requires consideration of the possible risks and benefits for both the woman and her fetus. For HIV-infected women, treatment decisions during pregnancy are complicated by a lack of information regarding the fetal effects of drugs and the effects of pregnancy on the efficacy of treatment.

Information about the effects of drugs on fetal development is usually limited, even for drugs have been in clinical use for many years. In recent years the Food and Drug Administration has required an assessment of fetal risk to be made during the drug approval process. The information available from animal and human experience results in classification of the drug on the basis of its potential to cause risk to the fetus (Table 2). The most commonly assigned class is C, indicating that adequate trials in pregnant women have not been performed. Other methods for studying fetal effects, including animal models, do not fully describe human reproduction and may in fact be misleading. Data from research using animals is commonly available and may be useful in guiding decisions. Caution is recommended, though, as animal data may come from a species with no relevance to human physiology or from a study using doses out of proportion to those used in the treatment of humans. Justification for evaluating new drugs in pregnant females is difficult unless the therapy is targeted at pathology associated with pregnancy.

How pregnancy changes the pharmacokinetics and pharmacodynamics and therapeutic value of a drug and to what degree, and whether those changes are consistent throughout the pregnancy, have not been well studied for most drugs, and neither have the adjustments that need to be made during the evolving pregnancy. These issues are especially important for drugs with a narrow therapeutic window, where failure to properly consider all factors may result in a toxic or subpotent dose.

The indirect benefit to the fetus resulting from improved maternal health must be considered. Will the use of a drug of indeterminant fetal toxicity indirectly benefit the fetus by stabilizing the health of the woman? This issue is probably most easily dealt with when the decision involves a life or death situation, where the woman (and subsequently the fetus) risks death without treatment. More often, however, the "correct" clinical decision is less obvious.

In the final analysis, moral, ethical, religious, and sometimes legal issues confound the decision-making process for both patient and practitioner and may evoke emotions as divergent and strong as those surrounding the abortion issue. The patient may choose to put herself at risk against the advice of her practitioner or, conversely, make a decision that clearly places the fetus at risk. The final choices must be shared by those who will live with the consequences

B. Specific Therapies

1. AZT

The package insert included with AZT places it in Category C: "animal studies demonstrate fetal risk but there are no human trials *or* neither human nor animal studies are available." The recommendation further states

Table 2 Treatment During Pregnancy

Drug	FDA pregnancy category	Use in serious disease[a]
Acyclovir	C	Yes
Amikacin	D	Traditionally avoided in early pregnancy
Amphotericin B	B	Yes
Ciprofloxacin	C	Avoid
Clindamycin	N/A	Yes
Clofazamine	C	No experience
Clotrimazole oral troche	C	Yes
Clotrimazole vaginal supp/cream	B	Yes
Dapsone	C	Yes
ddC	N/A	No experience
Didanosine (ddI)	N/A	No experience
Ethambutol	N/A	Yes
Fluconazole	C	No experience
Ganciclovir	C	No experience
Isoniazid	N/A	Yes
Ketoconazole	C	No experience
Pentamidine IV	N/A	Avoid in preference to alternatives
Pentamidine inhaled	C	Little systemic absorption; no experience
Primaquine	N/A	Avoid
Pyrazinamide (PZA)	N/A	Avoid
Pyrimethamine	C	Possibly
Rifampin	C	Yes
Sulfadiazine	N/A	Yes
Trimethoprim	C	Seldom indicated alone
Trimethoprim/sulfamethoxazole	C	Yes
Zidovudine (AZT)	C	Yes

[a]For life-threatening condition or serious indication.
N/A: Classification not available; A: controlled studies in women demonstrate no fetal risk; B: animal studies demonstrate no fetal risk, but there are no human trials, *or* animal studies demonstrate a risk not corroborated by human trials; C: animal studies demonstrate fetal risk but there are no human trials, *or* neither human nor animal studies are available; D: evidence exists for fetal risk in humans—benefit may outweigh the risk; X: evidence exists for fetal risk in humans—benefit clearly outweighed by risk.
Source: Reproduced from AIDSFILE (100).

that "it is not known whether zidovudine can cause fetal harm when administered to a pregnant woman or can affect reproductive capacity. Zidovudine should be given to pregnant women only if clearly needed." A registry of women who have by choice or inadvertently received AZT is kept by the drug manufacturers. To date, there has been no specific adverse effect to mother or child (82). Pharmacological studies in humans do not suggest excessive accumulation of AZT in the placenta or fetal tissue and Ob/Gyn specialists in HIV now strongly recommend AZT for women with fewer than 200 CD4 cells and many recommend AZT for those with 200-500 CD4 cells. There are regional differences of opinion in attempting to balance the issue of maternal benefit and potential fetal risk. When prescribed, doses are the same as in nongravid women (82).

2. PCP Prophylaxis

No prophylactic therapies have been endorsed or approved by the FDA for use in pregnancy. However, based on past experiences and the growing body of community practice dictated by necessity trimethoprim-sulfamethoxazole (TMPSMX) has become the standard PCP prophylactic regimen used in pregnancy and women (82,98). Although conventional wisdom suggests that TMPSMX should be avoided in the third trimester of pregnancy because of kernicterus, this has not been borne out, and TMPSMX can be used through delivery of those women who can tolerate it (82,98). Dapsone has been used in pregnant women who have dermatitis herpetiformis and leprosy, conditions that necessitate daily and long-term therapy with dapsone, without major problems (99). However, because of the risk of interference with dihydrofolate reductase, dapsone should be used with caution and necessitates a careful glucose-6-phosphate dehydrogenase evaluation before initiation. While aerosol pentamidine has the advantage of little systemic absorption, the pulmonary distribution in a woman with a gravid uterus is unknown; it has been less effective than TMPSMX in clinical trials, and aerosol pentamidine does not protect against extrapulmonary PCP.

PCP may be particularly severe in pregnancy (82,95). For treatment of active disease, TMPSMX is the most desirable therapeutic option. Intravenous pentamidine is to be avoided. Dapsone should be held in reserve until after careful risk/benefit assessment.

Treatment of other opportunistic infections in pregnancy may be particularly problematic, as indicated in Table 2 (100). Of 26 therapies for common opportunistic disorders or HIV disease that may occur during pregnancy, there are no drugs classified as Category A (demonstrated to pose no fetal risk in controlled trials in women). The clinician is left with a very difficult professional choice about treatment options. Even if extensive anecdotal experience suggests that a drug is well tolerated in the pregnant woman, the decision to use the drug must still be fully considered on an individual basis. The patient should be informed in simple terms about the state of knowledge and the best options. Table 2 indicates drugs by FDA pregnancy category and some very general guidelines for the use of these therapies in serious or life-threatening disease based mostly on anecdotal experience. Published guidelines in this emerging field are sparse; however, several excellent reviews address this issue as well as counseling and testing indications for pregnant women (82,101).

V. THE NATIONAL RESEARCH AGENDA FOR WOMEN INFECTED WITH HIV

A. Background

To address the many information gaps, the research agenda for HIV-infected women must be far reaching. The behavioral and social milieu in which specific studies are conducted creates special challenges for the implementation of clinical trials, and the success of these trials will require extensive collaboration among scientific disciplines and the development of partnerships with the communities of women for whom these trials are designed.

In December 1990, a 2-day conference on women and HIV infection was sponsored by the National Institutes of Health (NIH), with participants encompassing a wide gamut of health care professionals, women with HIV, social workers, government administrators, researchers, and activists. The conference steering committee framed recommendations (102) and presented them to the NIH AIDS Program Advisory Committee (APAC) on April 30, 1991, which endorsed the proposal and urged implementation. These recommendations are intended to serve as guidelines for future research throughout the public health system.

One major research need is a large-scale epidemiology and natural history study of HIV infection in women. The CDC has initiated a pilot program, and various components of the NIH and the Public Health Service are cooperating in combining efforts in such a project to ensure larger data sets that can provide answers to questions. Three areas are highlighted.

B. Natural History

A specific recommendation of this national conference is to conduct large-scale natural history studies to evaluate 1) the full spectrum of HIV-related illnesses and malignancies in women; 2) the relationship of immunostatus markers, e.g., CD4 cell count to conditions more common among women (e.g., esophageal candidiasis, bacterial pneumonia); 3) progression of precancerous reproductive organ and genital tract lesions; 4) relation of survival to surrogate markers in order to understand factors contributing to the phenomenon of shortened survival time in women; 5) culturally appropriate methodology; 6) the psychosocial needs of HIV-positive women and their family systems (traditional and nontraditional including lesbian women); and 7) adolescent psychosocial needs emphasizing suicide prevention and support strategies.

C. Transmission

The national conference proposed the following recommendations for transmission studies and HIV prevention to evaluate and identify 1) the role of coinfections and other cofactors of transmission, especially those potentially increasing transmission via the female genital tract; 2) better barrier/contraceptive methods and viricides under women's control; 3) behavioral interventions emphasizing the role of the male partner in primary prevention of STDs and HIV infection; 4) the effect of antiretrovirals on transmission factors in pregnant and nonpregnant women; 5) study issues of chemical dependency that underlie HIV risk behavior in women, including initiation, habituation, tolerance, and relapse and the relationships among chemical dependency, sexual behavior, seroprevalence, and unique HIV prevention needs of subgroups of women, e.g., preadolescents, lesbians, prison inmates; and 6) STD laboratory and clinical infrastructures for HIV/AIDS education and prevention outreach programs.

D. Clinical Therapeutics

Finally, specific recommendations involving the area of clinical therapeutics and related service needs were addressed to evaluate 1) the safety and efficacy in women of currently available and experimental HIV therapies, including alternative therapies; 2) the safety of antiretroviral drugs and therapies for opportunistic infections in pregnant women; 3) gender-specific clinical assessments, e.g., PAP smears, as part of routine evaluation procedure; 4) clinical trial eligibility criteria; recruitment and retention procedures to facilitate enrollment and follow-up of women; 6) interactions between HIV therapies and other prescribed and recreational agents; 7) inexpensive and accessible therapeutics that can be used reliably by women who must frequently manage multiple responsibilities, e.g., family and job, despite declining health; 8) perceptions of women regarding clinical trials and research; 9) how to improve woman-centered HIV case-finding activities that are directly linked to medical and social services and employ street and community outreach for HIV case finding; 10) the extent of health care service needs for HIV-infected women; 11) determinants of health care-seeking behavior in women; 12) the quality of HIV antibody testing and counseling in women from diverse backgrounds; and 13) adequacy of HIV/AIDS training of health care providers.

One of the concerns of the newly formed NIH Office of Research on Women's Health is the enrollment of women into all trials sponsored by the NIH and the inclusion of women of child-bearing age and even pregnant women in clinical trials, which is critical since the majority of such women candidates are of child-bearing age. The Division of AIDS (NIAID), sponsor of the ACTG, has recently endorsed a full scientific committee, which will address the growing needs of research relative to women infected with HIV. The Women's Health Committee has targeted four major goals for the committee work within the ATCG: 1) to participate in the development and design of HIV-associated clinical trials of the treatments for women, pregnant and nonpregnant; 2) to increase the participation of women in ACTG clinical trials and establish uniform criteria to ensure the inclusion of women; 3) to ensure that clinical trials evaluate gynecological health and incorporate appropriate gender-specific end points; and 4) to participate in the development and design of clinical trials to interrupt maternal-fetal transmission ensuring the protection of maternal and fetal health. The CPCRA (Community Program for Clinical Research on AIDS) is also sponsored by DAIDS. To date, 19.6% of 3713 subjects enrolled into its clinical trials and observational data base are women (103). The significant enrollment of women reflects the unique relationship between the primary care giver and patient upon which the CPCRA was developed.

A multidisciplinary research approach is imperative among different specialties of medicine and specific government agencies and the community care givers and clinical researchers. Biomedical, psychosocial, and behavioral research must all be addressed. As the face of AIDS becomes female, the challenge to push the research establishment beyond its present bounds is again echoed 10 years after the epidemic was recognized.

REFERENCES

1. Chu S, Buehler J, Berkelman R. Impact of the human immunodeficiency virus epidemic on mortality in women of reproductive age, United States. JAMA 1990; 264:225-9.

2. HIV/AIDS Surveillance Report: November 1991. Atlanta, GA: Centers for Disease Control, 1991.

3. Berkelman R, Fleming P, Chu S, et al. Women and AIDS: the increasing role of heterosexual transmission in the United States. Presented at Seventh International Conference on AIDS, June 1991, Florence, Italy.

4. Ellerbrock T, Bush T, Chamberland M, et al. Epidemiology of women with AIDS in the United States, 1981 through 1990: a comparison with heterosexual men with AIDS. JAMA 1991; 265:2971-5.

5. Kamb M, Otten M, Guerna F, et al. Extensive HIV seropositivity among heterosexuals in a STD clinic [Abstract]. Presented at Seventh International Conference on AIDS, June 1991, Florence, Italy. (W.C. 99).

6. San Francisco Department of Public Health Bureau of Epidemiology and Disease Control. Epidemiology of reportable STDs in San Francisco, 1985-1990. San Francisco Epidemiology Bulletin, 1991:7.

7. Homes K, Karon J, Kreiss J. The increasing frequency of heterosexually acquired AIDS in the United States: 1983-1988. Am J Public Health 1990; 80: 858-63.

8. Schoenbaum E, Hartel D, Friedland G. Crack use predicts incident HIV seroconversion [Abstract]. Presented at Sixth International Conference on AIDS, June 1990, San Francisco, CA. (Th.C. 103).

9. Padian N. Heterosexual transmission: infectivity and risks. In: Heterosexual transmission of AIDS, N Alexander, H Gabelnick, J Spieler, eds. New York: Wiley-Liss, 1990:25-34.

10. Padian N, Shiboski S, Jewell N. Female-to-male transmission of human immunodeficiency virus. JAMA 1991; 266:1664-8.

11. Cameron D, Simonsen N, D'Costa L, et al. Female to male transmission of human immunodeficiency virus type I: risk factors for seroconversion in men. Lancet 1989; 2:403-7.

12. Laga M, Taelman H, Canderstuyft P, et al. Advanced immunodeficiency as a risk factor for heterosexual transmission of HIV. AIDS 1989; 3:361-6.

13. Moore L, Padian N, Shiboski S, et al. Behavior change in a cohort of heterosexual couples with one HIV-infected partner [Abstract]. Presented at Seventh International Conference on AIDS, June 1991, Florence, Italy. (W.C. 103).

14. Moss G, Clemetson D, D'Costa L, et al. Despite safer sex practices after counseling, seroconversion is high among HIV serodiscordant couples in Nairobi, Kenya [Abstract]. Presented at Seventh International Conference on AIDS, June 1991, Florence, Italy. (W.C. 3119).

15. Ginerva M, Costigliola P, Richie E, et al. Rick factors in heterosexual transmission of HIV [Abstract]. Presented at Seventh International Conference on AIDS, June 1991, Florence, Italy. (W.C. 3111).

16. De Vincenzi I, Ancelle-Park R, for the European Community Study Group on heterosexual transmission of HIV. Follow-up of a European cohort of couples [Abstract]. Presented at Seventh International Conference on AIDS, June 1991, Florence, Italy. (M.C. 3028).

17. Marmor M, Weiss L, Lynden M, et al. Possible female-to-female transmission of human immunodeficiency virus. Ann Intern Med 1986; 105:969.

18. Musicco M, and the National Research Council of Italy. Incidence and risk factors of man to woman sexual HIV transmission: longitudinal study on 171 women steady partners of infected men [Abstract]. Presented at Seventh International Conference on AIDS, June 1991, Florence, Italy. (M.C. 4).

19. Padian N, Marquis L, Francis D, et al. Male-to-female transmission of human immunodeficiency virus. JAMA 1987; 258:788-90.

20. De Vincenzi I, Anvelle-Park P, and the European Study Group. Heterosexual transmission of HIV; follow-up of a European cohort of couples [Abstract]. Presented at Fifth International Conference on AIDS, June 1989, Montreal, Quebec. (M.C. 3028).

21. Padian N, Shiboski S, Jewell N. The effect of the number of exposures on the risk of heterosexual HIV transmission. J Infect Dis 1990; 161:883-7.

22. Anderson D, Politch J, Martinez A, et al. Prevalence and temporal variation of HIV-1 in semen [Abstract]. Presented at Sixth International Conference on AIDS, June 1990, San Francisco, CA. (Th.C. 553).

23. Fischl M, Fayne T, Flanaga S, et al. Seroprevalence and risks of HIV infections in spouses of persons infected with HIV [Abstract]. Presented at Fourth International Conference on AIDs, June 1988, Stockholm. (4060, p. 274).

24. Hellman N, Desmond-Hellman S, Nsubuga P, et al. Genital trauma during sex is a risk factor for HIV infection in Uganda [Abstract]. Presented at Seventh International Conference on AIDS, June 1991, Florence, Italy. (M.C. 3079).

25. Hellman N, Desmond-Hellman S, Nsubuga P, et al. Risk factors for HIV infection among Ugandan couples [Abstract]. Presented at Seventh International Conference on AIDS, June 1991, Florence, Italy. (M.C. 3080).

26. Plummer F, Simonsen N, Cameron D, et al. Cofactors in male-female transmission of human immunodeficiency virus type 1. J Infect Dis 1991; 163:233-9.

27. Moss G, Clemetson D, D'Costa L, et al. Association of cervical ectopy with heterosexual transmission of human immunodeficiency virus: results of a study of couples in Nairobi, Kenya. J Infect Dis 1991; 164:588-91.

28. Mussico M, for the Italian Partner's Study. Oral contraception, IUD, and condom use and man to woman sexual transmission of HIV infection [Abstract]. Presented at Sixth International Conference on AIDS, June 1990, San Francisco, CA. (Th.C. 584).

29. National Commission on AIDS. The twin epidemics of substance abuse and HIV. Washington DC, 1991.

30. Cohen JB. Why woman partners of drug users will continue to be at high risk for HIV infection. J Addic Res 1991; 10:99-110.

31. Stein Z. The need for methods women can use. AJPH 1990; 80:460-2.

32. Holman S, Berthaud M, Sunderland A, et al. Women infected with HIV: counseling and testing during pregnancy. Semin Perinatol 13:7-15, 1989.

33. Amaro H. Women's reproductive rights in the age of AIDS: new threats to informed choice. In: The genetic resource. Boston: Massachusetts Department of Public Health, 1990; 5(2):39-44.

34. Chirgwin K, DeHovitz JA, Dillon S, et al. HIV infection, genital ulcer disease, and crack cocaine use among patients attending a clinic for sexually transmitted diseases. AJPH 1991; 81:1576-9.

35. Weissman G. Working with pregnant women at high risk for HIV infection: outreach and prevention. Bull NY Acad Med 1991; 67:291-301.

36. NIAID/NIH & NIH Centers for Disease Control. Clin Courier 1991; 9(6):1-8.

37. Witt DJ, Craven DE, McCabe WR. Bacterial infections in adult patients with the acquired immune deficiency syndrome (AIDS) and AIDS-related complex. Am J Med 1987; 82:900-6.

38. Beral V, Peterman TA, Berkelman RL, Jaffe HW. Kaposi's sarcoma among persons with AIDS: a sexually-transmitted infection? Lancet 1990; 335:123-8.

39. Gail MH, Pluda JM, Rabkin CS, Biggar RJ, Geodert JJ, et al. Projections of the incidence of non-Hodgkin's lymphoma related to acquired immunodeficiency syndrome. JNCI 1991; 83:695-701.

40. Carpenter CJ, Mayer KH, Stein MD, Liebman BD, Fisher A, Fiore TC. Human immunodeficiency virus infection in North American women: experience with 200 cases and a review of the literature. Medicine 1991; 70:307-25.

41. Fischl MA, Richman DD, Grieco MH, et al. The efficacy of axidothymidine (ACT) in the treatment of patients with AIDS and AIDS-related complex: a double-blind, placebo-controlled study. N Engl J Med 1987; 317:185-91.

42. Volberding PA, Lagakos SW, Koch MA, et al. Zidovudine in asymptomatic human immunodeficiency virus infections: a controlled trial in persons with fewer than 500 CD4 positive cells per cubic millimeter. N Engl J Med 1990; 322:941-9.

43. Lagakos SW, Fischl MA, Stein DS, Lim L, Volberding P. Effects of zidovudine therapy in minority and other subpopulations with early HIV infection. JAMA 1991; 266:2709-12.

44. Easterbrook PJ, Kerylu JC, Creagh-Kirt T, Richman DD, Chaisson RE, et al. Racial and ethnic differences in outcome in zidovudine-treated patients with advanced HIV disease. JAMA 1991; 266:2713-8.

45. Centers for Disease Control. Guidelines for prophylaxis against *Pneumocystis carinii* pneumonia for persons infected with human immunodeficiency virus. MMWR 1989; 38:1-9.

46. NIAID State of the Art Conference, C Carpenter, Chair, March 1990: Recommendations for zidovudine: early infections. JAMA 1990; 2673:1606-9.

47. Graham NM, Nelson KE, Solomon L, Bonds M, Rizzo RT, et al. Prevalence of tuberculin positivity and skin test anergy in HIV-1 seropositive and seronegative intravenous drug users. JAMA 1991; 267:369-73.

48. Ness RB, Kelly JV, Killian CD. House staff recruitment to municipal and voluntary New York City residency programs during the AIDS epidemic. JAMA 1991; 266:2843-6.

49. Dahling JRA. Risk factors for condyloma accuminatum in women. Sex Transm Dis 1986; 13:16.

50. Oriel D. Genital human papillomavirus infection. In: Sexually transmitted diseases, Holmes KK et al., eds. New York: McGraw-Hill, 1990:433-41.

51. Pass F. Progress towards a new wart biology. J Invest Dermatol 1979; 70: 109-12.

52. Von Krogh G. Warts. Immunologic factors of prognostic significance. Int J Dermatol 1979; 8:195-201.

53. Rudlinger R, Grob R, Buchmann P, et al. Anogenital warts of the condyloma acuminatum type in HIV-positive patients. Dermatologica 1988; 176:277-81.

54. McMillan A, Bishop PE. Clinical course of anogenital warts in men infected with human immunodeficiency virus. Genitourin Med 1989; 65:225-8.

55. Greenspan D, de Villiers EM, Greenspan JS, et al. Unusual HPV types in oral warts in association with HIV infection. J Oral Pathol Med 1988; 17: 482-7.

56. Syrjanen S, Von Krogh G, Kellokoski J, Syrjanen K. Two different human papillomavirus (HPV) types associated with oral mucosal lesions in an HIV-seropositive man. J Oral Pathol Med 1989; 18:366-70.

57. de Villiers EM, Wagner D, Schneider A, et al. Human papilloma virus infections in women with and without abnormal cerivical cytology. Lancet 1987; 2:703-6.

58. J Reeves WC, Caussy D, Brinton LA, et al. Human papillomaviruses and cervical cancer in Latin America. N Engl J Med 1989; 320:1437-41.

59. Azocar J, Abad SMJ, Acosta H, et al. Prevalence of cervical dysplasia and HPV infection according to sexual behavior. Int J Cancer 1990; 45:622-5.

60. Carson LF, Twiggs LB, Fukushima M, et al. Human genital papilloma infections: an evaluation of immunologic competence in the neoplasia-papilloma syndrome. Am J Obstet Gynecol 1986; 155:784-9.

61. MacNab JCM, Walkinshaw SA, Cordiner JW, et al. Human papillomavirus in clinically and histologically normal tissue of patients with genital cancer. N Engl J Med 1986; 315:1052-8.

62. Daling JR, Weiss NS, Hislop TG, et al. Sexual practices, sexually transmitted diseases, and the incidence of anal cancer. N Engl J Med 1987; 317:973-7.

63. Crum CP, Mitao M, Levine RU and Silverstein S. Cervical papillomaviruses segregate within morphologically distinct precancerous lesions. J Virol 1985; 54:675-81.

64. Mitchell H, Drake M, Nedley G. Prospective evaluation of risk of cervical cancer after cytological evidence of human papilloma virus infection. Lancet 1986; i:573-5.

65. Palefsky J. Human papillomavirus infection among HIV-infected individuals: implications for development of malignant tumors. Hem/Onc Clin N Am 1991; 5:357-70.

66. Jablonska S, Dabrowski J, Jakubowicz K. Epidermodysplasia verruciformis as a model in studies on the role of papovaviruses in oncogenesis. Cancer Res 1972; 32:583-8.

67. Penn I. Cancers of the anogenital region in renal transplant recipients: an analysis of 65 cases. Cancer 1986; 8:61-6.

68. Berger TG, Sawchuk WS, Leonardi C, et al. Epidermodysplasia verruciformis-associated papillomavirus infection complicating human immunodeficiency virus disease. Br J Dermatol 1991; 124:79-83.

69. Frazer IH, Medley G, Crapper RM, et al. Association between anorectal dysplasia, human papillomavirus, and human immunodeficiency virus infection in homosexual men. Lancet 1986; ii:657-60.

70. Palefsky JM, Gonzales J, Greenblatt RM, et al. Prevalence of intrepithelial neoplasia and anal papillomavirus infection among immunosuppressed homosexual makes with group IV HIV disease. JAMA 1990; 263:2911.

71. Caussy D, Goedert JJ, Palefsky J, et al. Interaction of human immunodeficiency and papilloma viruses: association with anal epithelial abnormality in homosexual men. Int J Cancer 1990; 46:214-9.

72. Melbye M, Palefsky J, Gonzales, et al. Immune status as a determinant of human papillomavirus detection and its association with anal epithelial abnormalities. Ont J Cancer 1990; 46:203-6.

73. Law CLH, Qassim M, Thompson CH, et al. Factors associated with clinical and sub-clinical anal human papillomavirus infection in homosexual men. Genitourin Med 1991; 67:92-8.

74. Choward LC, Paterson-Brown S, Chan STF, et al. Squamous cell carcinoma of the anus in young homosexual men with T-helper cell depletion. Genitourin Med 1986; 62:393-5.

75. Ambros RA, Kurman RJ. Current concepts in the relationship of human papillomavirus infection to the pathogenesis and classification of precancerous squamous cell lesions of the uterine cervix. Sem Diag Path 1990; 7: 158-172.

76. Feingold AR, Vermund SH, Burk RD, et al. Cervical cytologic abnormalities and papillomavirus in women infected with human immunodeficiency virus. J AIDS 1990; 3:896-903.

77. Maiman M, Fruchter RG, Serur E, et al. Human immunodeficiency virus infection and cervical neoplasia. Gynecol Oncol 1990; 38:377-82.

78. Maiman M, Tarricons N, Viera J, et al. Colposcopic evaluation of human immunodeficiency virus seropositive women. Obstet Gynecol 1991; 78:84-8.

79. Rhoads JL, Wright C, Redfield RR, Burke DS. Chronic vaginal candidiasis in women with human immunodeficiency virus. JAMA 1987; 257:3105-7.

80. Imam W, Carpenter CJ, Mayer K, Fisher A, Stein M, Danforth SB. Hierarchial pattern of mucosal candida infections in HIV seropositive women. Am J Med 1990; 89:142-6.

81. Centers for Disease Control. 1991 revised classification system for HIV infection and expanded AIDS surveillance case definition for adolescents and adults (draft). HHS/PHS, Nov. 15, 1991.

82. Minkoff HL, DeHovitz JA. Care of women infected with human immunodeficiency virus. JAMA 1991; 266:2253-8.

83. Johnson RE, Nahmias AJ, Magder LS, et al. A seroepidemiologic survey of the prevalence of herpes simplex virus type 2 infection in the United States. N Engl J Med 1989; 321:7-12.

84. Quinn TC, Glasser D, Cannon RO, et al. Human immunodeficiency virus infection among patients attending clinics for sexually transmitted diseases. N Engl J Med 1988; 318:197-203.

85. Maier JA, Bergman A, Ross MG. Acquired immunodeficiency syndrome manifested by chronic primary herpes. Am J Obstet Gynecol 1986; 155:756-8.

86. Stone KM, Whittington WL. Treatment of genital herpes. Rev Infect Dis 1990; 12S:S610-9.

87. Safrin S, Assaykeen T, Follansbee S, Mills J. Foscarnet therapy for acyclovir-resistant mucocutaneous herpes simplex virus infection in 26 AIDS patients: preliminary data. J Infect Dis 1990; 161:1078-84.

88. Pepin J, Plummer FA, Brunham RC, et al. The interaction of HIV infection and other sexually transmitted diseases: an opportunity for intervention. AIDS 1989; 3:3-9.

89. Jessamine PG, Ronald AR. Chancroid and the role of genital ulcer disease in the spread of human retroviruses. Med Clin North Am 1990; 74:1417-31.

90. Piot P, Laga M. Genital ulcers, other sexually transmitted disease, and the sexual transmission of HIV. Br Med J 1989; 298:623-4.

91. Safrin S, Dattel BJ, Haver L, Sweet RL. Seroprevalence and epidemiologic correlates of infection in women with acute pelvic inflammatory disease. Obstet Gynecol 1990; 75:666-70.

92. Hoegsberg B, Abulafia O, Sedlis A, et al. Sexually transmitted diseases and human immunodeficiency virus infection among women with pelvic inflammatory diseases. Am J Obstet Gynecol 1990; 163:1135-9.

93. Brettle RP, Lee CLS. The natural history of HIV and AIDS in women. AIDS 1991; 5:1283-92.

94. Araneta MR, Lemp GF, Cohen JB, Derish PA, Carmona I, Clevenger AC. Survival trends among women with AIDS in San Francisco [Abstract]. Presented at Seventh International Conference on AIDS, Florence, Italy, June 16-21, 1991. (M.C. 3122).

95. Minkoff HL, Willoughby A, Mendez H, et al. Serious infections during pregnancy among women with advanced immunodeficiency virus infection. Am J Obstet Gynecol 1990; 162:30-4.

96. Schoenbaum E, Hartel D, Selwyn P, Klein R, Davenny K, et al. Risk factors for human immunodeficiency virus infection in intravenous drug users. N Engl J Med 1987; 147:104-8.

97. Carter RJ, Schoenbaum E, Robertson V, Klein R, Rogers M, et al. Knowledge of HIV antibody status and decisions to continue or terminate pregnancy among intravenous drug users. JAMA 1989; 261:3567-71.

98. Minkoff HL, Moreno J. Drug prophylaxis for human immunodeficiency virus infected pregnant women: ethical considerations. Am J Obstet Gynecol 1990; 163:1111-3.

99. Jacobus Pharmaceutical. Dapsone USP. Medical Economics Co., Crandall, NJ: Physicians' desk reference 1991:1107.

100. Coleman R. Treatment during pregnancy. AIDS File 1991; 5:6.

101. Working Group on HIV Testing of Pregnant Women and Newborns. HIV infection, pregnant women, and newborns. JAMA 1990; 264:2416-20.

102. NIAID/NIH. AIDS agenda, Summer, 1991, M. Warren, ed.

103. Cotton D, Feinberg J, Finkelstein D, ACTG SDAC. Participation of women in multicenter HIV clinical trials programs in the United States [Abstract]. VII International Conference on AIDS, Florence, Italy, June 1991. (Tu.D. 114).

Index

About the Editors

PAUL VOLBERDING is Professor of Medicine in Residence at the University of California, San Francisco. He also serves as Chief of the Medical Oncology Division, and Director of the AIDS Program of San Francisco General Hospital. A leading figure in AIDS research, Dr. Volberding has authored or coauthored more than 100 technical articles and abstracts and has coauthored and contributed chapters to more than 25 books and monographs. He served as Co-Chairperson of the VI International Conference on AIDS, held in June 1990, in San Francisco, California. He is the President of the International AIDS Society and is a member of the American Society of Clinical Oncology, the American Cancer Society, the American Society of Hematology, the American Federation for Clinical Research, and the Clinical Immunology Society, among other professional societies. Dr. Volberding received the B.A. degree (1971) from the University of Chicago in Illinois, and the M.D. degree (1975) from the University of Minnesota in Minneapolis.

MARK A. JACOBSON is Assistant Professor of Medicine in Residence, Divisions of AIDS, Infectious Diseases, and Clinical Pharmacology, Department of Medicine, University of California at San Francisco, and the Medical Service, San Francisco General Hospital, where he is also Director of Clinical Research for AIDS. An authority of AIDS research, Dr. Jacobson has authored many book chapters, articles, and abstracts in leading medical journals. He is a member of the National Institute of Allergy and Infectious Diseases AIDS Clinical Trials Group, where he serves as chair of the Cytomegalovirus Pathogen Study Group. He received the B.A. degree (1971) from the University of California, Berkeley, and the M.D. degree (1981) from the University of California, San Francisco.